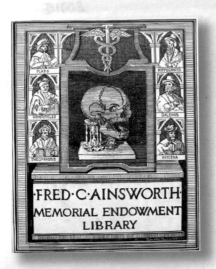

BORDEN'S
DREAM

The Walter Reed Army Medical Center
in Washington, D.C.

Mary W. Standlee

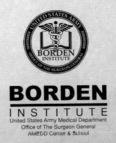

BORDEN
INSTITUTE
United States Army Medical Department
Office of The Surgeon General
AMEDD Center & School

B O R D E N   I N S T I T U T E

MARTHA K. LENHART, MD, PhD
COLONEL, , MC, US ARMY
DIRECTOR/EDITOR IN CHIEF

BRUCE G. MASTON
Layout Editor

DOUG WISE
Layout Editor

The opinions or assertions contained herein are the personal views of the authors and are not to be construed as doctrine of the Department of the Army or the Department of Defense.

Published by the Office of The Surgeon General, US Army
Borden Institute
Walter Reed Army Medical Center
Washington, DC 20307-5001

LIBRARY OF CONGRESS CATALOGING IN PUBLICATION DATA

Standlee, Mary W. (Mary Walker)
  Borden's dream / by Mary W. Standlee.
    p. cm.
  Includes bibliographical references and index.
  ISBN 978-0-9818228-4-6
  1. Walter Reed Army Medical Center—History. 2. United States—Armed Forces—Medical care—History. 3. Borden, William Cline, 1858-1934. 4. Doctors—United States—Biography. I. Borden Institute (U.S.) II. Title.
  UH474.5.W3S73 2009
  355.7'209753—dc22
                       2009010398

For sale by the Superintendent of Documents, U.S. Government Printing Office
Internet: bookstore.gpo.gov   Phone: toll free (866) 512-1800;   DC area (202) 512-1800
Fax: (202) 512-2104 Mail: Stop IDCC, Washington, DC 20402-0001

ISBN 978-0-9818228-4-6

CONTENTS

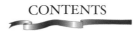

If you would understand anything,

observe its beginning and its development.

—Aristotle

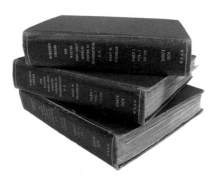

PREFACE
The Story of the Book

Publication of this book has been abandoned twice—its appearance now coincides with the abandonment of Walter Reed Army Medical Center (WRAMC), established over 100 years ago. The story begins in 1938 when Mary Walker Standlee began to collect anecdotes about WRAMC. She was a Texan, born in 1906. She left medical school at the University of Texas to marry First Lieutenant Earle Standlee, MC, USA.[1] He was a graduate of Baylor University School of Medicine and also a Texan. She accompanied him on service tours to Washington, the Philippines, Boston and New York, and on his return from World War II to Washington. He held senior staff positions in the Surgeon General's office and the Department of Defense. Promoted to Major General in 1952, he served as Far East Command Surgeon, U.S. Army forces in Japan, 1953–1957.[2] He retired on returning to the United States in 1957.[3] During the three years in Japan Standlee, with a Japanese collaborator, wrote The Great Pulse (Rutland, VT, Tuttle, 1959), a short monograph on the history of medicine, midwifery and obstetrics in Japan. She later wrote, "This I did . . . so that I would always have a good excuse for escaping the ladies luncheons."[4] Standlee notes in her foreword that she had been collecting Walter Reed "stories" and had begun an informal history in 1948. The book really began in 1950 when Brigadier General Paul S. Streit, MC, Commanding General, requested and partially funded the work. She did much of it on her own time as she was the "general's dogsbody, editing a nursing procedures manual, speech writing and 'ghosting' articles." (Foreword) She was also editing two histories of Army nursing, but neither was published.[5] The 399-page, 300-photograph manuscript reflects Standlee's vivid personality, for example, page 157: ". . . the topic for social conversation at Army dinner tables"; pages 160–161: "Twice told tales . . . wide circulation . . . "; pages 180, note 13 and 181, note 27: "Personal knowledge of the writer" and variously "Social conversations with . . . ." Chapter 3, "The Intermediate Host" (on the Walter Reed yellow fever study), led to extended correspondence with Dr. Phillip Hench of the Mayo Clinic (and Nobel Laureate). Hench collected Walter Reed material (now deposited at the University of Virginia), and sent her a detailed, single-spaced, 15-page letter of advice on 15 August 1961. This chapter was published earlier, in 1954, as a journal article.[6] Standlee's draft manuscript was circulated to a number of readers. In general the letters praise the text—but usually with a demur or two about what was said about the readers. There is no evidence that she altered any of the text. The final typed manuscript with photographs was prepared in four copies. The original was sent to the Office of the Surgeon General, one to the Walter Reed General Hospital library, one to the Borden family, and one Standlee kept. The manuscript was not published. In 1988 Colonel Mary Sarnecky, writing a history of the Army Nurse Corps, found an item in the National Archives labeled "Borden's Dream." She gave the call number to me; I filed it and resurrected it 20 years later for Colonel Lenhart, director of the Borden Institute. She and her staff found a treasure chest of letters (including mine) and other records in the National Archives, which I have used for this account. The reasons that the manuscript was not published are not fully obvious, but a story can now be suggested. In chapter 17, there are hints that Standlee and MG Streit had a falling out. The chapter does not have the analysis of WRAMC's commander found in all the other chapters. There are hints in three of her letters that she is preparing a new chapter 17 about MG Streit that might not be favorable.[7] Perhaps the best evidence that Streit stopped the publication is his letter of September 1974 to Colonel John Lada, Director of the Army Medical Department's Historical Unit. Noting that there was a re-awakening of interest in "Borden's Dream," he writes that "in the early 1950s I had some reservations about publication without some revisions, but I am now convinced that enough time has passed to remove my previous reservations. I write now to withdraw previous reservations and to urge you most strongly to publish Borden's Dream. It is a delightful memoir . . . I am most anxious to see Mrs. Standlee's volume in print."[8] In 1961 Standlee published a very short Part II to "Borden's Dream" on the Army Medical Library, which began as the Library of the Surgeon General's Office in 1836 and later evolved into the National Library of Medicine. Her account is brief, not as well documented as Part I, but has the same insouciant air and unique oral histories. The account covers the period from 1836 to 1956, when the Army turned over the library collections and responsibility to the U.S. Public Health Service and the National Library of Medicine began.[9] In 1974 the Commanding General of WRAMC, MG Robert Bernstein, MC, asked me to write a history of the medical center for the upcoming dedication of the new hospital building. I agreed, found the "Dream" manuscript in the hospital library and said, "Here is the history." I planned to edit and update the manuscript. I learned that General and Mrs. Standlee were alive and active in Texas. LTC Charles Simpson, MSC, USA (Ret.), was the Executive Officer of the Army Medical Deptartment Historical Unit and an old friend. He knew the Standlees "from the old days." When Mrs. Standlee agreed to my request to permit publication, I immediately asked him to help, especially with publishing the book. In fits and starts as time allowed I edited the chapters.[10] I described my editorial approach as "look at content and for documentation of facts, and then do an overall rough cut at format." Mrs. Standlee, who did not agree with some of my suggestions, commented, "You know the modern Army. I knew the 'old Army.' Let's not nitpick. In general, I think your suggestions are excellent."[11] However, she did comment after reviewing some of my later suggestions about "the blood on my ax. . . ."[12] In August 1976, after five years at the Walter Reed Army Institute of Research, I accepted a faculty position at the new Uniformed Services University of the Health Sciences medical school. I kept in touch with Standlee and the manuscript's situation through Simpson. By 1977 the Historical Unit had been absorbed by the U.S. Army Center of Military History. Charles Simpson died in 1982. His replacement, Dr. Jeffrey Greenhut, asked me about the "Dream." I sent all the material I had collected to him, discussed the issues, and lost track of the project. I discovered a year or so later that he had left the center, and "Borden's Dream" was not going to be published. COL Lenhart told me April 2008 that Robert Mohrman, the Walter Reed librarian, had brought the "Dream" to her attention, suggesting that publication might be germane as part of the commemoration of the closure of WRAMC, and she agreed. So there it is: a tale that begins in 1938 and ends 70 years later. A book that twice comes near to publication and fails each time. Finally, ironically, the first history of WRAMC is being published as the medical center is being closed. And Mary Walker Standlee? She passed away in 1985, twice disappointed by not having her work published. She would have wonderfully pithy comments on the reason her book appears at last. But the book is being published as she wanted. "I would not want anyone to update it to carry through later administrations. It represents the end of an era."[13] "I do not want the material updated. It is a 'period piece' and not Swedish Modern. Let's keep it that way."[14] This wonderful text is published exactly as she wrote it.

Emeritus Professor Robert J. T. Joy, MD, FACP
Department of Medical History
Colonel, MC, USA (Ret.)
Uniformed Services University of the Health Sciences

REFERENCES

Unless otherwise noted, all references are to an extensive collection of material at the National Archives and Records Administration, RG 112, Entry 1004, "Borden's Dream: (1936–1977)." Copies of this material are on file at the Borden Institute.

1. Telephone conversation, M.E. Condon-Rall and Robert Bueshler, grandson, April 2008.

2. File, General Officers, Medical Corps, Office of the Surgeon General of the Army.

3. Department of Defense Press Release, 23 April 1957.

4. Letter, Mary W. Standlee to Robert J.T. Joy, 26 July 1957.

5. Florence A. Blanchfield: The Army Nurse Corps in World War II, 2 vols and Organized Nursing and the Army in Three Wars, 4 vols. She was Chief of the Army Nurse Corps, 1943–1947. Manuscript copies are in the library, USUHS.

6. Mary W. Standlee, "Seeking the intermediate host," Mil. Surg. 115, 256–267, 1954.

7. Letters, Standlee to Joy, 11 February 1976, 11 March 1976, 20 June 1976.

8. Letter, Paul B. Streit to John Lada, 5 September 1974.

9. Wyndham D. Miles, A History of the National Library of Medicine, Washington, D.C., Public Health Service, 1982.

10. I was Deputy Director and then Director, Walter Reed Army Institute of Research.

11. Letter, Standlee to Joy, 11 February 1976: comment written on return of edited chapter 7.

12. Letter, Standlee to Joy, 11 March 1976.

13. Letter, Standlee to Joy, 26 July 1974.

14. Letter, Standlee to Joy, 17 August 1976.

PROLOGUE

If you peruse the history of Walter Reed Army Medical Center (WRAMC) on the hospital Web site,[1] the first entry is dated 1909, the date Walter Reed General Hospital was founded, and the second entry is dated 1972, when planning for the current hospital building began. Only two sentences between the two entries summarize what transpired in that 63-year period. At the WRAMC Medical Library, we have been asked more times than I can count where to find additional historical information about the intervening years. Aside from a chapter in a 1923 book about the US Army Medical Department,[2] when the hospital was only 14 years old, any detailed history or description of the development of this installation is hard to find (except perhaps in boxes in the National Archives). We are approaching two milestones in WRAMC's history: the centennial of its founding and the anticipated closing of the original site (for the planned integration of WRAMC with the National Naval Medical Center in Bethesda, Maryland). Closing the medical center without a published history would be a sad legacy of its 100-year history.

Fortunately, a record of the first 40 years of the medical center does exist. The little-known manuscript, called "Borden's Dream" after the surgeon whose concept it was to build this institution, started out as a collection of newspaper clippings and historical photographs by the hospital's first librarian, Mary E Schick. Intending to the use the collection as the basis for an institutional history, Schick continued to file materials but never found time to tackle the writing for the project. Instead, in 1943 she urged a younger member of the staff, Mary W Standlee, to write the story as an informal narrative history.[3,4] The story was finished in 1951, but Schick died shortly before the first draft was typed and never saw the finished product. It was deposited in the post library as a permanent documentary record.

Except for a copy donated to the author's alma mater, the University of Texas at Austin, and a few photocopied volumes distributed to military medical libraries, the book has never been made available to the public. It is known only to a few researchers as a source of historical information about WRAMC. When I came to work in the WRAMC library in 1997, I was briefed on the existence of this rare manuscript, but aside from trying to keep it intact and safely locked in a cabinet, we did nothing to preserve it. As the years passed, a number of the photographs and illustrations fell out or disappeared, and the ink slowly bled into the onion skin paper and became illegible. Clearly, something needed to be done to save this work for the future, but there were always more pressing issues.

When I took charge of the library in 2002, I decided it was time to correct this oversight. Inspired by the Library of Congress' American Dream project, I researched digitization as a means of not only preserving but also providing access to the document. There was much more work (and expense) involved than I had anticipated, however, but then a serendipitous meeting with the staff of the Borden Institute provided the answer. Over the last 5 years, first COL Dave Lounsbury and then his successor, COL Martha Lenhart, gave their wholehearted support to the project, and not only have we succeeded in preserving a digital copy of the original manuscript, but it has been formatted for publication for the first time.

As this icon of dedicated military medical care enters its second century, WRAMC finds itself once again crowded with soldiers wounded in combat. As in decades past, state-of-the-art care is being provided by a committed professional staff to men and women injured while serving our country. We hope that this book will help place the mission of this great hospital in the context of 100 years of honored service, as well as in a larger tradition of the Army medicine that dates to the founding days of the Republic.

Bob Mohrman
Librarian
Walter Reed Army Medical Center
June 2007

REFERENCES

1. 96 Years of Service: 1909–2005. Walter Reed Army Medical Center Web site. Available at: http://www.wramc.army.mil/welcome/History.htm. Accessed July 19, 2007.

2. Weed FW. The general hospital (permanent): Walter Reed General Hospital, Washington, DC; pre-war period. In: Ireland MW, ed. *Medical Department of the United States Army in World War.* Vol V. In: *Military Hospitals in the United States.* Washington, DC: Government Printing Office, 1923: Chap XV. Available at: http://history.amedd.army.mil/booksdocs/wwi/WRAMCWWI/WRGHWWI.html. Accessed July 19, 2007.

3. Standlee MW. The book lady (obituary of Mary E Schick). *Military Surgeon.* July 1952: 49.

4. Standlee MW. Borden's dream. Vol 1. Unpublished manuscript. 1952: i-ii.

PROLEGOMENON

Borden's Dream represents the culmination of years of work by Mary Standlee. It includes research, interviews, and interpretation by the author that provide insight into lesser known events in the history of the Walter Reed Army Medical Center. Although significant time has passed between completion of the manuscript and its publication, many of the situations, interactions, and reactions revealed within translate as familiar scenarios—lessons learned—still applicable today. Readers need to keep in mind that the manuscript content is original and unedited. In so noting, reflection on some of the contents may uncover circumstances that in their time went unremedied. No offense is intended by publishing this manuscript as originally written; rather, it is in keeping with the author's comment of more than fifty years ago that the book represents a "period piece" at the end of an era.

The publication is laid out with contemporary additions to the front matter – Preface, Prologue, and this introductory material, the Prolegomenon. The text of Mary Standlee's work begins with her Foreword on page xii and concludes at the Index on page 424. We have added a Postface after the Index that includes Major Borden's article: "The Walter Reed General Hospital of the United States Army, Mil Surg. 20-35, 1907," detailing his vision. Original suggested edits with hand written comments shared between Dr Joy and Mary Standlee (original materials now housed at the National Archives) and author information bring to a close the Postface.

And yet, this manuscript would remain unpublished today if not for the efforts and contributions of those acknowledged below.

Robert J. Mohrman —— as WRAMC librarian tasked with maintaining the manuscript and who sought preservation of this remarkable aging text and its images.

Bruce G. Maston —— who created the original design and layout that inspired further efforts toward publication of this work. His artistry and eye for imagery is extraordinary.

Sheryl Cohn Chiasson —— whose intrepid attention to detail resulted in the accurate transition of the original manuscript to the published text.

Dr. James Cox, Jr, COL, MC, USAF (Ret) —— who imparted energy, expertise and thoughtful input assuring our attention to detail in the final push to publication.

Dr. Chuck Callahan, COL, MC, USA (former WRAMC DCCS) —— wholeheartedly supported the publication efforts.

Dr. John Pierce, COL, MC, USA (Ret) —— as unwavering supporter of WRAMC history.

Dr. Robert Joy, COL, MC, USA (Ret) —— who earlier engaged the author, Mary Standlee, and more recently bridged the gap between initial efforts to publish the manuscript and its ultimate printing.

Martha K. Lenhart
Colonel, MC, US Army
Director, Borden Institute

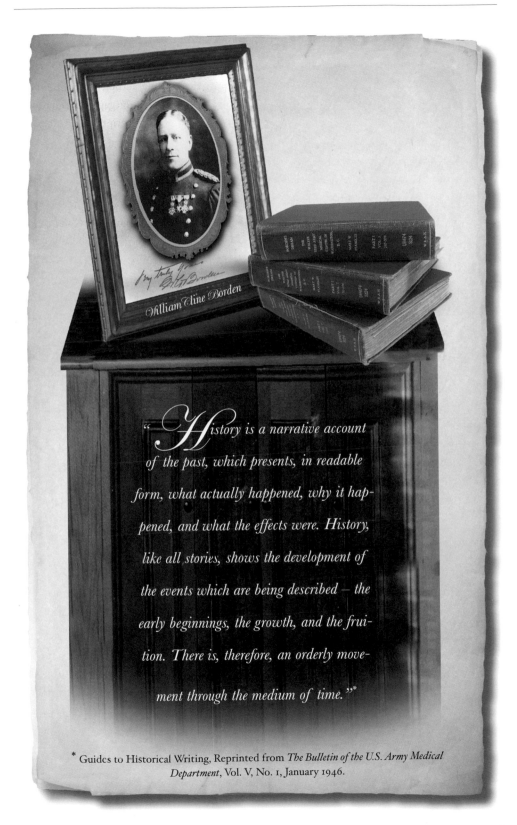

William Cline Borden

"*History* is a narrative account of the past, which presents, in readable form, what actually happened, why it happened, and what the effects were. History, like all stories, shows the development of the events which are being described — the early beginnings, the growth, and the fruition. There is, therefore, an orderly movement through the medium of time."*

* Guides to Historical Writing, Reprinted from *The Bulletin of the U.S. Army Medical Department*, Vol. V, No. 1, January 1946.

FOREWORD

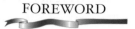

The life story of the Army Medical Center has long been of interest to the library staff of the Walter Reed Army Hospital, who have been obliged to answer many pertinent reference questions each year. The writer collected some of the human interest stories used in this manuscript as early as 1938, as by-products of social conversations with Miss Mary E. Schick, senior librarian, the most frequently consulted authority on Post history. General and Mrs. M.W. Ireland, as well as other distinguished members of the Medical Corps, had often asked Miss Schick to write the hospital story, but, contrary to the usual conception of a librarian as a sedentary person stamping the "date due" on an endless succession of books, her activities left no free time for so exacting a pastime as writing. Largely because of her insistence, in 1943 the writer began an informal narrative history, one which did not, however, discuss the growth of the Walter Reed Army Medical Center in context with the general development of the Army Medical Service. As word got around that a collection of "Post Lore" was being made there were many interested inquiries regarding the progress of the history, and in the summer of 1948 Colonel Clifford V. Morgan, then Deputy Post Commander of the Army Medical Center, urged that a permanent record of Post activities be prepared for local use. Unfortunately, the writer was not then free to devote the time necessary for completing the project.

In the late winter of 1950, Major General Paul H. Streit, the nineteenth Post Commander, was interested in the project and suggested that the writer develop an adequate history of the installation but disclaimed an ability to provide appropriated funds for what would be a possibly two-year project. The writer requested, in turn, at least a six-month period of subsidized research, the final history to be completed, as begun, on a non-pay status. No time limit was imposed, but in accordance with the policies established by the Historical Division of the Surgeon General's Office, the manuscript was to be properly coordinated with the broad aspects of the Medical Service history by individuals familiar with the Corps history, two copies of the finally assembled material, including some two hundred historical photographs, were to be deposited with the Post Library as a permanent documentary record.

Only two specific guideposts were proposed for developing the manuscript. The first was suggested by General Streit, who requested inclusion of biographical sketches of the eighteen former Post Commanders. The second requirement, consensus of several opinions and endorsed by the Commanding General, provided that a discussion of the hospital activities, Walter Reed Army Hospital, constitute the main theme of the story. Under the written terms of reference the writer became the final authority on the inclusion of any material presented in the volume. The agreements, both verbal and written, which encouraged completion of "Borden's Dream," are undoubtedly unusual; it is therefore appropriate here to acknowledge publicly a debt of gratitude to General Streit for his interest in and endorsement of an installation story of this scope. Sufficient material for an additional volume, "The Interrupted Dream," mainly dealing with the locator problems of the Army Medical Library and Museum, long proposed as part of the Walter Reed Army Medical Center, is organized and partially written but could not be completed prior to termination of General Streit's term as Post Commander, a goal toward which the writer has driven with stubborn determination.

It has been a pleasure as well as a privilege to recreate through interviews with former Army Medical Service personnel, and insofar as such personnel has been available, the individuality of some of the Post Commanders. The physical appearance of these men was familiar, for The Library has long maintained a chronological collection of their portraits. As individuals, the majority were unknown to the writer. In one or two instances the biographical sketches are meager past the point of acceptability, for contemporaries who knew the subjects well cannot be located. This is an unfortunate handicap, not an oversight. The writer has, however, accepted the familiar precept that the recording and interpretation of history "involves not only a clear conception and a lively explanation of events and characters, but a sound, enlightened theory of individual and national morality, a general philosophy of human life whereby to judge them and measure their efforts."

In 1935 a former executive officer of the Army Medical Center, Major (later Major General) Paul R. Hawley, unwittingly proposed a satisfactory maxim:

> *The Army Medical Center was, in the beginning, an idea. By slow and at times painful processes the institution has evolved to its present state. It is not yet complete; and no one man is responsible for all of the accomplishments thus far. Many distinguished officers have left indelible impressions upon these masses of brick and stone.*

The story of the Walter Reed Army Medical Center could not be encapsulated and set apart from the plans and policy program of the Army Medical Service, and so it has been necessary to include some general discussions which clarify the military hospital program. The reader should, therefore, fully understand the interrelationship of this installation to the Office of the Surgeon General, which prescribes the medical doctrine implemented in this and other Medical Service installations. The writer has made a conscientious attempt to keep this relationship in sight without detracting from the unusual development of the Army's most famous general hospital.

The majority of the photographs and illustrations were provided from the files of the Walter Reed Army Medical Center. However, Miss Helen Campbell and Mr. William C. Harris of the *Arts Section*, Catalogue Division of the Armed Forces Medical Library, not only assisted in the selection of some of the pictures, but with unfailing industry and cheerfulness they provided many "missing links." To Miss Josephine Cobb, Chief of the *Still Pictures Section*, National Archives, the writer owes a very special debt, for as a result of her interest in locating early pictures of the U.S. Army General Hospital, Washington Barracks, D.C., the writer made the acquaintance of Daniel L. Borden, M.D., who permitted the uncensored use of his father's personal records and papers, without which the story could not have been written.

The list of interested readers was long, and the writer has profited immeasurably from the careful comments and kindly criticisms offered for the improvement of the manuscript. Colonel James M. Phalen, M.C., ret., editor of *The Military Surgeon*, not only volunteered his services as editor but provided considerable first-hand information of a historical nature. Major General Charles R. Reynolds, M.C., ret., formerly a Surgeon General of the Army, likewise edited the manuscript with extreme care, providing for the writer some fifteen pages of laboriously hand-written notes to be used as supplementary material. Colonel J.F. Siler, M.C., ret., provided comprehensive and complete technical editing of such a high nature that the writer is unable properly to express appreciation for the time expended. Chapter III, "The Intermediate Host," has been the most difficult section of the book to write and would have presented nearly insurmountable obstacles without the unstinted editorial efforts of Philip S. Hench, M.D. of the Mayo Clinic, the outstanding civilian authority on Major Walter Reed and the Yellow Fever episode. Dr. Hench twice reviewed and corrected drafts of the chapter. As there are many published manuscripts on the strictly scientific aspects of the Yellow Fever experiment in Cuba, Chapter III was prepared as a medico-historical sketch of Walter Reed, the man, patron saint of the hospital and Center rather than as an evaluation of the scientist or his work.

More than one reviewer called to the writer's attention the fact that much of the credit for successful installation management is due the able executive officers of the hospital and center who so loyally supported their chiefs. Unfortunately, proper acknowledgment of the services of these men could not be made, for the framework of the military structure is such that the commanding officer alone is finally responsible to "higher authority" for the success or failure of his organization. Further, the criticism has been offered that the only claim to distinction for the majority of the hospital commanders evolves from their assignment to the installation. This, however, was the first assumption used in preparing the manuscript.

It is an indisputable fact that the military hospital management is unique, not only from the standpoint of the complex administration but because of the generally homogenous employment background of the patients. Like members of a guild, they belong to a specialized group. The doctors, nurses, attendants and even the civilian employees reflect the group mores. Government Issue, military orders, inspection, "chow call" and formation are all familiar words in the daily routine. The writer has, for many years, been impressed with the lack of interest in, and knowledge of military medical administration evidenced by the average civilian, layman or doctor. It is to be hoped, therefore, that the reader will gain cleared insight into the intricacies of a service so often taken for granted and an appreciation of the splendid men who have given their lives to its development.

Mary W. Standlee
29 Fenwick Road, Fort Monroe, Virginia
5 December 1952

ACKNOWLEDGMENTS

Lt. Col Jessie M. Braden, ANC, Ret.

Miss Clara Birmingham

Mrs. Montgomery Blair

Daniel L. Borden, M.D.

Colonel J.R. Darnall, M.C.

Colonel Chauncey Dovell, M.C., Ret.

Colonel James D. Fife, M.C., Ret.

Mrs. Leon Gardner

Miss Juanita Gould

Colonel James F. Hall, M.C., Ret.

Philip S. Hench, M.D.

Colonel John Huggins, M.C., Ret.

Colonel E.C. Jones, M.C., Ret.

Colonel H.W. Jones, M.C., Ret.

Mrs. J.R. Kean

Mr. Robert Kean

Portia B. Kernodle, PhD

Colonel James C. Kimbrough, M.C., Ret.

Major General N.T. Kirk, M.C., Ret.

Brig General Albert G. Love, M.C., Ret.

Major General George F. Lull, M.C., Ret.

Major General James C. Magee, M.C., Ret.

Major General Shelly U. Marietta, M.C., Ret.

Colonel Clifford V. Morgan, M.C.

Mrs. William Nichol

Colonel James M. Phalen, M.C., Ret.

Miss Frances Phillips

Major General Charles R. Reynolds, M.C., Ret.

Brig General Frederick F. Russell, M.C., Ret.

Miss Mary E. Schick

Colonel J.F. Siler, M.C., Ret.

Brig General James S. Simmons, M.C., Ret.

Mrs. Emmy Sommers

Brig General A.E. Truby, M.C., Ret.

Brig General Charles Walson, M.C., Ret.

TABLE OF CONTENTS

Chapter VII

Chapter VIII

Chapter IX

Chapter X

Chapter XI

Chapter XVI

Chapter XVII

ILLUSTRATIONS

APPENDIX

A Half Century Before

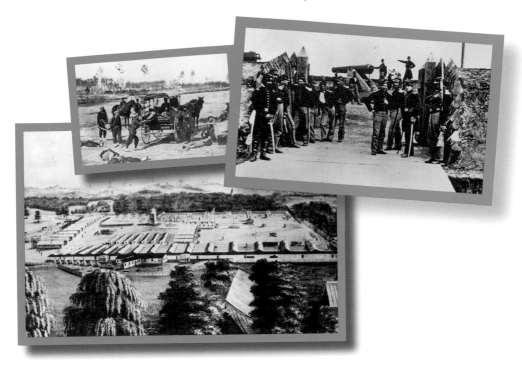

*"Country practitioners in green sashes
(became acquainted) with hygiene and vaccination."[1]*

A long stretch of historical thread connects the story of a military hospital and the women's reform movement, a thread thinly stretched across the century, for women are now so commonplace in public life as to be taken for granted. As a result men too often ignore the fact that by nature they are interested in trying new things, are by and large orderly planners as well as reformers. Moreover, women persevere, with more finesse than forthrightness, in behalf of their cause. If blocked, they eventually adjust their day dreaming to reality, and willy nilly progress is effected. But a hundred years ago most of the women were mainly concerned with home supremacy and serenely unaware that the hand that rocks only the cradle can't be too sure of ruling the world.

In 1847, when medical officers of the Army were at last accorded actual[2] military rank, Elizabeth Blackwell, an intrepid young feminist of the day, was finally admitted to Geneva Medical College, New York. She had been refused by better schools, and she was accepted at Geneva as the result of a practical joke.[3] There she was graduated in 1849—America's first woman physician.

An ambitious as well as an enterprising woman, Dr. Blackwell eventually became director of the New York Dispensary for Poor Women and Children, founded in 1855. Friend and admirer of the famous English nurse, Florence Nightingale, early in the Civil War she persuaded the lady managers of her infirmary that women listed as military nurses should qualify through a one-month training course in Bellevue Hospital, New York. Dr. Blackwell was ahead of her time, as Old Bellevue was not to have a recognized nurses' training school until 1873; it is not surprising that her proposal produced few "trained" nurses for the Army. On the other hand, the lady managers were members of a small group of enthusiastic and public spirited women who met in New York, April 25, 1861, to see what they could do to assist in winning the war. Unable to shoulder muskets and fight, they chose the only obvious course for a minority group, they organized and formed the Women's Central Association of Relief, which, with other interested welfare groups, evolved into the United States Sanitary Commission.[4]

Women who encourage men with ideas are legion and for the most part they remain anonymous. Men who encourage women with ideas are rare, but some secure sturdy seats in the halls of fame for their foresight. Such was the case of Henry W. Bellows, D.D., pastor of All Souls' Unitarian Church, New York. Undoubtedly well versed in the energetic ways of ladies' missionary societies, he advised the Women's Central Association not to duplicate any military relief activities which the Government could or would undertake for the soldiers.

History credits the Government with lack of interest in the relief movement. The President believed it a supernumerary organization; the War Department opposed it. The Medical Department was then a somnambulant and lethargic organization, probably as a result of the conservative influence of Thomas Lawson, Surgeon General since 1836, who died on May 15, 1861, the day before the welfare delegation arrived in Washington to plead its case. Historians differ on the reception accorded the committee. Some believed the "meddlesome civilians... (were received) with coldness, and discouraged... by evasion and delay."[5] Others credit Surgeon Robert C. Hood, a senior medical officer then serving as acting Surgeon General[6] as willingly[7] supporting the distinguished visitors in sanctioning "a commission of inquiry and advice in respect to the sanitary interests of the United States Forces."[8] The plan for a relief agency proposed on May 23, 1861, was approved by the President on June 13. Dr. Bellows became President of the Commission. Of the three Army representatives, Surgeon Wood represented the Medical Department, thus setting an organizational precedent for future relationships with the American National Red Cross.

There was neither preparation, organization nor precedent for such an activity, for even the British experiences in the Crimea were so recent that Dunant had not had time to arouse general interest in military relief work.[9] Thus amidst the chaos and disorderliness of the Civil War, the haphazard medical service and the poor state of medicine itself,[10] the planned orderliness of the Sanitary Commission stands out as a shining example of welfare work accomplished in spite of, not because of, federal responsibility for the wounded. Its early sponsors are largely forgotten, and the record accomplishments of the Commission overshadow Dr. Bellows. Individual women, however, such as Dorothea Dix, who became the Government's first superintendent of nurses, and Clara Barton, one of the few and certainly unknown "government girls" of her day, rose to spectacular fame. They earned immortality as humanitarians, nurses and relief workers, but Elizabeth Blackwell, M.D., having set nurse training as a goal for the military hospital service, was promptly forgotten. Nevertheless, in her small way she had begun a professional revolution, for the women who went to war in those days were dissatisfied with the conditions they found in the federal hospitals. And because they suffered vicariously with their friends and relations, they eventually set the house in order and took control of the situation. Of more immediate importance, the female-sponsored Sanitary Commission became politically powerful, and partially through its influence a long-standing policy of the Medical Department was set aside when a young man rather than an oldster was made Surgeon General.

Forecast For the Future

The unexpected death of Surgeon General Lawson established Surgeon Wood, a man of bureaucratic experience and inclination, of good family and allegedly notable political connections, as a candidate for the Surgeon Generalcy. When the President adhered to the custom of appointing the senior medical officer in the Corps to this position and named Clement L. Finley, Surgeon Wood continued to serve agreeably as the principal assistant. From the Surgeon General's office at Fifteenth Street and F Street, in Washington City,[11] medical service affairs were managed very much as usual. The appointment of military surgeons then was largely an activity of the state militia rather than of the Federal Government. The Surgeon General, a Colonel, fifty Surgeons, eighty-three assistant Surgeons and an indefinite number of stewards comprised the department. Two officers and five clerks comprised the staff of the Surgeon General's Office.[12]

The Medical Department, whose first regulations dealing with the duties of medical officers were published in 1814, as part of Army Regulations[13] was, in 1861, essentially "one of the coordinate branches of the general staff of the Army.... Its members were not permanently attached to any regiment or command, but their services were utilized wherever required."[14] Nor was there any distinction in the duties of surgeons and physicians, the term military surgeon, in the Army, connoting any licensed commissioned doctor. Regimental hospitals served the field troops, and the regimental surgeons were remarkably independent. The Surgeons were assigned regulated quantities of supplies, but many of the items were not only too bulky and cumbersome for use under combat conditions, but because of slow transportation they were often far in the rear of the supply train when needed.

From the standpoint of organization there was no sanitary service; hospital stewards were authorized under the Act of 16 August 1856 (11 Stat. 51), with an extra monetary allowance for duty performed as nurses. The uniform, during the Civil War period, was a variety of colors, and there are some who believe that its gay appearance depreciated the abilities of the wearers. General hospitals of sorts had been used in other American wars,[15] primarily as a place to accumulate the non-transportable wounded than as an effort to classify the sick, but no Army general hospital existed at the outbreak of the Civil War.[16] On August 3, 1861, the Congress authorized an increase in the number of medical officers and provided for the employment of medical cadets and female nurses.[17] The former were mainly students recruited to serve as dressers and assistants to the surgeons, and female nurses, in spite of Dr. Blackwell's foresight, were untrained.

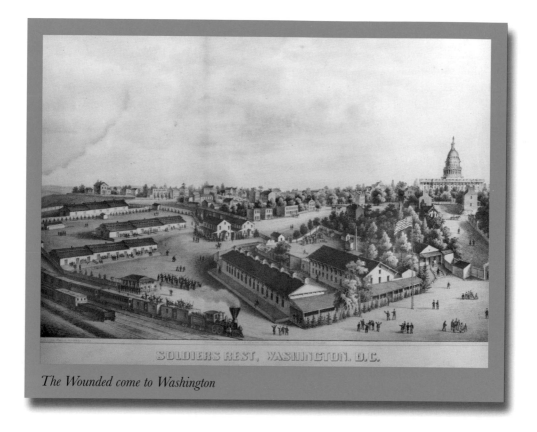

SOLDIER'S REST, WASHINGTON, D.C.

The Wounded come to Washington

The vicissitudes of war brought frequent changes in the military command, some of which inevitably affected Medical Department policies. In the summer of 1861, George B. McClellan succeeded McDowell as commander of all the troops in Washington City, and almost immediately he set about organizing and equipping the Army of the Potomac. An ambitious, autocratic and controversial figure, McClellan succeeded in undermining the waning official confidence in the military abilities of the aged Winfield Scott and supplanted him as general-in-chief, although Scott favored Henry W. Halleck as his successor.[18]

In spite of personal differences in temperament and politics, the President respected Edwin B. Stanton, a shrewd capital city lawyer, and appointed him to succeed Simon Cameron as War Secretary. Stanton, ruthless, irascible and domineering, initiated bureaucratic economies and set out to remodel the government services to his own specifications. Moreover, he attempted actively to direct the progress of the war. As his prestige and independence increased and McClellan's military procrastination brought a decrease in his popularity, the personal relationships of these two dynamic characters became strained to the breaking point.

The President, discouraged by his fractious and quarrelsome advisers, and the determined civilian management of the war, belatedly accepted Scott's recommendation of Halleck, who during the summer of 1862, came to the Capital as special military adviser and general-in-chief. Unknowingly, however, the President had supplanted one autocrat with another. Halleck was not a good field soldier in his own right, and in view of his many military shortcomings it was doubtless unavoidable that he gave no thought to improving the regimental medical service. Had he been either brilliant or a great leader, conditions might have improved, but as an arm chair strategist, a man "who marshaled files of paper and commanded ranks of facts"[19], he doubtless believed the two ambulances nominally assigned to a regiment during combat were sufficient, ignoring the fact that the Quartermaster had jurisdiction of vehicles and that when an Army lost its equipment and supplies there was no transportation for the wounded.[20] Halleck may have disliked McClellan, the young interloper, for any number of personal and official reasons, and he apparently translated his dislike into a veto of McClellan-sponsored men and policies. At any rate he was a negativistic man, and like the powerful Stanton, an unreasonable obstructionist.

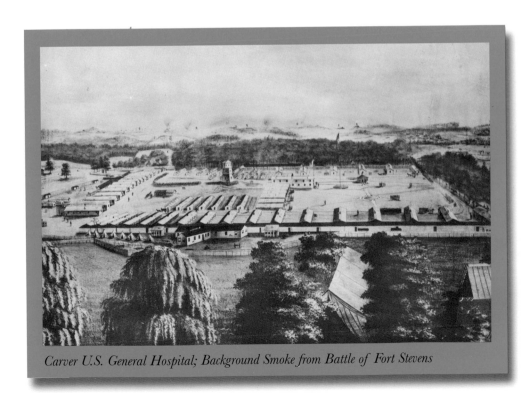

Carver U.S. General Hospital; Background Smoke from Battle of Fort Stevens

On April 7, 1862, a War Department order placed general hospitals under the Surgeon General's supervision, although clarification of the command responsibilities of medical officers, within their own sphere, was not obtained until after Presidential approval of the act establishing an organized ambulance service.[21]

General Finley, already sixty-four years old at the time of his appointment, found the combination of Stanton's irascibilities and the interference of the Sanitary Commission too much to bear, and applied for retirement on April 14, 1862. Again Surgeon Wood maneuvered to obtain appointment as Surgeon General. Again he was unsuccessful, for as a result of McClellan's patronage and the influence of some members of the Sanitary Commission, William Alexander Hammond, a young and energetic assistant surgeon, was appointed. Wood continued for a time in his position as principal assistant, but like many other older officers, he was embittered at having the traditional appointment of seniority ignored. The Capital was as usual a city of political intrigue and uncertain rumors, and Hammond, apparently believing Wood an obstructionist to any medical service reforms, had him reassigned.[22] In so doing he incurred Stanton's active dislike.[23] No doubt the fact that Hammond was the ill-fated McClellan's personal choice did nothing to encourage popularity with the equally dilatory and pompous Halleck.

Insofar as military hospitals were concerned, Washington City was unimportant until that spring of 1862 when Hammond was appointed. The Surgeon General's authority was confused by complicated organizational relationships with other Army Departments, and the new War Department order providing Medical Department supervision of the general hospitals was a mixed blessing, for it did not entail control of two of the basic services to patients – transportation of the wounded and food service. This oversight, plus the independence of the untrained regimental surgeons, created confusion in the hospitals. There was much absenteeism in the volunteer Army as a whole, composed largely of state militia, and Dr. Charles Tripler, McClellan's first Medical Director of the Army of the Potomac, believed that general hospitals were a general nuisance[24] to be endured rather than encouraged. In Washington, convenient haven for the federal wounded, hospitals, hotels and other public buildings were crowded with the casualties, and temporary hospitals were built as rapidly as possible. In location and operation some showed that the planners had little or no knowledge of public health and sanitation, and insofar as clinical medicine was concerned, asepsis and the microbiology of disease were unexplored fields. Volunteer surgeons and nurses arrived with the hordes of sightseers, office seekers and female camp followers, some of questionable repute. Many, failing to receive reimbursement for their expenses, returned home.[25]

The first field ambulances had been poor affairs, little more than crude carts, but when in need of transportation for supplies, Army commanders unhesitatingly appropriated them. In spite of the organization and devotion of the Sanitary Commission and other relief agencies to the welfare cause, many supplies and comforts destined for the regimental wounded were appropriated by the conveyors or delayed by poor transportation until spoiled. Men nurses had no hesitation in imbibing the "medicinal" liquors and, like the beverage, frequently failed to reach their destination.

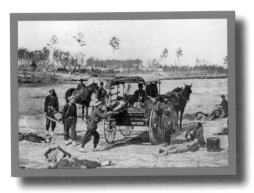

Civil War Ambulance (Brady Collection)

As one of his first official acts, the new Surgeon General replaced Dr. Tripler with Dr. Jonathan Letterman, thus providing McClellan, his patron, with an energetic young physician who recognized the factual needs of field medical organization.[26] The appointment, however, did not please War Secretary Stanton.[27] Dr. Letterman had already organized an ambulance corps and modified the field medical service extensively by August 2, 1862, when on August 21, Surgeon General Hammond presented independently, to the Secretary of War, a comprehensive plan for an organized hospital corps and ambulance company under Medical Department control. General Halleck, accustomed to the status quo as well as the tactical supremacy of line commanders, disapproved of granting Corps control to a technical service. The Surgeon General appealed the decision on September 7, but again the military commander disapproved.[28] Authorized by the drill-minded and orderly McClellan, it was fortunate that the Letterman plan was already in operation and would soon be adopted by other Commanders. Like many other meritorious plans, it survived, though not without a struggle.

Politics or Progress

Small and apparently inconsequential changes affect men's careers, and were the fabric of history unraveled, their personal ambitions, their successes and defeats would provide the warp and woof for the pattern. On May 2, 1862, Surgeon Joseph K. Barnes was ordered from the Department of Kansas to report to the Surgeon General in Washington and assigned as visiting physician to the military population of the city. In the following year he not only made the acquaintance but won the friendship and approval of the temperamental and vindictive Stanton, already at odds with the Surgeon General.

Medical inspectors were at a premium during this period, and by February 9, 1863, Barnes had been promoted to Lieutenant Colonel and occupied such a position; on August 10, 1863, he was advanced to the rank of Colonel and made a Medical Inspector General.[29] Stanton was especially interested in preventing waste of material as well as abuse of government contracts. Although of different temperaments the two men apparently had congenial interests. On the other hand, Barnes, a less dynamic figure than Hammond, may have been more pliable.

In late August 1863, much to his own surprise, Surgeon General Hammond was ordered to the Department of the South to inspect sanitary conditions; on September 3, Joseph K. Barnes was placed in charge of his office. General Hammond demanded restoration of his office or trial by court-martial. In view of Secretary Stanton's known dislike of him, the answer to his demands was predictable. He was court-martialed and dismissed, his honor remaining uncleared until 1878. On August 22, 1864, Barnes became Surgeon General in name as well as in fact, and during the remaining three years of Stanton's term, the medical service seemingly had his complete approval.[30]

The friction and controversy surrounding the Hammond administration make his short term appear extraordinarily successful, for many of the Medical Department's most outstanding and permanent achievements can be traced to his foresight and planning. The Act of Congress of June 30, 1834 (4 Stat 714) confirmed earlier provisions for the examination of medical officer candidates by a board of three officers, but General Hammond reorganized the boards and raised the standards. He introduced a new and more complete system of hospital reports; increased the number of items on the supply table; made provision for hospital clothing for patients, urged Medical Department autonomy in the construction of hospitals and transportation of supplies. Further, and of far-reaching consequence in the care of patients, he urged formation of a permanent hospital corps. He encouraged expansion of the Surgeon General's meager collection of professional books, begun in 1836, into a full-scale medical library. On May 21, 1862, he authorized the Army Medical Museum, for the preservation of pathological specimens collected during the war, and the Stanton-disapproved course in military medicine, scheduled for 1863-1864, undoubtedly had his sanction.

General Hammond was familiar with all aspects of the medical service during this period, and he recognized the importance of continuing a well supplied permanent or fixed general hospital as part of the peacetime medical service and planned to locate the institution in Washington. For, regardless of the fact that there were no clinical thermometers, none of the heart stimulants now in common usage, no general use of microscopes, no sterilization of instruments and dressings, and that unclean surgical practices increased the infection of wounds,[31] patients so hospitalized fared better than those treated in the extemporary regimental hospitals. Some of the welfare ideas first advocated by the Women's Central Relief Association were effected by Surgeon General Hammond, including the establishment of a "diet table",[32] in other words, special diets for invalids. As the first proponent of a centrally controlled medical service during a war, he paved the way, by his determined efforts, for reforms later effected by his successors.

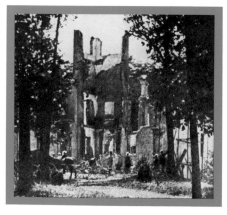

Blair House, Silver Spring, Md.; Destroyed by Confederates, 1864

As he said, "the hospital system had scarcely received any attention up until this time", and at one period "hospitals for over twenty thousand sick and wounded were established in Washington alone",[33] where during the war a total of forty-three hospitals were operative, with seven additional ones in Georgetown.[34] Soldier, teacher and progressive physician, Hammond was well aware of the poor professional preparation of many of the apprentice-trained doctors of his day who had "read" medicine with a proctor but practiced on the unsuspecting public – or the soldier. To many of them even the poor standards of the temporary military hospitals were a professional revelation, for here the "country practitioners in green sashes[35] (became acquainted) with hygiene and vaccination." There is little cause for surprise that in addition to a permanent general hospital in Washington City,[36] General Hammond favored establishing an Army Medical School for the orientation and post graduate instruction of medical officer candidates. Recommendations and accomplishments are, however, as far apart as dreams and reality. And Washington City, had it known of this future honor, then would have thought little of the proposal.

A Skirmish Is Called a Battle

Within the city proper the approach to the uncrowned Capitol was dusty or muddy, depending entirely on the season and the weather. Pennsylvania Avenue was for the most part tree shaded, although the double line of horse car tracks gave it the vague air of a metropolis. The cars were gaudy affairs, noisy and crowded.[37] The buildings, some of them public in the private sense of the word, were architecturally unexciting by present day standards. A well known bawdy house operated within a block of the President's Park,[38] and F Street, unpaved and sporting a mongrel architecture, hardly appeared cosmopolitan looking – or even urban. Although its pretentious boundaries were measured and its circumference extended thirty-seven miles, to the north the city outskirts reached only to Boundary Street or Florida Avenue, half-way to the Soldier's Home, where the President had a summer White House.

The road was not in existence in 1800, when Congress and the government departments moved to the city, but travelers now approached the city from the north along the Seventh Street Road, a turnpike connecting the gawky metropolis with the outlaying Maryland farming area. Authorization for the turnpike was granted between 1808 and 1810, when the Columbia Turnpike Company was chartered to build a highway, but since they delayed the work, the Washington and Rockville Turnpike Company undertook the job,[39] which was not completed until after 1819. According to some records the Congress gave a "Maryland Company" authority to build a turnpike to the District Line, to be known as the Rockville Road. There was another road to Rockville, through Tennelly town, so the new road was commonly referred to as the Seventh Street Turnpike and Seventh Street Road.[40] By 1822, it was noted as important,[41] although it was narrow and at times impassable.

By 1832, prosperous Methodists had erected Emory Chapel in the outlying section, about three miles from Boundary Street, and a half mile or so from Crystal Spring, from which the area took its name. The Chapel was the first community landmark of its kind; the lower part was built of log and served as a school, while the upper or church-half had separate galleries for its fifty-nine white and thirteen Negro members.

Some three miles beyond this settlement, on the Maryland side, Francis Preston Blair, editor of *The Washington Globe*, and his son Montgomery, later Postmaster General in the Lincoln cabinet, owned estates. It was probably because of the Blair influence that a plank road was laid on the turnpike in 1852, extending from Boundary Street to the District Line, for the older Blair retired in 1853 and moved from his Pennsylvania Avenue mansion to the Maryland estate. The engineering for this project consisted of embedding half-split trees, rounded side down, into the ordinary road base, with the pike depressed several inches below the road. Heavy teams were excluded, and doubtless as an effort to meet the cost of such a luxurious highway, a Toll House was erected a little to the north of the church but well above the Milk House Road (Shepherd Street), which connected this unpretentious area with Tennelly town (Cleveland Park) and Georgetown on the west and southwest.[42] Crystal Spring, Emory Chapel, rebuilt of brick in 1856, and in close proximity Moreland's Tavern,[43] with its handsome grove of tress, were the most important landmarks in the area. The rustic name of Crystal Spring was already falling into disuse prior to the Civil War, when this small link to urban activity was known first as Brighton, but later, because of confusion with a nearby Maryland town, as Brightwood. By 1860, the latter name was apparently better known then Crystal Spring, for here, at the reserve "Camp Brightwood", the death of a Union Soldier was noted November 16, 1861.[44]

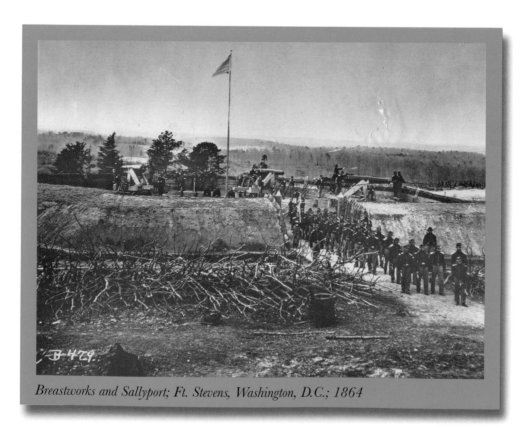

Breastworks and Sallyport; Ft. Stevens, Washington, D.C.; 1864

The Piney Branch of Rock Creek was an open stream and some of the large and prosperous farms in the area were owned by the Whites, Pierces, Shoemakers, the Klingles and the Bealls.[45] The Beall tract, know as Norway, included about 338 acres and extended north along "the old plank road" (to approximately Aspen Street) and adjoined the Lay farm.[46] When the new Emory Chapel was appropriated by the Union Troops, razed, and the bricks used to build Fort Stevens, the old log schoolhouse was converted into a guardhouse for unruly soldiers.[47] Moreland's Tavern was commandeered as headquarters for General Alexander McCook in 1864.[48]

A half mile to the north of Fort Stevens the turnpike was itself bisected by a deep ravine, later called Cameron's Creek, a small tributary of the Piney Branch of Rock Creek. All the land within two miles of the fort[49] was cleared during the war in order to prevent surprise attacks, but the section beyond Norway was generally wooded and rugged. In spite of such precautions, and the string of forts that rimmed the city, the Capital was not well protected during that hot July 1864. Levies of men were hard to come by, and a large number of the garrison troops had been deployed to active combat areas. Thus it was an excellent time for the rebels to attack. With a better intelligence system to aid them, or more perseverance, they might have succeeded in spite of the sultry heat and the fatigue induced by forced marches. When word circulated in the city that Rhodes' Division of General Jubal Early's rebel troops was moving south, the outlying defenses were hastily strengthened and "General Alexander McCook was assigned to command a reserve camp on Piney Branch Creek, midway between the city and Fort Stevens (on) the Seventh Street Road."[50] This was apparently Crystal Spring,[51] occupied by one company of the 150th Ohio regiment, two hundred and nine men if counting a battery of artillery and a few convalescent soldiers. And it was this meager support, occupying the adjacent rifle pits, that created the "white puffs of smoke (which) rose from the entrenched line of Federals in the valley, and from the groves and orchards and farmhouses where the Confederate sharpshooters were posted."[52]

There were fifteen or twenty thousand of Early's rebel veterans approaching the city by way of the Georgetown and Frederick Turnpike when the Union forces, panicky because of the unexpected invasion, began calling for re-enforcements. Preliminary skirmishes with Union troops in the outlying area to the northwest caused Early to turn his advance east in order to prevent the Union troops from making a stand at the natural defense of the deep Maryland channel of Rock Creek. He therefore turned off the main road at Rockville and moving east to the Seventh Street Road, entered it about Silver Spring, Maryland.[53] Spotters as well as evacuees fleeing from Rockville, Silver Spring and other Maryland towns warned of the advance, but in spite of the prospects of a battle, the usual curious spectators from Washington thronged the Seventh Street Road, anxious to view the battle from a safe place. Crowded by those going out and those going in to the city, the turnpike was a busy place.

The unpopular Halleck, ranking military man in the city,[54] apparently made no effort to restrict the sightseers, although re-enforcements were being sent to Fort Stevens as rapidly as word could be spread that the Capital was threatened. Men from the Army of the Potomac were brought in by train and boat, within three days some ten thousand of them. The main advance of Confederates halted on the outskirts, near the hastily abandoned house of Montgomery Blair, the Postmaster General, but a mile or so farther down the turnpike sharpshooters from Rhodes' Division occupied the Reeves House, to the East of Seventh Street Road. The cupolaed Lay House, on the west, with its giant tulip tree, provided excellent vantage points for sniping at occupants of the fort.[55] The President, no less curious than the other Washingtonians, ventured to the Fort and narrowly missed being a military casualty. Instead, a surgeon[56] standing by his side was killed by a sharpshooter's bullet, fired from a tall cherry tree in the rear of the Reeves House, a distance of about 900 yards.[57] In quick retaliation, thirty-six shots were fired from Fort Stevens and nearly as many from Fort De Russey, on the left and just across Rock Creek.

The Lay and Reeves houses were destroyed, and the giant tulip tree was damaged, but the sharpshooter, later wounded by an equally good Union marksman of his kind, died on the grounds of the Beall farm.[58] When Wheaton's men advanced to clear the rebels from their stronghold, Rhodes' men appeared from concealment in the ravine of Cameron's Creek and a short-range but important engagement

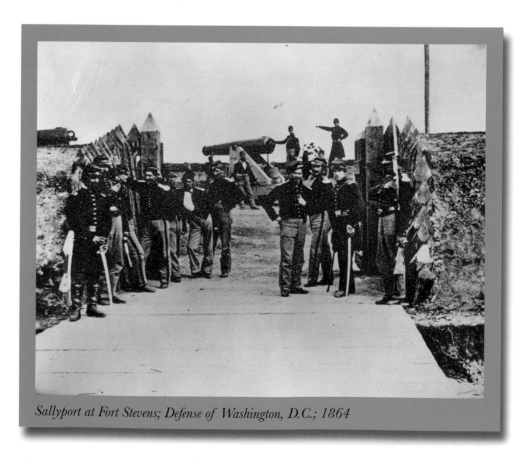

Sallyport at Fort Stevens; Defense of Washington, D.C.; 1864

took place. The outnumbered rebel forces withdrew during the night of July 12, leaving seventeen of their dead to be buried in the Episcopal graveyard at Woodside, Maryland, and one at Silver Spring. The Union men were buried in a hastily created cemetery to the east of Seventh Street Road, behind the Reeves House but on land which may have been part of Norway, as this tract was apparently bisected by the turnpike.

Brightwood area residents disapproved of the tollgate, so they organized and purchased a right-of-way around it and extending south to the approximate location of the Tavern, later known as Brightwood Club House[59] and still later the site of the Masonic Temple. The northern part of the meandering right-of-way became Piney Branch Road;[60] the southern part, crossed by Magnolia Avenue, renamed in turn Concord and Missouri Avenue, was renamed in accordance with the Capital planning, for the State of Colorado.

In time the Lay farm was sold to Thomas Carberry, Mayor of the District from 1822–1823. Still later it was sold to Ex-senator J. Donald Cameron,[61] whose ownership gave the small stream the name of Cameron's Creek. Alexander Shepherd purchased the land to the north and after he became famous Milk Ford Road was renamed for him. Military Road, cut through from the northwest section during the war, was the only one of the thoroughfares to retain its original name. The Crystal Spring Race Track (at Kennedy and Colorado) flourished until about 1860. Here the sports came from Washington, and families came on picnics. The fare by stage was seventy-five cents for the round trip, with one-half fare for children.[62] Saul's nursery, one of the finest of its kind in the country, dated from 1872, and by 1885 it consisted of some seventy-five acres and twenty greenhouses,[63] with the owner specializing in rare evergreens as well as fruit trees. The principal place lay between the turnpike and "Piney Branch Park", to the west.

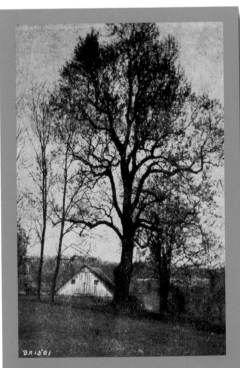

Sharpshooters Tree used by Confederates; Battle of Ft. Stevens

Carberry House, or the Lay Mansion, as it was more generally known, was rebuilt after the war and continued to be known as Norway until the early part of the twentieth century. It was a stately four-chimney house with a fashionable observatory on the roof and with spacious porches of which only the front remained in any state of repair. A double line of maples bordered the drive, concealing its decaying grandeur from the disinterested public traveling the turnpike. Few people knew and fewer would have cared that a privately owned clay and gravel road trailed off to an ironstone springhouse in the low southwest section of the grounds where passed a "rocky, tree-lined stream",[64] for Cameron's Creek rose close to the District Line west of Takoma and after describing a crooked course from northeast to southwest entered Rock Creek at the Military Road.

Bleak House, the Shepherd residence to the west of the Turnpike, was a mansion of historic proportions,[65] with a stone lodge for the gate-keeper located at the front of its spruce-line drive. These were the days when the rickety "Red Bird" stagecoach plied between Washington City and the suburb.[66]

When the Brightwood Citizens' Association was organized in 1891, the community began to make improvements. Horse racing was no longer the community sport; Boundary Street was still Boundary Street, not Florida Avenue, and the reliable old *Washington Star* warned its cycling readers that "It is true there are a number of streets extending beyond Boundary, but they lead nowhere, ending in wilds and wilderness".[67] By 1899 a venturesome capitalist had extended the District's street railroad from Rock

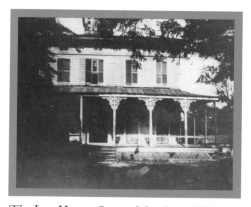

The Lay House; Once a Mansion of Historic Proportions

Creek Road to the village of Brightwood. Equipped with the discarded horses and bobtail cars of the metropolitan line of the B & O, the impatient patrons dubbed their public transportation system the GOP, "get-out-and-push", because of its frequent founderings en route. Takoma Park and North Takoma were disarticulated rural dependencies. The Brightwood postal service, one a "will-call" station in the crossroads store at Piney Branch Road and the turnpike, location of the tollgate, sported a letter carrier, complete with horse and sulky. The adolescent breastworks of Fort Stevens, and unimportant battleground where a President went to war in his carriage, evoked little interest from passers-by, for it had become a dumping ground for trash. The sharpshooter's tree had recovered from its barrage, concealing its battle scars with new growth; the ejected bullets from the rebel guns had settled deep in the soil at Norway. By 1901, when a second war provided dead heroes, the Brightwood Citizens' Association began sponsoring memorial services in the Union cemetery on Brightwood Avenue.[68]

References

1. P.M. Ashburn, *A History of the Medical Department of the United States Army*, Boston and New York, Houghton – Mifflin, 1929, pg. 213.

2. Relative rank accorded by Resolution of the Continental Congress, 3 Jan. 1781, see Harvey E. Brown (comp), *The Medical Department of the U.S. Army from 1775–1873*, SGO, Washington, D.C., 1873, pg. 61; definte military rank was accorded by Act 11 February 1847 (9 Stat. 124).

3. Elizabeth Blackwell, M.D., *Pioneer Work For Women*, N.Y., E.P. Dutton, 1914.

4. Kathrine Prescott Wormley, *The United States Sanitary Commission*, Boston, Little, Brown and Company, 1863, pg. 3-8; Albert G. Love, *The Geneva Red Cross Movement, European and American Influences on its Development*: A compilation with notes. *Army Medical Bulletin* No. 62, Special Issue, Carlisle Barracks, Pa.: M.F.S.S., May 1942. Reprinted, GPO, 1944.

5. Margaret Leech, *Reveille in Washington, 1860–1865*, New York and London, Harper and Brothers, ca 1941, pg 212.

6. James Mathew Phalen, *Chiefs of the Medical Department United States Army 1775–1940*. (published by the Army Medical Bulletin) pg. 39.

7. Love, *op cit*, pg. 11.

8. The Photographic History of the Civil War in Ten Volumes, Vol. VII, Prisons and Hospitals, pg. 330.

9. Jean Henri Dunant, Swiss citizen, is generally credited with the pioneer work in organizing military relief.

10. Leech, *op cit*, pg 204-233; Photographic History, *op cit*, Vol. VII; Ashburn, *op cit*, pg 68-93; James Tanner, *Experience of a Wounded Soldier at the Second Battle of Bull Run*. Reprint from Military Surgeon, Feb. 1927.

11. Leech, *op cit*, 189.

12. Love, *op cit*, pg. 10.

13. Roger Chew Weightman, *Military Laws and Rules and Regulations* for the Army of the United States, Washington City, 1814 (quoted).

14. Photographic History, *op cit*, pg 220.

15. One general and several regimental at Corpus Christi, Texas, in 1845. See Ashburn, *op cit*, pg 56.

16. Leech, *op cit*, pg 211.

17. 12 Stat, 288.

18. Leech, *op cit*, 179, 180.

19. Leech, *op cit*, page 180.

20. Louis Casper Duncan, Capt., MC, U.S. Army, *The Medical Department of the United States Army in the Civil War*, Washington, 1911, pg 2.

21. Photographic History, *op cit*, pg 310.

22. Photographic History... *op cit*, pg 334; Phalen, *op cit*, pg 43.

23. Leech, *op cit*, 216.

24. Ashburn, *op cit*, pg 70, 80.

25. Leech, *op cit*, pg 197.

26. Photographic History, *op cit*, pg 219.

27. Statement of Causes Which Led to the Dismissal of Surgeon General Hammond, pp, New York, 1864, pg 8.

28. Photographic History... *op cit*, pg 305-306.

29. Phalen, *op cit*, pg 48.

30. Phalen, *op cit*, pg 49.

31. George M. Sternberg, *The Functions of the Army Medical School*, address given at the annual commencement, 1902, American Medicine, Vol. III, No. 14, April 5, 1902, pg 547-551.

32. Hammond, *op cit*, pg 8.

33. *Statement of causes*... pg 11.

34. John Claggett Proctor, *Washington Star*, June 11, 1950.

35. Military identification for medical officer.

36. Phalen, *op cit*, pg 44.

37. Leech, *op cit*, 182-183.

38. Leech, *op cit*, pg 264, 267.

39. Proctor, *op cit*, Feb. 14, 1932.

40. *Ibid –Washington Star*, Jan. 31, 1937.

41. Proctor, *op cit*, Feb. 14, 1932.

42. Proctor, *op cit*, April 21, 1929.

43. Later location of the Masonic Temple.

44. Proctor, *op cit*, Jan. 31, 1937; Feb. 3, 1938.

45. *Ibid.*

46. Proctor, *op cit*, April 21, 1929.

47. Proctor, *op cit*, April 7, 1929.

48. Proctor, *op cit*, Feb. 13. 1938.

49. "With the Rambler", *Washington Star*, Apr. 9, 1916.

50. Leech, *op cit*, pg 336.

51. Proctor, *op cit*, Jan. 31, 1937.

52. Leech, *op cit*, pg 342.

53. Leech, *op cit*, pg 337.

54. *Ibid*, pg 342.

55. Annual Report, WRGH, 1919.

56. Leech, *op cit*, pg 343.

57. Annual Report, WRGH, 1919, pg 2.

58. Proctor, *Washington Star*, April 21, 1929.

59. Proctor, *op cit*, April 21, 1929.

60. Proctor, *op cit*, Feb. 13, 1938.

61. Proctor, *op cit*, April 21, 1929.

62. Proctor, *op cit*, April 7, 1929.

63. *Ibid.*

64. "With the Rambler", *Washington Star*, April 9, 1916.

65. Built about 1873, in the area between Alaska on the east; Holly on the north; Geranium on the south and 14th Street on the west. "With the Rambler", *Washington Star*, May 7, 1916.

66. *Public Improvements Secured in the Northern Section of the District of Columbia*, an address by Wm. Van Zandt Cox, Aug. 6, 1897, on file Washingtonia Sect., D.C. Public Library.

67. "On Suburban Rides", *Washington Star*, Jan. 29, 1896.

68. Proctor, *op cit*, Jan. 31, 1937.

Schooling for the Medical Department

1860–1901

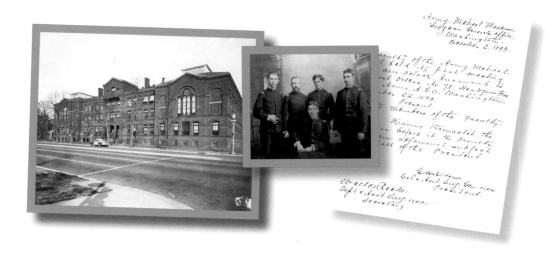

" Training, too, was needed to make an Army."[1]

A War Department Order of April 7, 1862, placed general hospitals under the Surgeon General's direction, but the right of medical officers to command, within their own sphere, was not settled until publication of General Order No. 306, December 27, 1864. By February 8, 1865, such control was extended to include hospital trains and hospital boats. The great temporary general hospitals of the Civil War period disappeared rapidly as the Army demobilized and by 1866 there were none.[2] The collection of professional reference books, begun in 1836 for The Surgeon General's convenience, was increased through reassignment of surplus funds remaining from the deactivated general hospitals, and in the fifteen-year period following the war, the collection began to assume the proportions as well as the name of The Surgeon General's Library.

The Army was concentrated at small stations in the West, South and Southwest, with the number of regular Army medical officers supplemented by contract surgeons. Newly appointed officers could anticipate at least two four-year assignments at such stations,[3] where life was rugged and news of medical progress in the outside world was slow to arrive. Changes were occurring which would have a profound effect on the military medical service, but not even the best of dreamers could visualize the future.

Three civilian training schools for nurses were opened in 1873, but no prophet seems to have noted as unusual the new trend toward orderly technical schooling for females. Medical education was destined for professional reform, and a few American doctors even then were interested in Lister's controversial germ theory of disease. Isolated as they were, frontier Army doctors had little time or inclination to question the old ways, and so George M. Sternberg, an Army surgeon who began an independent study of disinfectants in 1878, was unusual.[4] Such persistence required courage as well as foresight, for he was ridiculed by more functionary and less scholarly contemporaries.[5] Nevertheless, by 1884, the year that the Congress authorized limited medical care for the civilian dependents of military personnel,[6] and before disinfectants were in general use either in Europe or America, Army doctors were beginning to use antiseptic techniques in surgery.[7]

Able military medical assistants were needed in this new era of hospitalization, men with different training than that required of teamsters and packers, of cavalrymen and foot soldiers. On November 20, 1886, War Department General Order No. 86 authorized the instruction of corpsmen in first aid; the Act of March 1, 1887 (24 Stat. 435) established and permanently attached to the Medical Department of the Army, a Hospital Corps, whose uniform was still trimmed in the emerald green color used by the Civil War surgeons for the sashes of their full dress uniform. The United States, a procrastinator in ratifying the Geneva Treaty, had capitulated on March 1, 1882. By 1887 the Hospital Corpsmen were identified by a red cross mounted on a white arm band or brassard.[8] Likewise of major interest to the future structure of the medical service, on January 17, 1887, the Army and Navy General Hospital was opened in Hot Springs, Arkansas, with beds for sixteen officers and sixty-four enlisted men.[9]

Qualifying examinations had, since publication of the Medical Department Regulations of 1856, governed the promotion of corpsmen to acting hospital steward and steward, positions comparable to those held by non-commissioned officers of the line. War Department Order No. 56, August 11, 1887, promulgated rules and regulations. It would be many years, however, before the admission and departure of officers at general hospitals would be strictly controlled, for they continued, when they got chronic ailments, "to take a sick leave and wander off to be treated at their own expense, and often very poorly treated."[10] In fact prior to 1895, the sixteen-bed officer division received patients from October until June only.

By 1888, James E. Pilcher[11] had written the first Medical Department technical manual and similar manuals issued for some years thereafter included a section on Hospital Corps drill. Thus the post-Civil War period not only engendered a new interest in the care of the wounded, but for the Army medical service it was a period of organizational consciousness during which one of the first requisites "was to make the position of the medical officer such that he would place some value upon the retention of his office...."[12]

Hostilities against the Indians continued until about 1890, with the medical field soldiers performing their duties so satisfactorily that a detachment, or Company of Instruction, was organized at Ft. Riley, Kansas, in 1891. The military-minded young Captain John

Van R. Hoff was in command. Although in common use, the name Hospital Corps was not authorized officially for some ten years.[13] Securing satisfactory personnel for a stable and well-trained nursing service was an ever-present problem, as under the old system men detailed from the line received a higher rate of pay than those enlisting in the Medical Department. The Surgeon General was convinced that training the Hospital Corps was a major responsibility and that the organization must in "all particulars be a military one." Thus by 1892, three Companies of Instruction were in training at western posts, each with tentage and field hospital furniture. New recruits received practical instruction in first aid, nursing, cooking, administration, drill and other related duties, and after being trained some of the men were reassigned to small hospitals at garrisons and posts.[14] In spite of Congressional recognition, however, the medical soldier was destined to have difficulty in "winning his spurs", for now and then uncooperative Quartermasters decreed that mules were the only available mounts, hardly a dignified means of transportation when accompanying the more militant and clanking cavalry and artillery.

Militarily the United States was divided into eight Departments or areas of command by 1894: Department of the East; The Platte; Dakota; Missouri; Texas; California; Arizona and Columbia. The Columbia Department included the historic Washington Arsenal, renamed Washington Barracks in 1861.[15] Located at the confluence of the Po-tomac and Anacostia rivers and bounded on the east by James Creek Canal, the Barracks occupied some forty-four acres on Greenleaf's Point, used as a fort since 1797. Shops had appeared in the neighborhood in 1807, and by 1812 the fort was an important storage place for powder. Destroyed by the British in 1813, it was rebuilt in 1815, but destined for varied military uses – in 1826 as a penitentiary and during the Civil War as an ordnance and supply depot for the Army of the Potomac.[16]

The location was attractive though not especially healthful, for the ground was low, actually at sea level. Tonsillitis and rheumatic conditions affected the troops in winter and in the summer the humid Washington heat made the area uncomfortable. As if heat and humidity were not enough, the troops likewise suffered from the presence of "malarial exhalations in this locality (which accounted) for the prevalence of the disease". The James Creek Canal was still an open sewer in 1894, and the water was "foul smelling at all times". The animate theory of disease was not generally accepted and so the Surgeon General believed that the troops were fortunate that the river "bank next to the post (was) lined with a double row of poplars and willows, forming a dense screen of foliage which (did) much to intercept malarious exhalations".[17] True there were other health problems, for Washington City was still the naughty place of General Hammond's day, and in 1896 the Barracks "had a considerable excess of venereal cases and twice as much alcoholism as is ordinarily found at military posts,"[18] but neither of these afflictions could be considered seasonal scourges. It required more than poplars and willows to curb the exuberance of soldiers.

Line officers were responsible for recruitments and assignments but many were careless in their selection of men detailed to the Medical Department as nurses. And so the

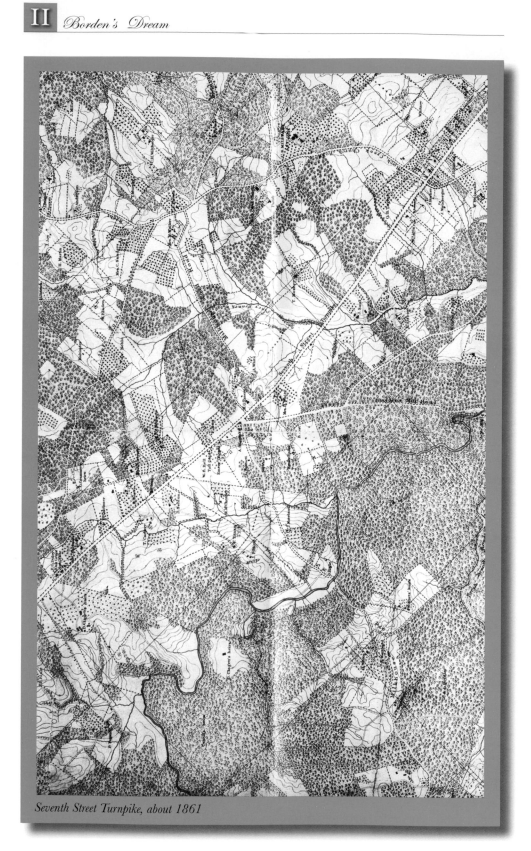

Seventh Street Turnpike, about 1861

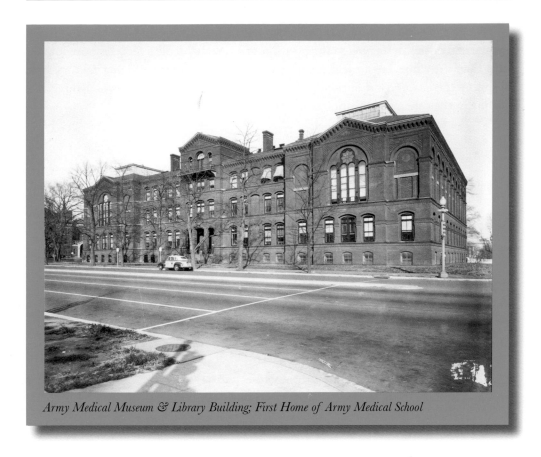

Army Medical Museum & Library Building: First Home of Army Medical School

doctors wasted valuable time training subordinates for semi-professional duties, only to have them reassigned at will. Moreover, assignments were not necessarily permanent, especially during war, as company (military) affairs frequently took precedence over care of the sick. The quality of enlisted personnel so assigned depended to a large extent on the tolerance or liking which company commanders bore their weaponless adjuncts, the doctors,[19] some of whom were heretical enough to urge that the soldier-attendants be dishonorably discharged for drunkenness rather than merely discipline, for "a drunken nurse in one minute of error may cause injury that can never be remedied."[20]

During this decade of apprenticeship, when the medical soldier was emerging as bonafide military personnel, his preceptor and sponsor, the medical officer, was being cultured by such men as Woodhull and Hoff.[21] Their contemporaries, when forced by circumstances to take a more general interest in sanitary matters affecting the health of the troops, would find that versatility in Army matters gained for them respect from line commanders inclined to ignore their professional recommendations if costly,[22] for many line commanders had the authoritarian's honest resentment of recommendations made by the uninitiated. Moreover, some evaluated the military surgeon in terms of a proper "bedside manner" and a willingness to be addressed as "doctor." Cured, or dead, they had no further use for him and seldom considered him a part of the Army.

Few of the grenadiers of that period agreed with the Surgeon General that "there are certain duties pertaining to the position of an Army Medical Officer more important than the clinical treatment of disease and injury."[23] But some young doctors took seriously the adapted inscription from an old sentry box in Gibraltar, which hung as a plaque in the office of many practicing physicians,

God and the doctor [24]
All men adore

In time of trouble
And no more;

For when war is over
And all things righted

God is neglected —
The old doctor slighted.

Militarily, it was time to improve the doctors' status. The only way to do it, according to Woodhull and Hoff, was to be both soldier and physician. It would require brilliant men to play such a role, for the prize would be large and the burden heavy.

The Army Medical School

While an organized field hospital service was acquiring a firm footing in training posts west of the Mississippi, Medical Department prestige was beginning a slow but sure climb in the East. The Army Medical Library and Museum were opened to "the medical profession at large, to scientific bodies and to professional students" by special act of Congress in 1892.[25] George M. Sternberg was appointed Surgeon General in 1893 and succeeded at last in establishing in Washington, the Army Medical School,[26] housed in the Museum Building, located at 7th and B, Southwest, which had sheltered the Surgeon General's[27] Library since 1888. Three of the principal activities planned for Hammond's quadrangular medical unit were now in existence; of the four, only the general hospital lacked authorization.

Three decades had passed since the proposal was made. Unless the Medical Department was willing to accept a secondary role in American medicine it was necessary to supplement the meager instruction in biological sciences, especially bacteriology and chemistry, then offered in the undergraduate medical schools.[28] Thus the School was established to instruct approved candidates for admission to the Medical Corps of the Army in their ever-widening responsibility as Medical Officers and in the basic sciences. Army physicians in and near the District of Columbia, and others who had sufficient leaves of absence, could be admitted to the four-month course under the same regula-

Memorandum recording first faculty meeting of the Army Medical School, October 2, 1893, signed by Walter Reed

tions governing the regular students. Four professors would be assigned from among the senior officers in or near Washington, and as many associate professors as necessary to provide practical laboratory instruction in the methods of sanitary analysis, microscopical technique, clinical microscopy, bacteriology, urine analysis, etc.

While designed for graduate instruction, it was a school in fact as well as name, for in addition to giving a course of lectures in property responsibility, the examination of recruits, certificates of discharge with disability (CDD) reports, rights, privileges and customs of the service etc., the President of the Faculty was responsible for discipline. Judging from the first class photographs, so sedate a group of young doctors could have had little time or inclination for pranks, for during the hours of class instruction they wore the stiff and uncomfortable uniform of their grade and in the laboratory, a black cambric gown.[29] As usual in military procedure, when the faculty held its first meeting, October 2, 1893, the junior professor served as secretary and recorder. The junior professor was, at this time, a little known but diligent student of microbiology, Captain and Assistant Surgeon, USA, Walter Reed, curator of pathology at the Army Medical Museum. Some of his first Army Commanders believed he had little scientific ability, and in 1890, when he began post-graduate clinical study at the newly opened but already influential Johns Hopkins hospital, he was told to leave the laboratories alone. It was Surgeon General Sternberg, apparently, who urged him to follow his own specialty, an interest he pursued as a commuter from Washington, often accompanied by Hospital Steward James Carroll, whose "peculiar aptitude for this type of work gained for him admission to the regular University courses."[30]

Like all faculties, the professors had a certain amount of school administration to contend with, and determining academic standing became an important issue when they gathered on the first Monday of the month to discuss academic problems. Captain Reed was obviously a congenital schoolmaster, for with the course hardly a month old he was the first professor to infringe on class time belonging to another. Serene and scholarly, he appropriated, apparently without apology, one hour of the time allotted to the Assistant Professor of Military Surgery and Instructor in Hospital Corps Drill.[31]

The students were undeniably members of a learned profession, and they seem to have had less aptitude, or perhaps less interest, in strictly military matters, for it took them until January 12, 1894 to become adapt at drilling a squad of litter bearers. The price of military proficiency had other drawbacks, for no matter what their progress on the ground, the budding young officers were at a disadvantage on a horse. As officers they could not indulge in the undignified comfort of mule-riding, and so early in the New Year 1894, the President of the Faculty learned that "five at least of the gentlemen still needed instruction" in equitation at the riding academy at Fort Myer, Virginia, where Saturday mornings were devoted to drill and riding.[32]

Military rank was fixed prior to attendance at the School, but the faculty believed this prevented competition and that the corps rank of new officers should be determined by the combined results of their school work and the findings of the Army Examining Board.[33] Alas for professional promotion, for rank and precedence, had academic standing been influenced by a correct seat in the McClellan saddle! There were only five students in the first class, gentlemen obviously predisposed to the use of carriages, but their lack of interest in equine anatomy was characteristic of many of their successors. A half-century later to some of the earlier "schoolboys":

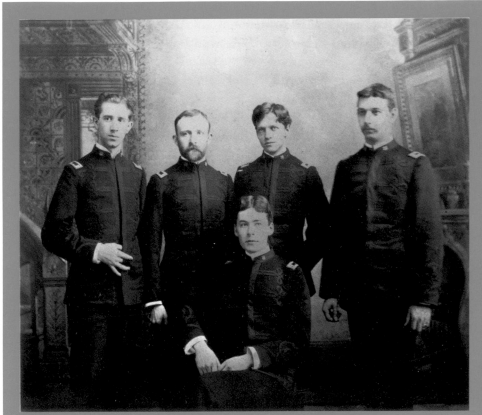

First Graduating Class; Army Medical School, 1894. Assistant Surgeons: T.S. Bratton, A.S. Porter, W.W. Quinton (Sitting), D.C. Howard, W.H. Wilson

… Memory of the riding hall exercises (was) better than of more important subjects. Of the class of forty, six or seven had never been on a horse before. Some were afraid to jump … and would collect on the side lines or find something wrong with their saddles. One, Collins, fell off his horse while he was standing still, and sprained his ankle. The ambulance was called, but as it was away, the soldiers loaded him in a trash cart and hauled him across the parade ground to the hospital.

George H.R. (High Ranking) Gosman was so short and his stomach was so large that he could not jump on the horse while it was standing still, much less while it was at a trot. His efforts were so amusing that the soldiers had great fun watching. He was good natured, and the more he laughed at himself the worse he got. On one occasion his fractious mount was misbehaving and H.R. dropped the reins. As he was unable to control the animal, he grabbed it around the neck and held on until the soldiers ran and caught him. At that point one of the bystanders suggested to the Doctor that he climb down the hind leg while the horse was standing still![134]

The curriculum for the first year was more or less arbitrarily established, but by the time the second session began, in the autumn of 1894, some of the younger professors were urging a broader program of instruction in pharmaceuticals, chemistry, involving the testing of drugs and determination of the specific gravity of urine, tests for sugar and albumin. Many of the new recruits for the Hospital Corps came from the eastern part of the United States, and so for convenience as well as economy a Company of Instruction was located at Washington Barracks during the year, with the men performing duties at the School and the recently built post hospital, where some received on-the-job training "in the preparation for" surgical operation. Some of the professors wanted to increase this training, but the President of the Faculty resisted, possibly because he thought the time wasted as the Department had a contract with Providence Hospital to care for "the support and treatment of ninety-five medical and surgical cases."[35] Captain Reed, supposedly shy and retiring with people, was on better terms with bacteria and stated his position firmly:

> *...Saying that in his department it would be of importance to give stewards and acting stewards, and the brighter members of the (Hospital) Corps instruction in the principles of antiseptics, and that it would be not only feasible but most important to instruct them practically in hand disinfection.*[36]

The physical condition of American military camps was improving steadily during these years, and the awakening public health consciousness of medical officers was an effective instrument in reform. Basic humanitarian principles as well as good sense influenced some of the new measures, as the (diet) ration was improved, summer weight clothing was issued to men stationed in the south, bathing and latrine facilities were increased and decent mattresses and sheets were being issued in the garrisons. The Medical Department was making improvements within the hospitals, with the Surgeon General recommending that men assigned to nursing duties wear "white linen blouses and pantaloons."[37] The age of experimental medicine was dawning, and the professional care of the military ill was to be accomplished in a scientific manner, for in 1895 Post Surgeons were "directed to set aside in their hospitals a special room as an operating room...."[38]

Medical problems likewise received professional consideration during the autumn of 1895. The President of the Faculty was concerned for the mental health of the Army and believed that "instruction in lunacy (was) of importance to the student officers, especially as melancholia was so common a disease in the service."[39] As was characteristic of government agencies, even the "Bureau of Melancholia" was slow in cooperating, and while the budding young medical officers waited for Dr. Godding of the Government Hospital for the Insane, built in 1855,[40] to deliver a series of lectures on lunacy, Dr. Robert Fletcher, distinguished scholar and then editor of the famous

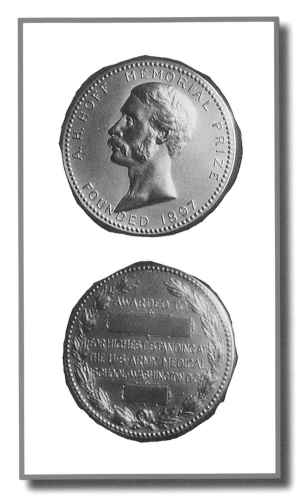

Hoff Memorial Prize Medal, 1897

Index — Catalogue, discussed elementary library techniques — the use of books and journals in the Library of the Surgeon General's Office.[41] It is worthy of note that whatever its other drawbacks and disabilities, the mental health of the Army as a whole failed to suffer markedly from the delay.

By 1896, three years after opening the School, the faculty decided that either the written or oral examinations could be used, with professional discretion. Captain Reed, whose scholarly lectures were salted with a certain amount of dry humor,[42] attacked the problem with enthusiasm and announced heartlessly that "the examination in his Department would cover the morning hours of the present week together with two mornings in the next."[43]

The incentive to excel, which the faculty believed deplorably lacking because rank was established prior to admittance, was coaxed by Lieutenant Colonel John Van R. Hoff, when the new session opened in 1897, for he offered to the best all-round man of the year a forty dollar[44] cash prize in honor of his medical-officer father. Early competition for the prize may not have been keen, or perhaps "the grind" was not as severe as the curriculum implied, for the students unanimously requested and were granted leave to attend the Army and Navy football game on November 26, 1897. However, with a real academic stimulus in view, the faculty determined to issue "Certificates of Proficiency" to students with average between 70-90, and "Proficiency With Honors" for grades of ninety and above.

A Prod to Scientific Awakening

The new-found interest in military medical training was interrupted by the Spanish-American War, the first war which found the Medical Department centrally organized, even if poorly equipped to perform its mission. There was no War Department general staff to correlate and coordinate military problems and inter-departmental relationships were complicated. Adequate financial support for a non-combatant arm of the service was hard to secure; supplies were poor, scarce, and the transfer of supplies still poorer; the Quartermaster was entirely responsible for the ration, and proper diets for the sick were not readily available. As in the Civil War, some newly uniformed civilian doctors were not only professionally unprepared but, lacking military training, they objected to discipline. Few had even the minimal administrative experience and knowledge of sanitation then being taught medical officers, and since they were unfamiliar with the vast requirements of a mobilization, some criticized the Medical Department freely.

Once again the women decided to go to war, this time with more determination, more publicity for their cause and a more knowledgeable basis for the freely voiced criticisms of camp sanitation and hospital management. In the interval since the Civil War, Clara Barton had organized the American National Red Cross, not without challenge, to be sure, but it was a going concern. Women welfare workers now had a recognized outlet for their energies, and the government had a humanitarian ally. Of more importance, the ally was able to act with an enviable degree of freedom and independence.

For the second time in less than half a century a woman physician took the initiative in sponsoring trained nurses for the Army. However, Dr. Anita Newcomb McGee, a prominent Washington physician, had an advantage which Dr. Blackwell lacked — she and her father were personal friends of General Sternberg.[45] Again in New York, the American National Red Cross Relief Committee formed a Women's Committee, an auxiliary which formed, in turn, an extremely active and influential subcommittee known as Auxiliary No. 3, or the Red Cross Society for Maintenance of Trained Nurses. The Auxiliary's two principal lay sponsors were Mrs. Whitelaw Reid and Mrs. Winthrop Cowdin, wealthy New York socialites, and its professional spokesmen included some of the most distinguished directors of nursing from New York hospitals. However, when both the national nursing organizations and the Auxiliary attempted to provide graduate nurses, they found the field controlled by the Hospital Corps of the Daughters of the American Revolution, with Dr. McGee installed as Superintendent of Nurses. There would be skirmishes among the skirtwearers as feminist challenged feminist, and until the nursing situation became acute, military commanders did not encourage the presence of female nurses in the camps.[46]

The Army was not alone in its conservative reaction to females, for in spite of the feminist movement then beginning to erupt in full force, the public had not endorsed wholeheartedly woman's new found freedom. The national Army was a hodgepodge of state militia. The Medical "Corps entered the war as a corps in name only, in reality an aggregation of post surgeons."[47] Its sentiments were the sentiments of the nation. Men familiar with rough camp life were not only unwilling to subject women to its trials but they were unwilling to add to their own burdens and responsibilities until defeated by conditions beyond their own control. Although the women viewed the disastrous epidemic condition in terms of the functional care of patients, the reluctance of some doctors to accepting them as military and professional colleagues encouraged some of the leaders in the nursing movement to believe the Medical Department was unwilling rather than unready to accept the distaff branch.[48]

The hospital-trained women nurses then under temporary contract to the government objected violently to the sanitary conditions of the camps; they criticized the care or lack of care offered by the hastily recruited corpsmen; they resented the supposition of soldier and officer that women could not adjust to camp life; the assumption of physicians and men nurses that they could not perform, within woman's natural sphere — nursing — the duties of nurses without special favors for their sex; many of the more robust ones endured hardships rather than complain. Camp life was a new experience, one without preamble or guidepost. As was to be expected, some nurses commented without hesitation on supposed military inefficiencies. Challenged as women, challenged as nurses, they in turn challenged in behalf of women's rights!

Fortunately, the war was short-lived. The new crop of Army doctors, riven by their own undefined problem, the medical officer versus the strictly medical practitioner, wasted no time on a psychosomatic diagnosis of aroused womanhood. Such a consideration was, after all, beyond their abilities in an era when they had not solved more factual health problems. The majority of the doctors were warm in their praise of the nurses' services, and such official encouragement instilled hope of a permanent place in the Army. The nurses were obedient aides, undemanding and anxious to be useful, for as the Surgeon General said "the systematically educated and trained nurse (was) developed by the medical profession...."[49]

Alcoholism and venereal disease were two of the principal health problems of the peacetime Army — reason enough, by nineteenth century standards, to protect American womanhood from the rigors of camp life. Prior to their replacement by contract nurses, eleven of the Red Cross — paid nurses were sent for relief work in the Philippines, shortly after the war. Both contract nurses and Red Cross nurses had served in Cuba and the United States, and one young nurse expressed the (post-war) situation graphically: "The sickness now among the men is dwindling down to just what the majority of the soldiers have, and just what, for that reason, the Army doctors say, a post hospital is no place for female nurses."[50] Nevertheless, a Congressional bill was already in the hopper to create a permanent Nurse Corps to replace the contract nurses appointed during the emergency. Corrected of some features objectionable to the Surgeon General, who earnestly desired to evade responsibility for its first defeat,[51] it passed, in 1901, and Eve entered the Army to stay.

The Army Medical School closed early in the spring of 1898, before recommendations for extending the course from four to five months could be effected.[52] Its students departed for "the front." Walter Reed, by then a major, was still in Washington when camp pollution from typhoid fever reached the proportions of a national scandal. There were few recognized sanitarians either in or out of the Army, and laboratory diagnosis of typhoid fever by stool and blood examination was an unused technique. Recognition of human carriers of this disease was nearly a decade away. As one of the three physicians composing the Typhoid Fever Board appointed by the Surgeon General, Major Reed eventually made important recommendations on what then was thought to be the spread as well as the etiology of the disease.[53] The monumental report prepared by this Board was a noteworthy scientific contribution both to public health and clinical medicine, and through his work Major Reed brought credit to the Army Medical School. For the Medical Department, much scientific work lay ahead; some of it would be more spectacular than any of its budding scientists had dreamed. Like twice told tales, the saga of military medicine during the otherwise gay nineties became a legend of heroic proportions. Although an advanced scholar for his day, even the Surgeon General was a baffled sanitarian. Cannily he qualified his observations and couched his comments on epidemics in vague terms:

> *Given certain conditions as to the environment of soldiers recently enlisted and assembled in camps of instruction and the prevalence of typhoid fever may be predicted with certainty.*[54]

References

1. Margaret Leech, *Reveille in Washington 1860–1865*, Harper & Brothers, New York and London, ca 1941, pg 107.

2. P.M. Ashburn, *A History of the Medical Department of the United States Army*, Boston and New York, Houghton-Mifflin Company, 1929, pg 88.

3. Ltr from "JM", Surgeon General, U.S. Army to S.F. Philipps, Senate Office Bldg. Washington, D.C., Jan. 10, 1890, SGO Folder 1430, War Records Div. Nat'l Archives.

4. Ashburn, *op cit*, pg 137.

5. Ashburn, *op cit*, pg 147, 148.

6. U.S. Statues at large, Chps. 217, 48th Congress, Sect. I, app. June 5, 1884; Act 5 July 1884 (23 Stat. 112).

7. Annual Report TSG to TSW, 1885, pg 27, 28.

8. Ashburn, *op cit*, pg 425.

9. James Mathew Phalen, *Chiefs of the Medical Department United States Army 1775–1940* (published by the Army Medical Bulletin) pg 60.

10. Biography of Gen. J.R. Kean, pg 96, Manuscript Copy, on file AML.

11. James E. Pilcher, the *Transportation of the Disabled... by Human Bearers*, Reprint from J. Mil. Serv. Ints. NY, 1888; *Ibid, An Exercise in the Extemporization of Litters from Rifles and Gunslings* Rept. from Boston M & SG, 1888.

12. Phalen, *op cit*, pg 29.

13. Phalen, *op cit*, pg 68.

14. Annual Report TSG... 1891–1892, pg 10-16.

15. General Order No. 40, May 12, 1881, changed name from Washington Arsenal to Washington Barracks, Telephone information provided by Miss Charlotte Greenwood, Ref. Lib., NWC, Dec. 6, 1950.

16. Charles J. Sullivan (comp) *Army Posts and Towns...* Burlington Free Press Printing, 1926, pg 46; *Arsenal in Old Days*, Washington Post, July 14, 1901.

17. Annual Report TSG... 1893–1894, pg 58, 59.

18. Annual Report TSG... 1895–1896, pg 19.

19. Kean, *loc-cit*.

20. Annual Report, TSG... 1891–1892, pg 14.

21. Ashburn, *op cit*, pg 156.

22. Kean, *op cit*, pg 128; Interview, Major General Orlando Ward, Chf. Office of Military History, WDSS.

23. Annual Report TSG... 1893–1894, pg 15.

24. The word doctor substituted for soldier.

25. James C. Magee, TSG, Memorandum, Reference, Army Medical Library and Museum Bldg., April 27, 1940 (prep. By Love) 631.-1 SGO Judge Thompson's file.

26. General Orders No. 51, Hdq. of the Army, AGO, Washington, June 24, 1893.

27. Information provided by Brig. Gen. Raymond Dart, M.C. (telephone) March 8, 1950.

28. Based on interviews with: J.R. Kean, B.G., M.C., Ret'd., Nov. 1946, Dec. 11, 1947, Apr. 17, 1950; J.M. Phalen, Col., M.C., Ret'd., April 19, 1950; A.G. Love, B.G., M.C., Ret'd., April 5, 1950; R.U. Patterson, M.G., M.C., Ret'd., Aug. 24, 29, 1950; A.E. Truby, B.G., M.C., Ret'd., Jun. 27-28, 1950.

29. Records of the Army Medical School, Oct. 2, 1893 – April 10, 1905, First to Ninth Session incl., original on file AMS, AMC.

30. *Ibid*. General Order No. 78 — Sept. 22, 1893, named faculty — Colonel Chas. H. Alden, Ass't Surgeon General, Pres; Lt. Col. Wm. H. Forwood, Deputy Surgeon General (Mil. Surgery); Maj. Charles Smart, Surgeon, Mil. Med. & Director of the chem. laboratory; John S. Billings later took over Prof. of Mil. Hyg; Capt. Walter Reed, Asst. Surg. professor of clinical and sanitary microscopy and director of the pathological laboratory; Capt. John M. Cabell, Asst. Surg., Asst. Professor of military surgery and instructor in Hospital Corps drill; Dr. Hurd's unpublished MS "First Quarter Century of the Johns Hopkins Hospital," apparently extracted from notes on *Welch's pupils* in folder "Welch as Scientist... Teacher and Speaker." Collection of the Inst. of Hist. of Med., Welch Medical Library, Baltimore, Md.

31. Minutes... AMS, (on file Office of the Commandant), Nov. 6, 1893.

32. Minutes... Jan. 12, 1894, *op cit.*

33. Minutes... March 6, 1894, *op cit.*

34. Ltr from Col. Jas. D. Fife, M.C., Ret'd, to the writer, Jan. 11, 1951 (edited).

35. Annual Report TSG... 1895-1896, pg 10.

36. Minutes... AMS, October 15, 1894, *op cit.*

37. Annual Report TSG... 1893-1894, pg 15-19.

38. Annual Report TSG... 1895-1896, pg 7.

39. Minutes... AMS, October 30, 1895, *op cit.*

40. Act 3 March 1855 (10 Stat. 682) built for use of Army & Navy personnel of the U.S. and D.C.; name changed to St. Elizabeths Hospital by Act 1 July 1916 (39 Stat. 309).

41. Minutes... AMS, Nov. 7, 1895, *op cit.*

42. Interview with Maj. Gen. Robert U. Patterson, Aug. 24, 29, 1950.

43. Minutes... AMS, March 2, 1896, *op cit.*

44. Minutes... AMS, Dec. 6, 1897, *op cit.*

45. Florence A. Blanchfield, *Organized Nursing and the Army in Three Wars*, MSS on file Historical Division, SGO.

46. Ashburn, *op cit*, pg 175, 176.

47. Ashburn, *op cit*, pg 218.

48. Florence A. Blanchfield, *Organized Nursing and the Army in Three Wars*, MSS on file Historical Division, SGO; History of WAC organization in World War II (unpublished) MSS by Miss Mattie Treadwell, on file WDSS.

49. Annual Report TSG... 1899, pg 24.

50. Ltr from Lida G. Starr to Mrs. Whitelaw Reid, Feb. 22, 1899, written en route to the Philippines. Files of Auxiliary No. 3, Archives, ANRC.

51. Ltr from George M. Sternberg, TSG to Mrs. Winthrop Cowdin, March 13, 1899, File, Auxiliary No. 3, Archives, ANRC.

52. Annual Report TSG... 1897–1898, pg 22.

53. Ashburn, *op cit*, 161-182.

54. George M. Sternberg, M.D., LLD., *The Functions of the Army Medical School*, American Medicine, Vol. III, No. 14, April 5, 1902, pg 547-551.

The Intermediate Host

1899–1902

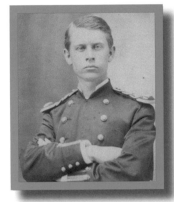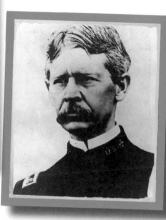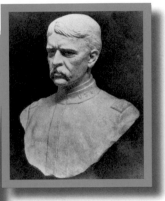

*"...and being dead it is an obligation of his friends
to see that his scientific achievements are not forgotten."[1]*

When so progressive a scientist as Surgeon General Sternberg believed "that certain conditions of environment" encouraged epidemic typhoid fever in camps but overlooked the solution, men with less technical knowledge could hardly be expected to have the correct answer to the even more puzzling riddle of yellow fever, scourge of the American tropics for more than two hundred years. The cause of this seasonal menace confused the doctors, but it was not yet the age of experimental medicine and so they did little more than write scholarly essays or engage in medico-literary battles. Few were able to buttress their personal opinions with any sort of laboratory strategy.[2]

In the late eighteenth century the Irish-born John Crawford, by then a Baltimore resident, favored the animate theory of fever transmission; less than fifty years later American-born Josiah Clark Nott of Birmingham, Alabama, hinted that the mosquito might be the guilty executioner. Concurrently a Venezuelan physician-naturalist actually named the mosquito as the culprit. Even Texas, that allegedly remote frontier of illiteracy, produced its Greensville Dowell, who publicly stated in 1876 that the mosquito might be associated with malaria and yellow fever.[3] None of these men substantiated their theories by laboratory diagnosis. Ross, a Britisher long stationed in India, became an expert on malaria and solved the principle of mosquito transmission of that disease,[4] while the etiology of yellow fever was still a tantalizing medical mystery.

In 1881 courtly, contentious Dr. Carlos Finlay of Havana delivered a scientific paper before the Royal Academy of Havana on *The Mosquito Hypothetically Considered as the Agent of Transmission of Yellow Fever*. Few if any of Dr. Finley's contemporaries gave his theories the consideration they deserved. And such is the resistance to new ideas, if not self-propounded, that in time the good doctor was considered senile or visionary — or both.[5]

Sternberg tried to solve the riddle, but, like the others, he failed. An immune, having suffered an attack in 1875, by 1879 he was considered something of an authority, and he was assigned to work with the Havana Yellow Fever Commission. By 1890 he had reported voluminously on yellow fever, proposing *Bacillus X* as the infectious agent. Like his predecessors he failed to solve the riddle. And Sternberg was reputedly the Medical Department's best qualified research worker[6] and authority on yellow fever.

Many distinguished physicians confused yellow fever and febrile icterus or Weil's Disease, and in the decade prior to the Spanish-American War, several new theories of transmission were published. In 1897 Guiseppi Sanarelli announced that *Bacillus icteroides* was the real culprit. Had the Army's Surgeon General not sired *Bacillus X*, been a bacteriologist of note and an author, there is no reason to suppose that the controversial *Bacillus icteroides* would have become an immediate subject for official investigation. The Johns Hopkins Hospital Medical Society meetings were notable affairs, and at one of the meetings early in 1898, General Sternberg reviewed his own work on yellow fever. Dr. William Henry Welch, the outstanding bacteriologist of the period called attention to the trustworthiness of his work and commended Sternberg's caution in accepting the *Bacillus icteroides*, a weak point in the evidence being the small number of cases examined.[7] It was therefore Sternberg the scientist rather than Sternberg the Surgeon General, who disputed Sanarelli's claims and set Walter Reed and James Carroll of the laboratory staff at the Army Medical School to investigating the problem. Sternberg and Reed had both studied with Dr. Welch and so their mutual professional interests lessened the gulf which military rank so often interposes between military men of different ages. The Surgeon General therefore followed their investigation carefully, both as adviser and friend.

This effort was not so much an attempt to solve the puzzle of yellow fever as an attempt to prove that Sanarelli had not found something new which Sternberg had overlooked. The fact that some doctors from the Marine Hospital Service[8] accepted the new theory doubtless made the disproof more challenging. By early spring of 1899, the Army investigators were convinced that Sanarelli's sensational bacillus was in reality a lowly member of the hog cholera family.[9] Moreover, Sternberg's *Bacillus X* was a little known variety of the Colon Bacillus.[10] In the meantime Dr. Henry R. Carter had studied the disease during the yellow fever epidemics of 1893, 1897, 1898 and 1899. Carter not only supported the theory of mosquito transmission, but he proposed the period of extrinsic incubation.[11] The earlier works on the malarial mosquito were, of course, published records. Like the base to a pyramid, they provided a sound structure for more ambitious undertakings. The channel was already chartered for a willing investigator, and Reed used Carter's findings as an index.[12] His careful preparations for controlled experimentation, without which the previously proposed mosquito–transmission theory could have remained disputable, would catapult him into a position of immortal fame.

Itinerant Scientist

The scientific maunderings on the etiology of yellow fever could have dragged along at a deliberate and scholarly pace but for a single catalytic agent–the Spanish-American War. Sanitary conditions in the hastily built camps became a national scandal; as usual, the deaths from diseases exceeded the number of combat dead. After the war the Medical Department, along with the Quartermaster, Commissary and other non-combatant arms, faced a soul-searching administrative investigation from the Congress.[13] Everything medical was investigated–diets, nursing, clothing, transportation and doctors.

Yellow fever was considered endemic in American continental stations in the south, such as Key West Barracks, Florida, and so the disease was clinically familiar to some of the young medical officers[14] stationed in Cuba with the occupation troops. The unsanitary conditions which permitted the spread of typhoid fever had no apparent relationship to the frequent outbreaks of yellow fever, but in May 1899 the Surgeon General sent Major Reed to Puerto Principe to investigate, among other medical service problems what was presumed to be an outbreak of malaria but which proved to be typhoid. The Major remained in Cuba almost two weeks, but not long enough to see any yellow fever cases, for the epidemic did not begin in earnest until July. When the fever began it was particularly virulent, and within a few weeks nearly one hundred cases were reported, with a twenty per cent mortality.[15] Perniciosa the Cubans called it, and it was well named, for the effects were violent, usually deadly to the victims. Troop morale was undermined, for the disease struck indiscriminately and without warning. Thus there was considerable uneasiness among the American doctors as well as the line commanders, stalked as they were by death–or another medical scandal.

In March and April 1900, Reed was again in Cuba and housed at the bachelor officers' quarters at Columbia Barracks, while he investigated a germicide then being made in Havana.[16] Dr. Jesse W. Lazear was then in Cuba as a result of a special request from that Department to the Surgeon General's Office for a bacteriologist. He was serving as a Contract Surgeon in charge of the laboratory at the Station Hospital, Camp Columbia, and so Dr. Reed may have met him for the first time, their mutual interests assuring their later professional association. It is possible that Major Reed may have requested General Sternberg to order him back to Cuba for a thorough study of yellow fever. It is more than probable, however, that Sternberg, the scientist, was still mindful of Dr. Welch's earlier criticism of Sanarelli's work, that is, the small number of cases studied, and that he was quick to see the advantages of a large-scale investigation when the severe outbreak of yellow fever occurred at Marianao on May 19. At any rate, on May 23, he appointed a Yellow Fever Board to study the situation.

Reed and Carroll had published their findings on Sanarelli's bacillus in the *Medical News* of April 29 and September 9, 1899; the Cuban, Aristides Agramonte, had worked on the same problem, likewise publishing his findings in the *Medical News* of February 10, 1900. He had been employed by the New York Board of Health as a bacteriologist; he was an immune and valuable, and so the Surgeon General had appointed him as Contract Surgeon and assigned him to the Army Laboratory in Havana. These three were named as members of the board, which was to "act under general instructions to be communicated to Major Reed by the Surgeon General of the Army."[17] Reed had already made contact with Dr. L. O. Howard, an entomologist with the Department of Agriculture, Washington, D.C. As Dr. Lazear had studied the mosquito-transmission of malaria at Hopkins,[18] where he was "dearly loved," he had been recommended for appointment as Army Contract Surgeon by Dr. Welch. It was only natural, therefore, that he become a fourth member of the Yellow Fever Board. Later, as the controversy raged over the individual contribution made by the several members of the board, Dr. Welch expressed his opinion that Dr. Lazear was "more broadly educated clinically and pathologically than any other man upon the commission."[19] In time the fact that Welch recommended Lazear was disputed, but Kean, an eye-witness to some of the historic events of this period, sincerely believed that he

> *had been selected by Reed on (Welch's) advice (and had) to come to Cuba as a member of the Yellow Fever Board which General Sternberg had planned… Lazear's special qualification was his familiarity with mosquitoes, as he had studied the mosquito transmission of malaria in Italy.*[20]

The exact nature of Dr. Lazear's alleged European studies may be open to dispute,[21] but his entomological training at Hopkins, where he worked with Dr. William Sydney Thayer "in the cultivation of the malaria parasite in anopholes maculipennis" was certainly of the best. Thus, like General Sternberg, the doctors Reed, Carroll and Lazear were all Welch-trained men, and the great doctor followed their scientific efforts with enthusiasm. Dr. Welch publicly credited General Sternberg, "who had previously so completely exhausted the purely bacteriologic study of yellow fever it was possible for the commission to follow the new direction which proved so fruitful," with the idea of creating the board. Nevertheless, Dr. Welch himself offered cogent advice to the Army group, including a suggestion that Major Reed test the filtrate of the blood of a yellow fever patient.[22] Some years later Kean, when preparing official documents for the record, noted that "Professor Welch was Dr. Reed's teacher in bacteriology and was his intimate and confidential friend, with whom he consulted about the details of the work in Cuba,"[23] although this point has likewise been disputed.

In view of the close interchange of information between the Hopkins doctors and the Army Medical School Staff, and the marked influence of the former group on professional activities of the Medical Department for more than forty years, this appears to be an incontestable point. Doctors Reed[24] and Carroll arrived from the United States on June 25, 1900, and so it was Dr. Agramonte, later prosector of the board,[25] who identified the yellow fever epidemic which raged at Pinar del Rio in July.[26] On arrival, Reed and Lazear confirmed the diagnosis; moreover, Major Reed apparently made certain personal observations at about this time that convinced him that the disease was not transmitted through personal contacts or femites. He took little interest at first in the mosquito theory, but, according to Dr. Welch, he "later became somewhat interested in Finlay, who had happened on the right mosquito."[27] Still, as a careful scientist, it was necessary, as his later experiments indicate, that he prove this point conclusively; and he was, certainly for the time being, unwilling to give up the idea that femites be disinfected as a precaution.[28]

Dr. Carroll was not especially hopeful of results from experiments with mosquitoes but Lazear, the entomologist, was enthusiastic. Still, "Reed outlined a masterly plan of action which was heartily approved by his colleagues." In July 1900, after entirely disproving Sanarelli's claims, the investigators began breeding mosquitoes[29] for testing Dr. Finlay's theory by making secret attempts at human inoculation of volunteers whose names were not reported by the Board.[30] Dr. Finlay had provided Major Reed with "eggs of the *Stegomyia calopus* which he specifically stated were those of the mosquito which conveyed the disease, and the first experiments of the board were made with mosquitoes grown from these eggs."[31]

Major Reed was ordered to return to the United States, departing on August 2, apparently in order to complete the report of the Typhoid Fever Board which unexpectedly devolved upon him. Dr. Carroll, as the senior contract surgeon, was technically responsible for seeing that Reed's carefully planned work was carried out during his absence. All of the men worked in harmony, "doing their special duties,"[32] in other words they performed independent assignments, and much progress was made in this two-month period, with Lazear producing the first conclusive evidence of the culpability of the mosquito. Carroll volunteered as a human subject, was inoculated by Lazear, developed a severe case of yellow fever and

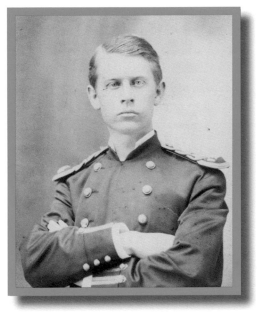

The Young Doctor, Walter Reed

nearly died. Nevertheless, he is credited with directing the work as planned "and in which he was so successful that when Dr. Reed returned... he found the preliminary experiments completely finished and the material for his report upon them ready for him."

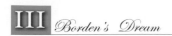

Dr. Lazear failed to contract the disease when first submitting to the bite of a previously infected mosquito; therefore, he may have believed himself an immune for he permitted an unidentified stray mosquito to infect him. Some authoritative research workers credit Lazear with more scientific curiosity than sheer carelessness in the matter, and forty years later proposed that "It was his sole purpose to identify the mosquito not only as to species but as to stage of infectivity."[33] Major Reed apparently did not know that Lazear had no life insurance and he is supposed to have believed that the entomologist was self-innoculated and therefore afraid to reveal the circumstances lest his family be deprived. It was apparently after Lazear's death that Reed wanted to be a human subject, for Dr. Welch as well as the Surgeon General advised against this.[34]

Although Carroll was nominally director of the work in Major Reed's absence it was apparently Lazear's records that proved the mosquito-transmission theory indisputably. The *Culex fasciatus*, otherwise stegomyia and *Aedes aegypti*, now determined as the transmitter of yellow fever, was doomed for extinction. Benevolent, stubborn Dr. Carlos Finlay proposed the theory; Carter proposed the modus operandi; clever, methodical laboratory-minded Dr. Lazear demonstrated the principle. The details of the study were yet to be assembled, the interpretation made. Reed, Carroll and Agramonte prepared the conclusion in two stages.

Carroll, a contract surgeon, had about seven years of experience in bacteriological and pathological work at the time he became a member of the Yellow Fever Board. Some believed that no more efficient an assistant could have been found for Reed, and that Carroll was not given appropriate credit for his participation in the work, especially in the second phase.[35] He was, however, considered only a technician by Regular Army doctors, one who, until Reed's death in 1902, worked entirely under his direction.[36] Sternberg retired in 1902, and after Reed's death surviving members of the Yellow Fever Board made more specific claims for individual credit,[37] claims which, perhaps in order to secure more adequate compensation for the heroes, Major Kean endorsed in 1906, as he prepared an official record for Surgeon General O'Reilly's signature:

> *Dr. Carroll was Dr. Reed's truest assistant and coadjutor from the inception of the work which resulted in the discovery of the method of propagation of yellow fever.... The third series of experiments were performed by Dr. Carroll alone, Dr. Reed having been refused permission to return to Cuba to complete his work.[38]*

Concurrently, Dr. Welch wrote the Secretary of War that he was in a position to know "that the original ideas embodied in this work" were Reed's.[39] Privately, however, he appeared to believed that Carroll deserved more credit than was actually accorded him, for he developed yellow fever under strictly controlled conditions. Thus there was early partisanship in giving credit for the work.

Only two years later, after Carroll died in 1908, the Medical Society of Johns Hopkins Hospital heard an appraisal of James Carroll made by his friends and teachers.[40]

Dr. Welch, the greatest American bacteriologist of his time, teacher of the four, Sternberg, Reed, Carroll, and Lazear, said that "Carroll was the most heroic in this work, as he was the first victim. Reed was the leader in fact and name, but Carroll was well trained for the work. A virile, manly and courageous type willing to sacrifice his life! The most heroic of all the members." General Sternberg, who also participated, said "The laboratory work was done mainly by Carroll and important additions were made by his individual work." In later years writers embellished[41] the facts with statements that Carroll "chiefly conducted the accurate and flawless experiments upon which the final conclusions were based." When Dr. John Hemmeter, a Hopkins associate of the period, included an unusually pro-Carroll version of the yellow fever episode in his book of historical essays the erudite Dr. Fielding H. Garrison, of the Army Medical Library, former associate of Reed's, declined to write the foreword if "that perfectly preposterous and misleading article" was included.[42]

Other Medical Department officers, some of whom were friends, and others, near-contemporaries, were convinced that Major Reed was the master mind of this controversial scientific exploit and they resented the "sentimental legend" fostered by the Hopkins group, apparently, they believed, primarily because Carroll was a graduate of the school. He was admittedly a competent histologist, but the Army group believed he, like Dr. Agramonte in later years, claimed undue credit for some responsibilities in the work. Dr. Welch had said that Lazear was the best prepared member of the board.

> *If the Baltimore post-mortem experts must root for somebody other than Reed, said one of the Army men, then why not root for Lazear? How strange is fact alongside the built-up legend? Reed gave credit to everyone of his associates in his initial paper on the yellow fever work, establishing priority, and it is well known among the Army files of his time and the enlisted men who were in Cuba with him, that he was the only one, except Carlos Finlay, who believed in the mosquito hypothesis until it was demonstrated.[43]*

The "initial paper" was mainly written by Major Reed, who studied Lazear's careful notes as he prepared the official announcement of the successful work of the Yellow Fever Board. He was excited over the unexpected and probably sooner-than-expected results. With a remarkable show of haste for so deliberate a man, within two weeks of his October 1900 return to Cuba, he was again en route to the United States,[44] for he believed British scientists were on the verge of announcing a similar interpretation of the etiology of yellow fever. The complete answer had not been found, but the course was laid; the horizon was in sight. Some non-military critics and popular writers have claimed that Walter Reed was not especially original as microbe hunters go,[45] and that his assignment to investigate yellow fever was "a big order considering who the man Walter Reed was, it was altogether too big an order."[46] Some associates of the great scientist asserted that "the notion of Reed as a pietist and prayerful brother is another sentimental legend... he was a bit humorless perhaps, except in the usual Army way,... but a very fair and square gentleman." Army medical officers, staunch in their loyalty, contend that the official record of his successive and successful investigations sustain his fame.

These were not scientific times and so the answer to such carping lies not in denial but in the affirmative results of the work. As a careful investigator and analyst he needs no defense. Like the *Culex fasciatus*, he was, fortunately for the western hemisphere, a scientific "intermediate host." The board's sensational conclusions were presented to the world in October 1900: *The Etiology of Yellow Fever, A Preliminary Note*, of which *The Philadelphia Medical Journal* noted:

> *If the observations of Major Reed are confirmed, even though the specific germ of yellow fever be not immediately discovered, there shall have been shed upon this most fatal disease a new flood of light....* [47]

Accepting the mosquito as the only agent of transmission and establishing its life cycle were only the initial steps, for the negative conclusion reached after the fact must be substantiated. In an attempt to disprove the proof, to provide a controlled experiment in a truly scientific way the clinical investigations were renewed after publication of the preliminary studies, investigations both spectacular and disagreeable. By February 1901, the scientific world knew the problem could be licked.[48] Yellow fever was proved to be in the virus field, and yellow fever was on its way out.

Setting the Stage for Martyrdom

The post hospital, Washington Barracks, D.C., became a U.S. Army General Hospital during the Spanish-American War, and Major William Cline Borden Reported as Commandant and operating surgeon shortly after hostilities ceased. In accordance with the Surgeon General's policy of using medical officers in and near the District of Columbia as faculty members, he was named instructor in military surgery when the Army Medical School reopened in the autumn of 1901. Major Borden was an unusual man, and he epitomized the new concept of medical officer versus Army doctor then developing as a result of the new interest in field medicine and sanitation. A man of precise habits[49] and distinct military bearing, he was both energetic and determined, and his professional versatility had earned for him some distinction as a research worker, inventor and author. Like General Sternberg, he showed an early interest in histology and bacteriology, and he occasionally communicated with his friend, Major Reed, on subjects of mutual interest. In 1887, he published a scientific paper on "An Extemporized Section Flattener." This paper was followed in 1899 by another on "The Origin and Development of the Fat Cell of the Frog," and by 1891 he had attacked a public health problem with equal vigor, publishing vital statistics on an Apache Indian community.

As if his professional thirst knew no bounds, he soon published an article on "Practical Photomicrography by Use of the Oil Lamp." By the time war came he had experimented with static X-ray machines. In 1899 he wrote, as a government project, the first American textbook on X-ray.[50] A rare combination of dreamer and realist, Major Borden was uncommonly able to translate his theories into practical accomplishments. There were, therefore, at least two independent research workers of widely different temperaments on the faculty when the Army Medical School reopened in 1901—Reed and Borden. Of the two, the latter had a more catholic list of publications to his credit. He had not only been more concerned with administration than had Major Reed, but the Surgeon General had not charged him with responsibility for evaluating special medical service problems, such as water purifiers, hog cholera bacilli and mosquitoes.[51] Fate, however, had not decreed professional immortality for Major Borden, or in fact immortality of any kind.

Majors Reed and Borden were busy men during the 1901–1902 session of the School, for in addition to their other duties they were lecturing at Columbian Medical College (George Washington). In Reed's case, the new-found fame imposed such obligations as attendance at out-of-town professional meetings,[52] and writing. He was a quiet man and lived modestly with his wife and young daughter at 1603-19th Street, where he occasionally entertained students. This was an undertaking of some importance, for the class of 1901 was the largest that had been admitted to the School and twenty doctors were graduated. The faculty was inclined to celebrate so memorable an occasion and graduated the group in true academic style, recording the irrelevant facts that buying a die, to make a seal, and securing sufficient ribbon trimming for the diplomas required an outlay of $5.70.[53]

Major Reed was considered a good teacher, one well prepared for his assignment. Gentle, soft-spoken, with an excellent command of English and a well concealed sense of humor, his lectures were almost text-like in perfection.[54] He had as good scientific training as the Army had to offer at that time and his students were properly impressed with his fame, considering it an honor to sit in his classes.[55]

The Medical Corps was tremendously proud of him. He had not only topped Surgeon General Sternberg's scientific record but he had become an international savior of public health. His friends agreed unanimously that he was courteous, blameless, mild, logical, conscientious, thorough, temperate and of a strong moral nature.[56] In addition to these positive traits he had a rare gift for analysis, orderly and logical methods or procedure and the ability to see a task to completion.

Nature supposedly has a way of predisposing man's fate, or so some students of the occult sciences claim, and it is possible that in the autumn of 1901, the clinical case of Walter Reed, Major-Surgeon, United States Army, was entering the last phase in which man-made intervention could avail. The century was less than a year old, but it was the beginning of a new era of medicine. Three decades later the lay public would share intimately the professional knowledge of its doctors, would be coached through campaign and cautious confidence to be wary of the onset of insidious diseases, would be warned in sibilant radio whispers to see its dentist twice a year. But medical tolerance as well as medical knowledge was strictly limited in 1901. According to the opinion of some,

Fragments of Letter from Walter Reed to William Cline Borden, 1894

Walter Reed was the victim of his own fame, for where less busy men than he might have heeded warnings of physical catastrophe he procrastinated. Less famous men than he would undoubtedly have received the immediate surgical disposition[57] accorded a "routine" case, but as doctor versus doctor, his own evaluation of his illness prevailed.

Case History

Dr. Reed had not been a well man for nearly two years. In fact, he had never been robust, and his associates in Cuba noted his poor physical condition in 1900. Some thought he "was suffering from chronic appendicitis and that this condition, which he did not recognize, was responsible for his being so careful of himself, especially his diet..."[58] for he "had to eat sparingly"[59]; others believed the warm weather and poorer refrigeration in Cuba accounted for his sudden distaste for meat.[60] He was then thin and inclined to be dyspeptic,[61] quite unlike the sixteen-year-old youth who left the farm to study medicine so brilliantly at the University of Virginia. Close friends who saw him frequently during 1901 noted that he seemed unduly exhausted that year and that he had indigestion. The responsibility for inoculating human subjects with yellow fever had depressed him during the Cuban experiment, and he had noted his melancholia for the Surgeon General,[62] unknowingly providing notes for his clinical history.

Although only fifty-one years of age in the autumn of 1902, "mental exertion was becoming strangely painful to the alert mind."[63] He was "in the prime of his life; but tired, so tired,"[64] in spite of resting at his summer home in Pennsylvania during the long vacation. He was nervous;[65] when school reopened he came home each evening mentally and physically exhausted, and his family noted his rapid deterioration with considerable alarm. By his own account he was "a very sick man;"[66] still, he failed to seek professional advice, as he struggled against cumulative and insurmountable physical odds.

On November 1, 1902, the recently appointed Surgeon General O'Reilly, detailed him temporarily and in addition to his other duties as Librarian of the Army Medical Library,[67] an assignment long coveted.[68] It is doubtful that he actively participated in the functions of this office, for taciturn, a worrier, "nervous and rundown,"[69] by November 12 Walter Reed was too ill to leave his bed. No longer able to evade professional consultation, two days later he consulted his friend and associate, Major Borden, who knew that he believed himself a sufferer from acute indigestion, intestinal colic or chronic

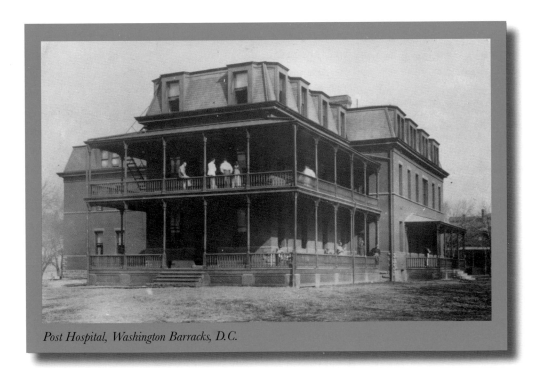

Post Hospital, Washington Barracks, D.C.

appendicitis, popular diagnosis for inexplicable abdominal pains. When his prognosis continued poor, Borden insisted on surgery. The faculty of the Army Medical School met routinely at 4 p.m. on Monday, November 17; all of the members were present except Walter Reed, who was already a postoperative patient in the Army General Hospital, Washington Barracks.

The patient had little or no fever at the time of operation, and his pulse was nearly normal. Further, he answered the anesthetist's routine inquiry about false teeth with an indignant "No."[70] Neither his surgeon nor the select group of doctors, including the Surgeon General, who flanked the operating table anticipated any extraordinary complications.[71] Much to their surprise, the appendiceal stump and the attached caecum were necrotic. The appendix was surprisingly large, "rather like a large carrot; four or five inches long; about three quarters of an inch in diameter at the largest part. It seemed to be thick and indurated from prolonged inflammation."[72] Even the surrounding tissue was highly inflamed, with the lumen obliterated in places.[73] "The wall of the caecum was infiltrated and necrotic; this gave trouble by the tearing out of the stitches."[74]

A new school of surgical technique was developing at this time, with many of the conservative older doctors believing that a long clean wound was necessary in order to bare the surgical field. However, younger and more adventurous men were beginning to advocate the McBurney muscle-splitting method, propounding the modern theory that a small wound insured a more rapid convalescence. Major Borden advocated this method and used it in operating on Major Reed for what was presumed to be an uncomplicated case of appendicitis. Initially a small incision was made which, after examination of the appendix, was extended. The dissected specimen, later viewed by the students, apparently failed to confirm some opinions[75] that a pus pocket had ruptured during surgery.

In spite of the fact that the offending area was walled off and the wound was well cleaned, trouble lay ahead. Dr. Borden was surprised at the "condition (which had) existed with a temperature not over 100.6 at any time and (at the) comparatively insignificant symptoms, showing what serious pathologic changes may be present with slight symptoms."[76] He predicted sloughing and that a fecal fistula would form. The appendix was ligated, the only possible course in view of the necrosis, and the wound was closed with a drain. Within five days the surgeon's dire prophesy was fulfilled.[77] Inasmuch as the operation was performed on Monday and not on Saturday, the usual day for surgical demonstration for the students of the School, they were not at their customary observation post on the raised step-dais. Nevertheless, the technical details of the operation were explained[78] for as professor or case history, the students were interested in all that befall the now famous man. Their professional opinion was not sought, for by that time the clinical interpretation was a fait accompli, for better men than they had solemnly subscribed to a primary diagnosis of chronic appendicitis. On the sixth postoperative day the patient died of peritonitis, then Major Borden's only fatality following an appendectomy;[79] asthenia was reported as the immediate cause of death.[80]

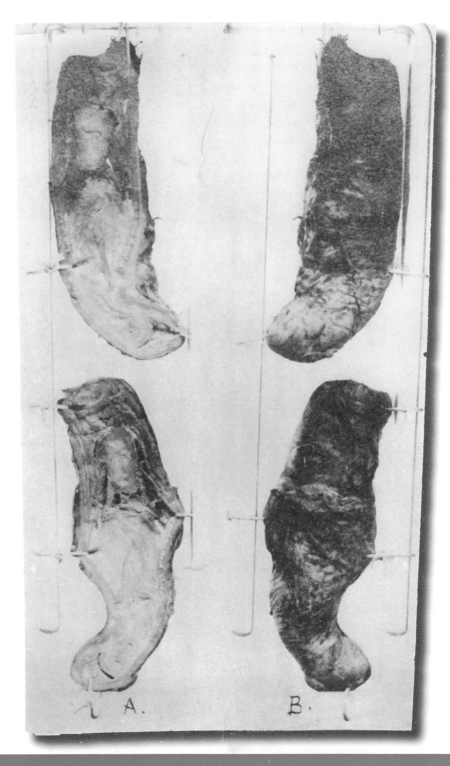

Walter Reed's Appendix; Reprint, Washington's Medical Annals, Vol. I, No. 6, Jan. 1903

Officially it was Major Borden's "painful duty" to advise the Surgeon General of the death; the Surgeon General, in forwarding the information to the Adjutant General, recalled that Walter Reed's services were almost priceless and that his "qualities as a man so endeared him to his associates that they (felt)... his loss as a personal calamity."[81] It was one of life's tragedies that the patient was a scientific hero, for otherwise surgical death following a ruptured appendix would have passed without especial note. As it was, some of the Reed admirers severely criticized Dr. Borden's surgical technique.[82] Lacking objectivity, they were never able to consider the death in context with other attendant physical symptoms. Yet as a definitive diagnosis "chronic appendicitis," medical nomenclature of the gay nineties, has like Sternberg's *Bacillus X* and Sanarellis's *Bacillus icteroides*, disappeared into a professional oblivion all its own.

Apart from the spectacular control of epidemics, which followed the work of the Yellow Fever Board, two factors assisted in immortalizing Walter Reed. Unlike the combat services, the Medical Department then had few publicized heroes, and his untimely death at the peak of his career, established him as a martyr. Secondly, solving the epidemiology of yellow fever was indisputably a major accomplishment, and as chairman of the board, he had received unprecedented scientific recognition.

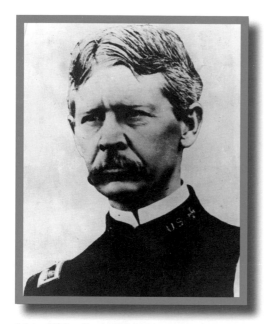

Major Walter Reed, 1902

Post-humous Recognition

Kean, Gorgas and Reed were associated in the sanitary reclamations in Cuba, with Kean and Gorgas gaining distinction as a result of the work done by the Yellow Fever Board. It was Reed who instructed Kean in the social creed of the military set when he moved his family to Washington in 1902, the requirements of which were a residence above Pennsylvania Avenue and West of Seventh Street Road, an account at the Riggs National Bank and membership in the Army and Navy Club.[83] It was for Major Gorgas that the Reeds were entertaining on the night Walter Reed became too ill to leave his bed; it was Kean who carved for him at the family dinner table as he lay abed upstairs.[84] It was Gorgas who inherited the military vacancy for a lieutenant colonelcy established for Walter Reed, senior major in the Medical Corps, when he died on the eve of promotion. Although Kean, McCaw and Ireland came in time to resent the favors[85] and publicity which followed Gorgas's prominent position, Gorgas likewise memorialized Walter Reed.[86] Thus friendship bound the past and the future.

If Major Reed was melancholy over his responsibility for human life while in Cuba, he was no less moody and discouraged in the autumn of 1901, for he believed "persons in authority" were trying to depreciate his accomplishments.[87] Sternberg was openly claiming credit in the work and Reed resented his inability to contest the point with his superior officer. He was inclined, perhaps because of his poor health, to give up his commission in the Army, and it was Dr. Welch who assured him the facts spoke for themselves and that he should remain in the Medical Corps, advice for which he was later grateful. Psychosomatic medicine was an undreamed of professional field at this time, but his professional friends undoubtedly knew that his troubled state of mind affected his health.[88]

Socially, professionally and militarily Sternberg's position was secure, and the Medical Corps was proud of his past accomplishments and indulgent in regard to his claims. There was, however, a recognizable but rarely acknowledged professional schism between Regular Army Medical Officers and the Contract Surgeons, and many of the latter group, unable to pass the rigid examination of the Army Examining Board,[89] became capable hirelings of the former group. Some considered them the sort of substantial men who

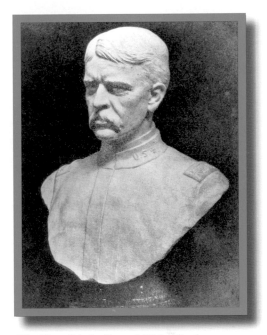

The Hans Schuler Bust of Walter Reed

acquitted themselves well and raised themselves "in the esteem of the volunteer medical officers, who, in the early days of the war, did not consider them good enough to share in their mess."[90] Carroll and Agramonte were Contract Surgeons; they were not members of the clan, the Regular Army. In Carroll's case, the fact that he was a self-educated enlisted man was never overlooked, regardless of Dr. Welch's praise. There had long been controversy over Ross' work in India, for some believed he had started the whole program.[91] Some of Reed's friends familiar with the chronological record of the military experiment believed therefore, that Carroll's and Argramonte's claims for belated scientific recognition, made *after* the death of Lazear and Reed, placed an exaggerated evaluation on their work.[92] The claims of Carter, Ross and Sternberg could not be ignored, for they had pioneered in the mosquito work. But as the Army Board had woven the scientifically loose strings left by these men into a solid mat of facts, Reed's friends, particularly the gallant southerner, Jefferson Randolph Kean, had accepted any threat to his immortality as a personal challenge.

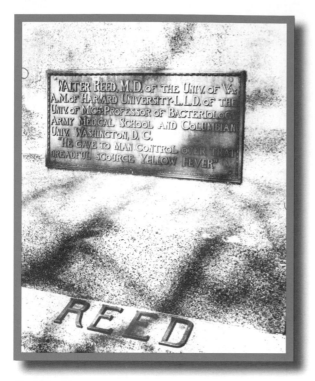

Reed Headstone

The yellow fever experiment was a familiar discussion during 1901 and 1902, and articles appeared in such publications as the *Medical News*, the *Transactions of the Association of American Physicians* and the *Popular Science Monthly*. During the summer of 1903 the *Bulletin of the Johns Hopkins Hospital* announced that a meeting had been held to arrange a suitable memorial. The Walter Reed Memorial Association was therefore formed and endorsed by many distinguished citizens, some of whom favored a public monument but chose the more humanitarian course of assigning to the Reed dependent family the interest from the privately subscribed monies. For as Ross said later "the wealthy American people allowed him to (die) without any adequate bonus or reward, and actually in a state of apprehension regarding the future of his wife and daughter."[93] In 1904, authorized by the Association, Major Walter D. McCaw, librarian of the Army Medical Library, prepared a memorial pamphlet designed to secure funds for the endowment, and Major Kean prepared a comparable sketch.[94] Again as a direct result of the Association's interest, Hans Schuler of Baltimore was paid $1,000.00 for a white Italian marble bust of "Walter Reed, doctor in uniform."[95]

In 1906, during the height of the controversy, Dr. Howard Kelly of the Hopkins faculty and one-time professional associate of Walter Reed, conferred with Major Kean when writing the sentimental biography,[96] *Walter Reed and Yellow Fever*. The McCaw *Memoir* was already in circulation, and some of the material for Kean's Senate Document 822, *Yellow Fever* a compilation of various notes, was in the making.[97] Dr. Welch had assured Reed that time would establish him securely and indisputably in the halls of scientific fame; as Kean his faithful friend, recorded a decade later he "being dead, it is an obligation of his friends to see that his scientific achievements are not forgotten."

References

1. Ltr from J.R. Kean, Lt. Col., M.C., to Dr. Guy L. Kiefer, Health Officer, Detroit, Michigan, Dec. 17, 1912, File 19928, War Records Division, Nat'l Archives.

2. Josiah C. Trent, M.D., ed., "Thumbnail Sketches of Eminent Physicians," *North Carolina Med. Journal*, Vol 7, 1946 (reprint) pg 1-7.

3. *Ibid*, pg. 24.

4. Ronald Ross, *Memoirs*, London, John Murray, 1923, pg 426.

5. Carlos Edwardo Finlay, *Carlos Finlay and Yellow Fever*, Oxford Univ. Press, 1940, pg. 94.

6. Martha Sternberg, *George M. Sternberg a biography*, Chicago, American Medical Association, 1920.

7. Ltr. from Geo. H. Torney, TSG to Hon. Robert L. Owen, United States Senate, April 29, 1910. (quoted) pg 24-30, Senate Doc. 822, 61st Congress, 3rd Session, Washington, GPO, 1911; Johns Hopkins Hosp. Bulletin, Vol. 9, 1898, pg 119.

8. Albert E. Truby, *Memoirs of Walter Reed, The Yellow Fever Episode*, New York, Paul B. Hoeber, Inc. 1943, pg 38.

9. Walter Reed, M.D.... and James Carroll, M.D., "... Bacillus Icteroides and Bacillus Choleral Suis – A Preliminary Note." (Reprint) from *Medical News*, April 29, 1899.

10. John C. Hemmeter, *Master Minds of Medicine*, New York Med. Life Press, 1927, pg 301 (article first appeared in *Janus*, 1908).

11. Hemmeter, *op cit*, pg 337-345.

12. Truby, *op cit*, pg 91.

13. The Dodge Commission.

14. Biography of General J.R. Kean, Manuscript on file, Army Medical Library, Washington, D.C.; Truby, *op cit*, pg 39.

15. Kean, *op cit*, pg 128.

16. Truby, *op cit*, pg 74-76; as per SO 51, Par. 16. March 2, 1900, to investigate, specifically, electro-zone. From W.R. Station and Duty Reports, SGO, War Rec. Div., Nat'l Archives, Wash., D.C.

17. Par. 34, SO 122, AGO, Washington, May 24, 1900; Maj. James Carroll, M.D., U.S.A. addresses by Dr. H.A. Kelly; W.H. Welch; W.S. Thayer; Surg. Gen. Sternberg, U.S.A.; H.H. Donnally; A.F.A. King; S. Ruffin; C.E. Munroe; and J.O. Skinner. *Bull. of Johns Hopkins Hospital*, 19: 202, pg. 8.

18. JAMA, October 13, 1900.

19. Ltr P.S. Hench, M.D., to writer, August 4, 1951 credits Welch as having secured the appt. as C.S.; For Welch's opinion of Lazear see *Bull. JHH*, 19: 202, pg 6.

20. Kean, *op cit*, pg 62.

21. Lazear traveled in Europe from May to September 1890 and in the company of his Mother from October 1894 to late August 1895. Hench to writer August 4, 1951; Morris Fishbein, *A History of the American Medical Association 1847 to 1947*, W.B. Saunders, 1947, pg 775.

22. J.A.M.A., 1910, vol. 54, pg 1326; Howard A. Kelly, *Walter Reed and Yellow Fever*, N.Y., Mc-Clure, Phillips & Co., 1906, pg 66; *Bull. JHH, op cit.*, pg 7.

23. Senate Document 822, 61st Congress, 3rd Session, *Yellow Fever*, a compilation of various publilcations, GPO, 1911, pg 20.

24. Reed had been in Cuba at least twice previously on other missions.

25. Kean, *op cit*, pg 62.

26. Truby, *op cit*, pg 94, 95.

27. Dr. L.F. Barker's notes on talks with William Henry Welch during his last illness, (Ap. 2, 1934), Collection of Inst. of Hist. of Med., Welch Med. Library; Kean, *op cit*, pg 63; Truby, *op cit*, pg 96; *Bull. JHH, op cit* (Dr. Kelly's statement)

28. Kean, *op cit*, pg 67.

29. *Bulletin, loc cit*; Ltr from A.E. Truby to writer, May 26, 1951.

30. Philip S. Hench, M.D., *Conquerors of Yellow Fever*, an address given at Cleveland, Ohio, June 21, 1941, (pp). On file, Library, WRGH.

31. Senate Doc. 822, *op cit*, pg 233.

32. Ltr from A.E. Truby, Brig. Gen., Ret. to the writer, May 26, 1951.

33. Dr. Hench has reached this conclusion through interviews with Dr. Agramonte's daughter (1939), John Moran, and a study of Lazear's letters to his wife. Ltr to writer, *op cit*. Ross, *op cit*, pg 425; Truby, *op cit*, pg 123-126; Hemmeter, *op cit*, pg 331; Hench, *op cit*, pg 5, quotes Truby as "interpreting" the source of Lazear's infection. Kean, a senior officer to Truby at the time, an intimate of Reed and Lazear, failed to mention this interpretation to the writer; he invariably said that Truby was a younger man than he and probably recalled more incidental details. Walter Reed was the subject of several interviews.

34. Dr. Phillip S. Hench, "Walter Reed and the Conquest of Yellow Fever": an illustrated address, delivered before the Fourth International Congresses on Tropical Medicine and Malaria, Washington, May 12, 1948, (pam) pg 51; Dr. L.F. Barker's *Notes, op cit*.

35. *Bull. JHH, op cit*; (Dr. Welch); Detailed report from 1st Lt. James Carroll to TSG, Aug. 16, 1906. File 19928, War Rec. Div., Nat'l Archives.

36. Interview with Love, Truby and Phalen, *op cit*; Carroll succeeded Reed at the Army Medical School. Carroll was considered a careful and thorough laboratory technician. Interview with Charles Stanley White, M.D., May 2, 1951.

37. Hench ltr, *op cit*.

38. Senate Document, *op cit*, pg 21.

39. Senate Doc., *op cit*, pg 20; Dr. L.F. Barker's *Notes, op cit*; *Bull. JHH*, Vol 19: 202, pg 1-12.

40. *Bull. JHH, op cit*, pg 1-12; Hemmeter, *Janus*, 1908, pg 59, likewise a Hopkins man, apparently used this meeting as a source for his quotations.

41. Hemmeter, *op cit*, pg 308.

42. Trent, *op cit*, pg 17; Ltr F.H. Garrison to H.L. Mencken from Ft. Santiago, Manila, P.I., Ap. 28, 1924, Collection of Inst. of The Hist. of Med., Welch Med. Library, Baltimore. Md.

43. Interview with Brig. Gen. Albert G. Love, M.C., Ret., Feb. 13, 1951; Truby and Kean Int's; Ltr Fielding H. Garrison to H.W. Mencken frm Ft. Santiago, Manila, P.I., Apr. 28, 1929; Coll. Inst. Hist. of Med., Welch Med. Lib., Balt., Md.

44. Truby, *op cit*, pg 128; "The Etiology of Yellow Fever, A Preliminary Note." *Philadelphia Medical Journal* v. VI, Phil., 1900. (Reed et al).

45. Paul de Kruif, *Microbe Hunters*, New York, Harcourt, Brace & Co., 1926, pg 322. (These conclusions were based on examination of the scientific publications. Ltr from Paul de Kruif to the writer March 29, 1951.)

46. *Ibid*, pg 313; Ltr. Garrison to Mencken, *op cit*.

47. Editorial, *Phil. Med. Jrn.* Vol. VI, No. 17, October 27, 1900, pg 761.

48. *The Etiology of Yellow Fever – an additional note*. Read at the Pan-American Medical Congress in Havana, Feb. 6, 1901.

49. Personal scrapbook of William Cline Borden, covering his entire military career, on file office of Dr. Daniel L. Borden, Washington, D.C.

50. Daniel L. Borden, M.D., "William Cline Borden, 1858-1934," *Medical Annals of the District of Columbia*, Vol. V, September and October 1936.

51. Senate Document 822, *op cit*, pg 44 credits Reed with 21 single articles printed between 1892 and 1902, and app. nine collaborative articles. Of these articles ten were on yellow fever; three or four dealt with typhoid, two with malaria, two with erysipelas etc.; with the exception of an article on electrozone, the subjects were infectious diseases and laboratory examinations. The writer has presently a list of some twenty-one articles prepared by Dr. Borden.

52. SGO Folder 19928, War Rec. Div., Nat'l Archives.

53. Minutes... April 3, 1902.

54. Interview with Charles Stanley White, M.D., May 2, 1951, one-time student of Walter Reed. Dr. White was the anesthetist when Major Borden operated on the scientist.

55. Interview with Major Gen. Robert U. Patterson, Ret., Aug. 24, 1950; Kelly, *op cit*, pg 238-240.

56. DeKruif, *op cit*, pg 311-333; Kean, Love, Truby & Phalen, *op cit*.

57. White interview, *op cit*.

58. Truby, *op cit*, pg 199, 200.

59. Laura Wood, *Walter Reed Doctor in Uniform*, New York, Julian Messner, Inc. 1943, pg 226.

60.   Interview with Brig. Gen. Albert E. Truby, MC, Ret., June 27-28, 1950.

61.   Interview with Brig. Gen. Albert G. Love, April 5, 1950.

62.   Wood, *op cit*, pg 247.

63.   Wood, *op cit*, pg 252.

64.   De Kruif *op cit*... pg 333.

65.   W.C. Borden, M.D. ... *History of Doctor Walter Reed's Illness from Appendicitis*, Reported with Specimen, by request, to the Medical Society of the District of Columbia, Nov. 19, 1902. Reprint, Washington Medical Annals, Vol. I, No. 6, Jan. 1903.

66.   Howard A. Kelly, *op cit*, pg 245.

67.   SGO 19928, War Records Div., Nat'l Archives.

68.   *Hist. of the Assoc. of Military Surgeon in the U.S., 1891–1941*; Washington, The Ass. of Mil. Surgeon, 1941, pg 31.

69.   Borden, *op cit*, pg 7.

70.   White interview, *op cit*.

71.   Kean interview, Nov. 1946.

72.   Ltr from Col. James D. Fife, MC, Ret, to the writer, Jan. 11, 1951; White interview, *op cit*.

73.   Borden *op cit*, pg 7.

74.   W.C. Borden, M.C.... *History of Doctor Walter Reed's Illness From Appendicitis*, *op cit*.

75.   Fife, *op cit*.

76.   Borden, *op cit*.

77.   Kean, *op cit*; Kelly, *op cit*, 246–248.

78.   Interview with Col. James D. Fife, May 26, 1950.

79.   Daniel L. Borden, *op cit*, pg 8.

80.   Memo to TAG from W.C. Borden, Surgeon, U.S.A. Gen. Hosp., Washington Barracks, D.C., Nov. 23, 1902, SGO 19928, War Rec. Div., Nat'l Archives.

81.   1st Ind. To above s/O'Reilly.

82.   Based on confidential interviews.

83. Interview with Brig. Gen. J.R. Kean, November 1946; Laura Wood, *Walter Reed Doctor in Uniform*, quotes a slightly different version of this account, names Woodward and Lothrop instead of the Army and Navy Club (pg. 252).

84. Interview... Kean, Nov. 1946.

85. Interview Brig. Gen. Albert G. Love, M.C., Ret., Feb. 13, 1951.

86. William Crawford Gorgas, *Sanitation in Panama*, NY and London, D. Appleton and Co., 1915.

87. Kelly, *op cit*, pg 242; Martha Sternberg, *op cit*; George M. Sternberg in *The Popular Science Monthly*, Vol 19, May to Oct 1901.

88. Dr. L.F. Barker's Notes on talks with William Henry Welch during his last illness, Par 7, *Walter Reed*, Ap. 2, 1934; Collection, *op cit*.

89. Interview with Brig. Gen. Albert G. Love, M.C., Ret., Feb. 13, 1951.

90. Annual Report TSG... 1899, pg 54.

91. See ext. from State Med. Ass. of Texas, 1904, pg 42, in SGO 19928, War Rec. Div., Nat'l Archives.

92. Truby, Love, Phalen, Kean, *op cit*; Garrison Ltr to Mencken, *op cit*.

93. Ross, *op cit*, pg 426; For a great many years an unknown donor supplemented the Memorial Association's fund by $100 a month. Interview with Mrs. Merritte W. Ireland, May 14, 1950.

94. Jefferson R. Kean... *Sketch of the Life of Major Walter Reed...* (nd) pg 14-16, Senate Doc. 822.

95. Minutes of Meeting of the Managers of the Walter Reed Memorial Association, April 27, 1904; Dec. 20, 1904; Jan. 20, 1905, borrowed from the Secretary.

96. Interview... Kean, July 19, 1950.

97. Senate Document 822, pg. 199; Ltr from A.E. Truby, May 26, 1951. General Truby states in part that "Senate Document 822, 1911 has long been "my Bible" in this work. It was thrown together hurriedly by... Gen. Kean, so there were many errors, but by correspondence I know the correct answer to most of them...."

In Defense of a Dream

1903–1905

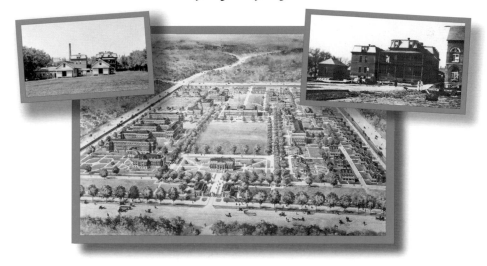

*"We… have to be ready to meet any
emergency that may arise anywhere, at any time."[1]*

The Proposal

The Spanish-American war brought many changes to the Medical Department; some were gradual, extending over a period of years; the effects of others were felt almost immediately. The gap between personnel requirements and manpower assignments never seemed to close, and as the mobile field hospitals organized to accompany the armies to the front became immobilized with typhoid cases, the nursing service problem became critical. In an effort partially to meet the deficit in nurses, the time-in-grade service for promotion of assistant hospital stewards was decreased from twelve to three months, and many willing but untrained corpsmen undertook the grave responsibilities of nurses.

Traditionally, the Army shrank or expanded according to Congressional whimsy and the current enthusiasm for economy. The Medical Department, less spectacular than the combat branches and thus considered less obviously necessary, hung with precarious footing on the fringe of Army appropriations. The Act of March 1, 1887, excluded the Hospital Corps from the effective strength of the Army, but when the Regular Army increased to 65,000 men in March 1899, the Hospital Corps complement barely escaped inclusion in the total manpower allowances. There were still insufficient corpsmen to meet the nursing requirements, which coincided with the increased number of military hospitals, and so by July 1, 1899, one hundred thirty-seven of the two hundred and two contract nurses remaining in the service were assigned to duty outside the United States.[2]

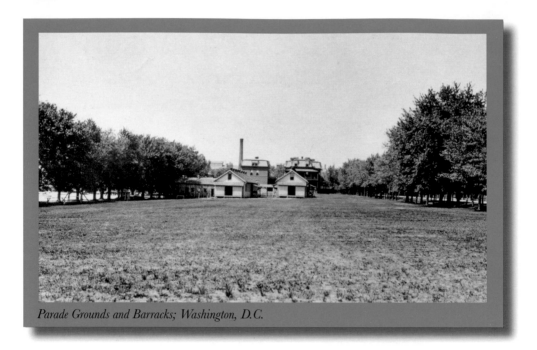

Parade Grounds and Barracks; Washington, D.C.

Like the Army Medical School program for doctors, formal training for the Companies of Instruction was curtailed during the war, and the corpsmen received instruction as practical nurses after detail to the temporary general hospitals. As these hospitals were not only overcrowded but lacked uniformity in organization, nursing service standards were open to improvement. Further, the on-the-job training program for men nurses coincided with the interests and opinions of the respective hospital commanders, with only the instruction in cooking "intrusted to civilian cooks or to female nurses in charge of the diet kitchen."

The corpsmen trained at Washington Barracks were more fortunate than some, for Major E.L. Munson, like Woodhull, Hoff, Clyde Ford and more recently Major F.R. Keefer, was intensely interested in military medical training. Under his general supervision, a three-week course of twelve progressive lessons in cookery was given by a female nurse who for undisclosed "local reasons" was classed as a civilian rather than as a contract nurse.[3] The feminine influence was pervasive, and since the corpsmen were supposed to do emergency cooking only, they were taught to prepare "the various articles of the several rations, so as to render them more delicate, appetizing, and suitable for the use of the sick". In true military fashion, however, the students attended cookery class in squads of ten to eighteen men. As a reward for culinary proficiency the more apt ones were detailed for "a short tour of duty in the general kitchen," to some, no doubt, a dubious recognition of merit. The company commander at Washington Barracks boasted proudly of the display of interest in cooking but may have failed to correlate the masculine enthusiasm for this feminine pursuit to the novel circumstance of having an instructress in charge of the class. As a matter of record for social anthropologists, the Surgeon General had predicted that the presence of female nurses in a male domain would be both disrupting and disturbing. Major Munson solved the behavior problem by the simple expedient of assigning "...an acting hospital steward during each hour of instruction."[4]

General Order No. 3, January 8, 1900, removed the Company of Instruction, Washington Barracks, from line control and attached it to the hospital. This arrangement not only provided more freedom in detailing the men to hospital and school duties, but it obviated minor clashes of authority between the hospital commander, Major Borden, and the post line commander who lived in close proximity on the military reservation.[5] The little hospital provided a basement room for Corps drill exercises during inclement weather, but otherwise there was little outward change in the military routine. In 1901, the Medical Department adopted maroon as its official color instead of green, and after February, the hospital corpsmen wore regulation Medical Department insignia. The Red Cross arm brassard was designated for use only during war.

Some 5,000 men then were in the Corps, few of whom had the careful training of the pre-war period. "To be sure," said the Surgeon General when advocating a four-month training course for the seven reactivated Companies of Instruction, the men were "no worse off... than the men in other branches of the service, but their individual responsibility (was) so much greater that lack of training became more apparent."[6] Further, the Corps was so loosely organized at this time, that the company commanders found some difficulty in transferring the medical soldier and his descriptive list, his complete service record, to new stations and having both arrive in good order.[7]

Fifty-nine members of the female Nurse Corps were on duty at military hospitals in the United States during 1901, the year the Army Nurse Corps received Congressional authorization. Many corpsmen resented the nurses' attempts at hospital supervision and military authority, but there was a decided improvement in the attitude of the average Army doctor toward the new professional allies. Only two years previously some of the more conservative officers had agreed that where women were concerned "as a rule their behavior was satisfactory and their work commendable, but they were an expensive luxury as they received more wages than the men of the hospital corps and required much waiting on."[8] Now, although the Surgeon General had not changed his opinion that their presence was "not considered desirable at post hospitals under ordinary conditions," the United States Army Hospital at Presidio of San Francisco, established in 1847, had forty-three. As the Presidio served as a staging area for the Philippines, it did not reflect the true pattern of other military hospitals, for neither the large Army and Navy Hospital at Hot Springs, Arkansas, nor the very active U.S. Army General Hospital at Washington Barracks, vanguard of the national capital, employed females for bedside nursing.[9]

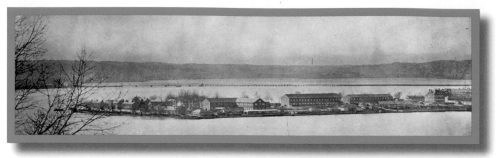

Greenleaf's Point, Washington Arsenal Grounds

Insofar as Washington Barracks was concerned, not only was there no housing for female nurses, but Company No. 1 at ease found dismal surroundings, for it was quartered in temporary wooden pavilions built during the war and already in need of repair.[10] Major Borden was not unmindful of the technical deficiencies of the corpsmen who worked in his hospital, and he commented in his usual direct manner on the fact that "a large number of recruits (had) never seen the interior of a hospital, and the great majority of them (had) not the faintest idea of how to care for the sick."[11]

Concurrently, new technical positions were being opened to the Hospital Corps, for contract Dental Surgeons were appointed in 1901, and each dental surgeon was authorized a corpsmen or acting hospital steward as an assistant. As a result of the occupation

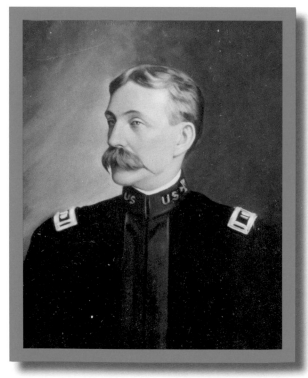

of Cuba, Puerto Rico and the Philippines, men were returning to the United States with strange tropical diseases which required special investigation. Tropical service was, therefore, not only presumed to affect the teeth, but the Surgeon General reported that servicemen were constantly "being discharged on account of their inability to properly masticate the Army ration." This was the identical ration with which the Medical Department strove to tempt the jaded appetites of the sick by rendering it more "delicate, appetizing and suitable," through subsidies from the Hospital Fund.[12]

Portrait of Captain John S. Marshall; First Dental Officer, U.S.A.

Many factors encouraged Major Borden's concern over the requirements for a larger hospital in or near the city of Washington. During 1902, he admitted 544 patients to the U.S. Army General Hospital, ninety-one of which were operative surgical cases.[13] With the building in bad condition and the wards crowded, he found it difficult to keep the operating room in the proper antiseptic condition. The low-lying tidal land of Greenleaf's Point was hot and humid in the summer, an unpleasant and unhealthy place when domiciling sick patients in tents or wooden pavilions. Moreover, he had found the teaching and demonstration facilities to be poor, altogether unsatisfactory for the instruction in surgery staged for the Army Medical School students.[14]

And so he prospected in the metropolitan area, searching for a suitable location for his hospital, if and when Congress could be persuaded to part with the funds. As the Army Medical Examining Board used the clinical case material available at the Barnes Hospital, U.S. Soldiers' Home, for examining candidates for Medical Corps commissions, he considered the advisability of a location proximal to Barnes Hospital. On the other hand, the northwest section of Washington was, as Major Reed had said, more exclusive. Therefore, in the course of his perigrinations the enthusiastic doctor considered the advisability of purchasing lands "fronting on Connecticut Avenue beyond Rock Creek bridge or elsewhere...."[15] In any case the idea of a new general hospital had caught firm hold, and he was desperately in earnest when pleading for an institution with professional facilities beyond the requirements of a post hospital, an institution staffed by personnel with clinical training exceeding the qualifications of the average doctor assigned to garrison duty.

Such an institution would, he believed, save personnel for the Army if a suitable place could be provided for the observation and careful examination of officers ordered before the retiring boards. Moreover, he was as fully convinced that general hospital administrators required training as he was that some special diagnostic apparatus and some medical and surgical procedures were peculiar to the military medical service. The lessons learned at such humiliating cost in the Spanish-American War were still vivid, and so he not only urged the advantage of hospital extension in time of war, but he proposed that the military attending surgeon for the city of Washington be attached to the institution as a visiting surgeon. This, he contended, insured the controlled treatment and final disposition of military personnel by Medical Officers. Cunningly, he pointed to the obvious economic advantage on the one hand, while on the other he noted that the added case load would broaden the clinical training of Army doctors.[16]

Dr. Borden's own experience with alleged administrative interference at Washington Barracks rankled, and he objected strongly to supervision by lay military commanders. And so as if to clinch the arguement for the defense, he used effectively and forcefully the principle of exclusive command of the general hospitals by medical officers reporting direct to the Surgeon General. Within these military medical cases, professional autonomy would be supreme. Many of the good doctor's associates believed him an idle dreamer, and some, perhaps, would have been openly critical had he not been known as the physician to Presidents. Others hinted that he was politically successful because he had known Cleveland,[17] and that having once X-rayed Teddy Roosevelt's knee[18] he had obtained the listening ear of politicians.

The Lively Dreamer

The Army Appropriation Act for 1903 brought the Hospital Corps closer identification with the Army as well as some changes in pay and grade. The titles of Steward and Acting Steward were replaced by Sergeant, first class, and Sergeant; the grade of Corporal was created for men showing leadership qualities but lacking the technical knowledge required to pass examinations to higher grades.

The Companies of Instruction were gradually gaining respectful recognition from other service branches, and the Medical Officers concerned with the training and management of men urged a standardized training program and revised drill regulations. Company No. 1 at Washington Barracks was by then something of a showpiece, and small smartly trained cadres frequently represented the Medical Department at public ceremonies, where the "numerous public exhibitions... excited considerable interest in Hospital Corps instruction and in the new field organization and equipment of the Medical Department."[19] The annual encampment of the Pennsylvania National Guard, held at Gettysburg, Pennsylvania, during the summer months, provided an excellent opportunity to test both the organization and equipment. Accompanied by three four-mule wagons carrying the equipment for a twelve-bed regimental hospital, the men usually made the eighty-six mile march from Washington in seven days.

A pack mule accompanied the entourage, primarily as a means of teaching the field medical soldier proficiency in packing,[20] but the two-horse ambulance served practical as well as demonstration purposes, for many untrained recruits became blister-casualties on the march. As a rule the eighteen miles from Washington to Rockville represented a one-day march, but on occasion the cadre made its first camp a little north of Fort Stevens, on the wooded ridges of the Norway tract,[21] part of which was then owned by the Shepherd family. By 1903, the summer demonstrations at Gettysburg were such a conspicuous success that Company No. 1 was sent as far afield as West Point, Kentucky (later Fort Knox, Kentucky), then to Fort Riley, Kansas, where it manned a Field Hospital and an Ambulance Company.[22] Securing the right number and the right kind of personnel was, however, an ever present problem, and scarcely a year later the proud company Commander bemoaned the fact that the quality of new recruits did not equal the opportunities and advantages afforded to members of the Hospital Corps.[23]

The Army War College was planned and organized in 1900 by the Secretary of War, Elihu Root, as a temporary substitute for the controversial General Staff then under study but not authorized until 1903. The college was scheduled for relocation from Jackson Place, in the heart of the city, to Washington Barracks.[24]

One of the Staff concepts provided for a four-year detail system for all staff officers, followed by duty with troops. This proposal met with opposition from firmly entrenched bureau heads who controlled national military policy under the old tenure system. The individualistic General Frederick C. Ainsworth, a one-time medical officer in charge of the Division of Records and Pensions in the Surgeon General's Office, had become sufficiently well known as an able administrator to be appointed as the Adjutant General, official record keeper for the Army. He was independent, autocratic[25] and influential with the Congress but so adroit a politician that this fact was not generally recognized.[26] General Ainsworth was decidedly anti-Staff, and he not only objected to but resisted all efforts to coordinate the activities and functions of his office with other War Department bureaus. Although his resistance to Staff authority and attempts to by-pass its organizational channels may have served as a blueprint for later generations of anti-Staff medical officers, he was otherwise an efficient and loyal officer. A model record keeper, General Ainsworth believed that the most minute and seemingly insignificant information should be recorded on the service record or descriptive list. As the instigator of modern personnel methods, he undoubtedly influenced administrators in other branches of the service to accept his system.

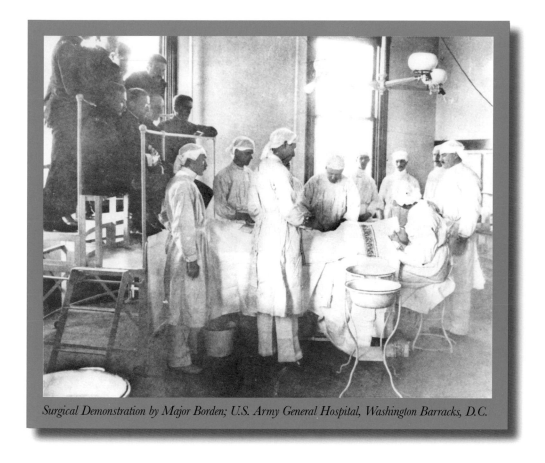

Surgical Demonstration by Major Borden; U.S. Army General Hospital, Washington Barracks, D.C.

Surgeon General Robert Maitland O'Reilly was not a spectacular successor to the professionally outstanding General Sternberg, but he was a conservative and agreeable man who endorsed sound policies. Any lack of aggressiveness was offset by his pleasant dignified manner and his quiet plodding along a course bounded by the Dodge Commission's recommendations and the enthusiasm of his young satellites for administrative innovations. Field medical officers were conscious of their lack of prestige with line officers, with whom seniority, rank and responsibility were nearly synonymous terms, and they were determined to overcome the military handicap which doctors, as technicians, met constantly in the highly organized caste system fostered by the Army.[27]

While General O'Reilly made an excellent impression on Congressional Committees, he would not personally lobby for special interest programs.[28] And so he detailed energetic young doctors to key office positions and held them responsible for the office management. The resourceful and aggressive Major Borden was offered the influential position of executive officer, but as his primary interest lay in the professional field he declined, saying he preferred being the "power behind the throne."[29] Although Borden had a personal career plan toward which he worked, there were a good many would-be powers in those days, and he soon found that he had a friendly rival in his alternate, Dr. Jefferson Randolph Kean, who was appointed executive officer and became one of General O'Reilly's principal advisers.

The two young doctors were opposite in type, temperament and interests. The suave and adroit Kean was already well known as a practical sanitarian and "trouble shooter" for the Department, but at this time he was intensely interested in establishing a personnel section in General O'Reilly's office, supervised by a doctor rather than the autocratic civilian Chief Clerk. Further, he disapproved of the allegedly patronage-ridden system of the National Guard and militia appointments and favored formation of an Officers' Reserve Corps which would guarantee a roster of professional men not only familiar with military medical problems but quickly available in time of war.[30] A great deal of Kean's recent service had been in the tropics, and he had come to believe that the medical officer made a better show of authority in effecting sanitary reforms when addressed by a military title, for "doctor" was a self-limiting functional term which restricted the holder to an advisory or service role.[31] Kean agreed heartily with Theodore Roosevelt's opinion that medical officers must "supplement in (their) calling the work of the surgeon with the work of the administrator."[32] It was during this period, therefore, that medical officers began abandoning their professional title, adopting, almost to the point of a fetish, the military form of address.

Captain Charles Lynch, Medical Corps, was assigned to the General Staff in 1904. Moreover, Major Kean was well known to William Howard Taft, who succeeded Elihu Root as Secretary of War in 1904, and he was therefore a politically formidable liaison between the Surgeon General's Office and the groping, struggling War Department General Staff. Further, since line officers had objected to granting to doctors rank above the grade of First Lieutenant, he was fully aware of the necessity of securing "military" i.e., line approval and support of medical service programs if the Medical Officer was to have recognition and prestige instead of sufferance. The plans for organizing the Army were under study, and *Borden's Dream*, an Army Medical Center incorporating a hospital, school, library and museum, did not then seem as important to him as actual military status. Well aware that General O'Reilly admired and trusted Dr. Borden's judgment, Kean not only left nothing to change but prepared

With much care and after consultation with (his) comrades, and especially with Major William C. Borden of whose shrewdness and good judgment the Surgeon General had a very high opinion, a formal document which (was) called the "Brief," which set forth the whole question of the personnel needs of the Medical Department.[33]

Several of the currently influential Medical Corps officers in and around Washington during that year had participated in the intervention in Cuba, including Major Merritte W. Ireland, endorsed by Kean as the first personnel officer of the newly created division. Ireland, like Kean, was personable, sociable and brilliant, and he collected a vast array of facts on the members of his Corps as he established the 201 files, or individual service records, of his brother officers. A man known for his phenomenally keen memory, he was likewise known for his loyalty to his supporters.[34]

The Medical Corps was not only small at this time but the individual abilities of its members were usually well known. Further, the standards for acceptability as fixed by the Army Medical Examining Boards were so high that only the hardiest academic and professional contenders received commissions. The grueling preliminary examinations posed by the Board in such general subjects as mathematics, history, geography, general literature, Latin grammar, Latin prose, English grammar, anatomy, physiology, chemistry, physics, materia medica and therapeutics and normal histology eliminated approximately eighty per cent of the candidates prior to examination in the clinical subjects. As a rule Army Medical School faculty members served as examiners in their special subjects. The faculty had deliberated for years over any advantages to be gained from fixing military rank *after* attendance at the School and in addition to the grades submitted by the Examining Boards but it was not until 1904 that the Surgeon General finally endorsed a change in policy.[35] The faculty changed in 1903, as the nucleus of the group of young officers destined to influence Medical Department policy for the next quarter of a century gradually began to gather in Washington. Majors Kean and Ireland, in the Surgeon General's Office, were politically the most important members of the group at this time, but Walter D. McCaw, James D. Glennan and the chemist, Carl R. Darnall, became staunch members of the faction later known affectionately as "The Ireland Gang." Darnall, as the junior faculty member and junior examiner, often acted as Secretary to the Examining Boards, and so it fell on him, "Old Wooden Face" as his contemporaries fondly called him, to announce the dismissal of unsuccessful candidates for Medical Corps Commission. "Doctor," the chemist would announce gravely, "the Board believes you should discontinue your examination at this time and return next year when you are better prepared."[36]

With Pen and Scalpel

One of the more awesome members of the 1903 faculty, and of course a member of the Examining Board, was the fiery Major William H. Arthur, detailed as Surgeon at Barnes Hospital, U.S. Soldiers' Home. Arthur not only resented Dr. Kean's popularity with Taft, but there seems to have been some professional competition with his surgical colleague at Washington Barracks, Dr. Borden, who, during the 1902–1903 session was "professor of military surgery, demonstrator in operations on the cadaver and in surgical clinics," but during 1903 and 1904, undertook instruction in X-ray work along with his duties as professor of military surgery. Arthur, the grenadier, whose exacting examinations in anatomy spelled defeat for more than one frightened young candidate for a commission, taught the "duties of Medical Officers" during 1904, and surprisingly the instructors noted "a few trifling lapses in deportment" among the dignified students.[37]

Deviations in behavior were not only practically unheard of prior to the Spanish-American war, but the caustic, letter-writing Arthur was a strict disciplinarian. While still only a Captain, he had reduced the number of cases of alcoholism at Vancouver Barracks by treating his patients as for acute poisoning, which after all it was. The treatment was simple but effective — either voluntary or enforced introduction of the stomach pump, followed by a bowl of hot beef broth weighted with cayenne pepper.

After an hour of rest, reported the intrepid doctor, the patient was "generally able, however unwilling, to do his duty."[38] This treatment was apparently reserved for the

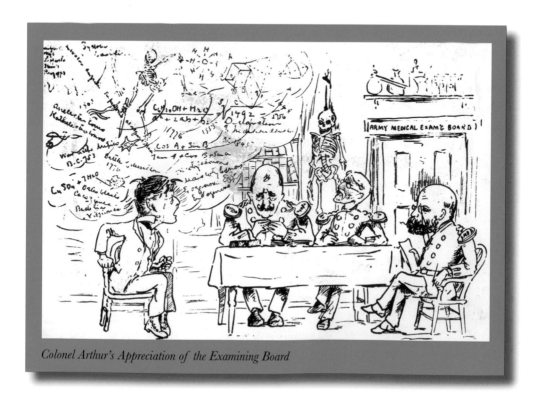

Colonel Arthur's Appreciation of the Examining Board

soldiers, but there is no reason to suppose that the plump, high-tempered, impulsive, fierce[39] major was less timorous in dealing with others. As commanding officer of the First Reserve Hospital, Manila, in 1902 he witnessed the Army's first strike by female nurses who objected to washing dishes on an officers' ward.[40] A man of strong convictions he completely disapproved of admitting the troublesome women to the disciplined military hierarchy.

As clever with pencil as with pen, Dr. Arthur amused himself and his contemporaries with timely sketches, and a popular depiction of a shivering young candidate facing the grim ordeal of the Army Examining Board had wide circulation through the Corps. As a hospital ship's surgeon during the Spanish-American War, he had had service in Cuban Waters; and well aware of the poor preparation of the militia for field duty, he caricatured Teddy Roosevelt as carrying a limp officer in his arms.[41] Indefatigable and fearless, Arthur the anatomist and surgeon took calculated risks which more timorous surgeons avoided, and in a ten-month period at Barnes, he operated on sixty-five old men, twenty-two of whom averaged more than seventy years. In reporting his exploits, in 1904 he advised his colleagues to be less conservative in attempting geriatric surgery.[42]

The Army Medical School admitted larger classes than before the war and Captain F.P. Reynolds, commanding officer of Company No. I, at the Barracks, reported enthusiastically that since the most important duties of medical officers came within the range of organization and administration, student officers should have rotating training in the various departments of a general hospital in order to learn intimately all of the management problems.[43] Dr. Borden was now urging the Surgeon General to support his plans for a large general hospital, and having decided that if the Surgeon General wouldn't set aggressively to secure his heart's desire he would take matters in his own hands, he openly sought Congressional funds. Then with his usual vigor, he began sketching his "dream," and when General O'Reilly returned from a vacation in Europe he found that Borden had completed a set of plans for a modified colonial hospital.[44] Each of these versatile young doctors exerted considerable influence on the Surgeon General and each pressed him for support. Borden had given Kean his best efforts when assisting with the "Brief," submitted to the Staff on December 26, 1903.[45] He was doubtless as discouraged as its author that neither the Reserve Corps nor the right and privileges of legal address by unqualified military title was granted until 1908. In the meantime, however, he pursued every advantage to secure his own project.

"Sketch plans are now in course of preparation for such a hospital, the establishment of which means so much to the Medical Department and the Army at large that it is hard to express the disappointment felt at failure to obtain the requisite appropriations from the last Congress,"[46] wrote its defender in 1903. The long planned construction work at Washington Barracks was well under way, with the War College and Engineer Schools planning to locate new buildings on the old hospital site.

The problem of adequate space was troubling Dr. Borden, busy in his dilapidated little hospital at Washington Barracks, where he admitted 542 cases during the year

1903 and performed "116 of the more important operations," forty-five of which were for various kinds of hernias and fourteen were appendectomies.[47] Nevertheless, he still found time to urge construction of a new hospital. In reemphasizing his opinion to the Surgeon General, he included a more telling argument than usual, for he estimated that as a result of the successful operations performed at Washington Barracks since September 8, 1898, thirty-one completely incapacitated officers were restored to active duty. According to Dr. Borden's fiscal juggling, the Government was thus saved an annual $60,000.00 in retired pay. Similarly, some 216 surgically treated enlisted men were restored to duty whose pensions would have equaled $28,000 annually. Thus the combined savings would, according to the enthusiastic Borden, cause a new and larger hospital to pay for itself many times over.[48] The Surgeon was fortunate in his official relationship with the Surgeon General, and in 1904 they collaborated on a section for W.W. Kean's fourth edition of the *American Textbook of Surgery*. The chances are that the senior officer, a man busy with official duties, accepted this credit without embarrassment, and that Dr. Borden did practically all of the actual work.

His close association with the Surgeon General may have accounted for the temerity with which he had Marsh and Peter, architects, develop the sketch plans; on the other hand, he may have hoped that the handsome watercolor drawing of the military medical post,[49] similar in style to the structures at Washington Barracks, would inspire confidence in the actualities of his undertaking. An improvement on the military hospitals of the day, the main building was designed to house seventy-five patients and was modern to the point of being lighted "...mainly by electricity." Cannily he proposed "that with a suitable place for locating the Library, and with the members of the medical profes-

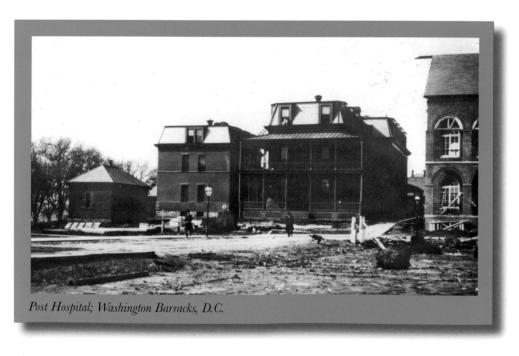

Post Hospital; Washington Barracks, D.C.

sion advocating it, a proper building (would) be erected" on the site.[50] His ideas were not slow aborning, and while he waited for his project to receive full approbation with both Congress and his colleagues, he prepared, in 1904, a classic summary of the vital responsibilities of the Medical Department to the Army as a whole. Familiarity with the technical limitations of untrained corpsmen and the military insufficiency of young doctors had impressed Dr. Borden with the necessity for training adequate to prepare officers to meet the myriad responsibilities of an understaffed and overworked department. Thus the individual as well as the Army must be mobile, versatile and willing. "A man who devotes his life to a military service," he wrote shortly after assisting Kean with his "Brief", "becomes a military specialist, in that he devotes his time and attention to so perfecting himself in knowledge relating to military matters that he can be an effective unit in that complex body known as the Army."[51]

Although not officially approved Congressional lobbying had its advantage, and so Dr. Borden haunted the Capitol during these years, discouraged but not relinquishing hope for financial support for the general hospital. Assistance came unexpectedly as a result of his professional interest in an aged Civil War amputee, doorkeeper of the Senate, whom he admitted as a patient in the hospital at the Barracks. The old soldier had suffered the effects of unskilled orthopedic surgery for more than forty years, and in gratitude for his surgical rehabilitation he confided to Major Borden the name of a senator known to be interested in District of Columbia real estate and whose Congressional proposals usually received favorable support.[52]

Primarily as a result of William Cline Borden's efforts, the bill laid before Congress in 1902 and again in 1905 was finally passed, and the Medical Department was authorized an appropriation of $100,000 to purchase ground and $200,000 for building a general hospital. Political life in the national capital must have been less strenuous in 1905 than in 1950, for official Washington served more tea and fewer cocktails. By chance, the Bordens were having an "at home" on the day public announcement of the Congressional appropriations for a general hospital was made. The shocked and incredulous disbelief of his professional colleagues, who had labored at their behind-the-scenes efforts for other measures, gave the party an air of tension which the amused Major Borden blandly ignored.[53]

The Secretary of War appointed a Board to select the site for the hospital, which must be near a railroad, have a streetcar facilities, water mains and sewers, be well drained and provide expansion for temporary pavilions in time of war. The Norway tract to the north of the city, facing the now finely macadamized Brightwood Avenue, cycling delight of the social set, answered all the requirements, including the interested Senator's approval. The metropolitan line of the Baltimore and Ohio Railroad passed within a quarter of a mile, in Takoma Park, "and on the west of Sixteenth Street (was) Rock Creek Park with its high ridges where temporary camps (could) be placed, if such (were) required."[54] Geographically, the 43$\frac{1}{2}$ acres purchased May 20, 1905 consisted of practically five elevations and part of the low ravine bounding Cameron's Creek.

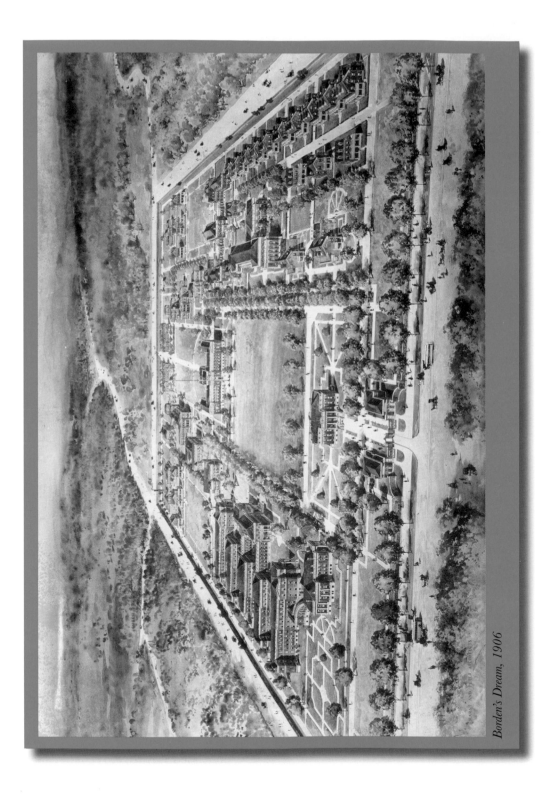

Borden's Dream, 1906

A professional controversy raged after Major Reed's death, as partisan adversaries defended the claims of the various participants to fame and the relative merits of "Finlay versus Reed, Reed versus Carroll, Agramonte and Lazear versus the others and, in a lesser way, Kissinger versus Moran."[55] In some instances public-spirited citizens had proposed that the Congress erect a national monument to the scientist, but no action was taken although the Washington parks bore mute testimonials to lesser men.

Only the Walter Reed Memorial Association[56] took an active interest in immortalizing the yellow fever episode, and within that group it was Kean, possessor of a detailed knowledge of the fact and access to the official records, who personally answered many of the letters which established indisputably Major Reed as the principal investigator responsible for this work. By 1906, *Borden's Dream* had assumed an identity of its own. The Walter Reed U.S. Army Hospital was no longer a nebulous plan, and although the Congress had not seen fit to immortalize the great scientist, Kean, the military surgeon, the sanitarian, the proud member of a proud profession, could visualize the great hospital of the future, and he believed it "a nobler monument than any which a sculptor could create in bronze or marble."[57]

References

1. Ltr from Florence A. Blanchfield, Col, ANC, to Hon. Margaret Chase Smith, M.C., 18 July 1945, SPMC 211 nurses.

2. Annual Report TSG... 1899, pg 20-25.

3. Annual Rpt... 1900, pg 25.

4. *Ibid*, 1899, pg 23.

5. Daniel L. Borden, *op cit*, pg 8; Major Wm. C. Borden, "The Walter Reed General Hospital," *The Military Surgeon*, Vol. 20, 1907, pg 20-35.

6. Annual Report... 1901, pg 39.

7. *Ibid*.

8. Annual Report... 1899, pg 52.

9. Annual Report... 1901, pg 62.

10. Annual Report... 1904, pg 127.

11. Wm. C. Borden, *op cit*, pg 29.

12. The equivalent was established by John Morgan, M.D. in 1776. The fund is two-stage: local in the respective hospitals, accumulated from unused diets and other sources, it is audited but non-appropriated; centrally, i.e., the Surgeon General's Office, from local surpluses and from hospitals that have closed. There are certain prescribed limitations on its use.

13.   Annual Rpt... 1902, pg 135.

14.   On May 6, 1775, Second Provisional Congress of Massachusetts Bay required a committee to examine prospective Surgeons; in 1814 Army Regulations provided that no candidate should thereafter be app. who had not received a diploma from a reputable school *or* exami-nation of an Army Medical Board; Act 30 June 1834 (4 Stat. 714) prescribed examinations for medical officers; Act of 23 April 1908 (35 Stat. 66) prescribed boards; unchanged by 4 June 1920 Amendment to Nat'l Def. Act of 3 June 1916. See George Albert Scheirer, *Chronological Table...* Med. Dept., U.S. Army 1755-1947, on file HD, SGO.

15.   Annual Report... 1902, pg 136.

16.   *Ibid*, pg 138.

17.   Interview with Brig. Gen. J.R. Kean, MC, Ret., Nov. 1946.

18.   Daniel L. Borden, *op cit*, pg 7.

19.   Annual Report... 1903, pg 35.

20.   Annual Report... 1902, pg 37.

21.   Interview with Lt. Col. Herbert H. Dean, MAC, Ret., April 12, 1950.

22.   Annual Report... 1903, pg 35.

23.   *Ibid*, 1904, pg 21.

24.   Otto L. Nelson, *National Security and the General Staff*, Washington, Inf. Journal Press, ca 1946, pg 79; The law authorizing the Staff was enacted Feb. 14, 1903, effective Aug. 15, 1903.

25.   Otto L. Nelson, *op cit*, pg 89.

26.   P.M. Ashburn, *A History of the Medical Department of the United States Army*, Boston and New York, Houghton-Mifflin, 1929, pg 213.

27.   Kean, April 17, 1950.

28.   *Ibid*.

29.   *Ibid*; Ltr from R.M. O'Reilly to "My dear Borden" written from Overbrook, Penna., 3 Sept. 1902, four days prior to assuming TSG, filed in W.C. Borden's Scrapbook.

30.   Kean, Nov. 1946.

31.   After 1908 Medical officer were no longer required to qualify their rank i.e. Major Surgeon etc.

32.   Address by President Theodore Roosevelt (11th Annual Meeting of Ass. of Mil. Surgeons *Jrn. of the Military Surgeon*, 1902, XI, pg 45.

33.   The Biography of Gen. J.R. Kean, MSS on file AML, Wash., D.C., pg 82.

34. Based on confidential interviews.

35. Annual Report... 1904, pg 13, 14.

36. Interview with Col. John Huggins, MC. Ret., April 20, 1950.

37. Annual Report... 1903, pg 12.

38. Annual Report... 1896, pg 43.

39. Interview with Col. James F. Hall, MC, Ret., April 17, 1950.

40. Annual Rpt... 1902, pg 144; "Nurses Refuse To Wash Dishes," clipping from Manila newspaper, Jan. 20, 1902. Folder 80 289, War Rec. Div., Nat'l Archives; Huggins, *op cit.*

41. Interview with Col. James D. Fife, M.C., Ret., May 26, 1950.

42. Annual Report... 1904, pg 116.

43. Minutes AMS, Oct. 22, 1903.

44. Kean, November 1946.

45. Kean, MSS, pg 82.

46. Annual Report... TSG, 1903, pg 125-126.

47. *Ibid*, pg 125.

48. Annual Report... 1903, pg 126.

49. Interview with Col. John Huggins, M.C., Ret., April 20, 1950. The drawing was so large it cost $30 to frame.

50. Major Wm. C. Borden, *op cit.*

51. W.C. Borden, M.D., *Relation of the Medical Department of the United States Army to the Profession.* Reprint from Medicine, Wm. A. Warren, publisher, Jan. 1904, pg. 4.

52. Daniel L. Borden, *op cit*, pg 9.

53. Annual Rpt... 1905, pg 146; *Med. Dept. of the U.S. Army in the World War*, Vol. V, "Military Hospitals in the United States," pg 273; Telephone conversation with Daniel L. Borden, M.D., 4 January 1951.

54. Maj. Wm. C. Borden, *op cit.*

55. Ltr from P.S. Hench, M.D. to the writer, April 16, 1951.

56. Walter D. McCaw, *Walter Reed a Memoir*, Washington, D.C., pub. by Walter Reed Memorial Ass., 1904.

57. Kean, MSS, *op cit*, pg 94.

Professional Training for Medical Personnel

1906–1912

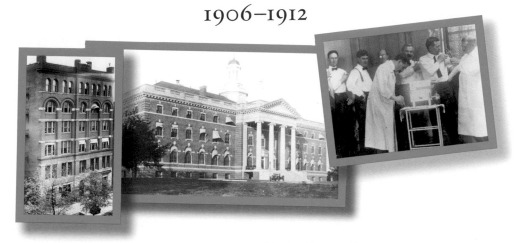

*"The man who thinks his whole
duty is done when he treats the sick is mistaken."[1]*

Life at Washington Barracks moved in its usual pleasant groove in 1906, and during the year 521 patients were admitted to the little hospital, sixty of whom underwent major surgical operations.[2] Venereal disease continued to lead as the principal cause of military hospital admission, discharge and non-effectives,[3] with the Infantry having the highest rate per organization and the Hospital Corps the lowest.[4] The latter small group was afflicted with manpower problems at this time, for under the three-year enlistment program about one third of the Corps was lost annually. The Surgeon General attributed the current lack of interest to ease in obtaining civilian employment "and the general prosperity of the working classes."[5] Nevertheless, the Army was becoming more stringent in its selection policies, with medical officers rather than the more lenient civilian doctors examining prospective recruits and screening those who might in time advance claims against the government for questionable line of duty defects.[6]

At Washington Barracks, Company "A" moved from its cramped and insanitary quarters in the lower end of the post to a frame building abandoned by the engineers, but the new comforts were short-lived, for on October 2, 1906 the personnel was assigned to constitute the complement for Field Hospital No. 2 of the Cuban Expeditionary Brigade. On October 4, the Acting Secretary of War authorized Company "C" as a replacement.[7] The old barracks buildings were due to be razed, and as Walter Reed U.S. Army General Hospital then was under construction, the Surgeon General proposed meeting the housing shortage with a new barracks and school building as part of the general hospital unit.

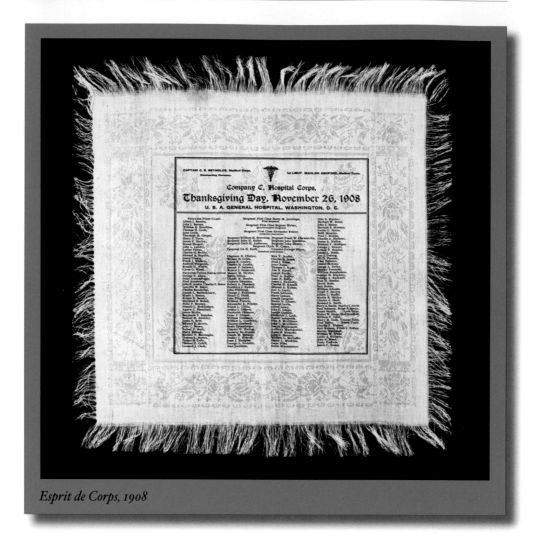

Esprit de Corps, 1908

Attractive accommodations for enlisted men, possibly as a means of offsetting discontent, were beginning to interest the Surgeon General by this time, and his meditations on the necessity for minimizing the difference in the material comforts afforded officers and enlisted men is one of the first faint indications of the philosophy of identification so evident in the findings proposed by the Doolittle Board after World War II. For, said the Surgeon General in relation to the proposed barracks construction of 1908,

> *It is now generally conceded by sanitarians that all plumbing fixtures should be open and exposed as freely as possible to light and air. Officers would not bathe nearly so frequently if they had to go down into a dark, damp and often cold cellar to take a bath, and enlisted men are much the same sort of animal.[8]*

Personnel shortages were not restricted to the Hospital Corps, for a year later the Medical Corps discovered there were not only many position vacancies for junior officers, but "no applications were received from the (young doctors from the) medical centers of the country...." The increased emphasis on use of Regular Army medical officers in the recruiting service, on examining and retiring boards and on the larger military posts was not only straining the personnel resources to the utmost, but hospitalization in general hospitals was becoming popular, a condition which created new requirements for experienced medical officers. This increased the cost of the hospitalization program somewhat, for in addition to equipping the hospitals and providing the staff "the government (was) put to considerable expense in transferring patients to general hospitals...."[9]

The Surgeon General, Kean and Ireland believed that passage of the Medical Department Reorganization Bill and an increase in the pay of doctors would solve the manpower shortage. Yet in spite of the active support of the President, Secretaries Root and Taft, the Chief of Staff and the General Staff, the bill still hung in the balance. In the meantime the Department found it necessary to employ a large number of civilian doctors "... men without military training, with but little knowledge of the special sanitary duties of medical officers in the field and whose professional efficiency (was) below that demanded of the commissioned medical officer."[10] As easy solution to the lack of interest in Medical Corps assignments, some blamed the existing of unfavorable legislation.[11]

The lack of interest in the military which always besets the Army following a war had not only set in, but the changed status of students decreased the number of applications for the course at the Army Medical School after 1900. In 1907 ten of the eleven student applicants completed the course. The faculty attempted to meet some of the academic problems by recommending modification of the preliminary and final examinations,[12] for it was well aware that "the Army Medical Service (had) lost much of its attraction for the bright young graduates from (the) best Medical Schools." Concurrently with the disinterest in military medical service the peacetime hospitalization requirements were increasing.

Major Borden was one of the better known military surgeons of his time, and the inpatient census at the U.S. Army General Hospital mounted steadily. Administration was burdensome, for the building was old and the struggle to keep the plant and utilities in adequate repair was recorded annually. Of the 395 patients admitted during 1907, sixty-one had major operations, a heavy case load, for the surgeon was a slow and methodical technician.[13] He was not too busy, however, to defend staunchly the economic advantages to the government of close observation of patients over a prolonged period.

Major Borden frequently represented the Surgeon General on inspection trips involving the construction and administration of both civilian and military hospitals,[14] and so he was, during this period, probably the best informed medical officer on the subject of hospital construction. Consequently he watched with interest the development of Walter Reed, on which he had lavished so much time and attention. He had not only "planned the Walter Reed Hospital, and was chiefly instrumental in getting through Congress the appropriation for it,"[15] noted Kean, the thoughtful recorder, but he hoped, with all the pride of accomplishment, actually to be the first commanding officer. He had, however, been stationed in Washington since 1898.[16] Under the four-year detail system he was not only some three years overdue for reassignment, but some of his contemporaries were jealous of his firm entrenchment with Congress,[17] afraid, perhaps, that he might become a contender for the Surgeon Generalcy. The newly organized person-

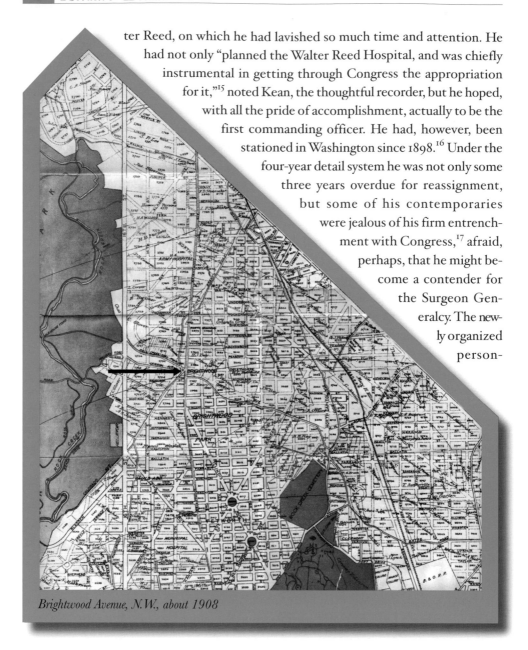

Brightwood Avenue, N.W., about 1908

nel division of that office was controlled by the astute Major Ireland, and, as the Surgeon General admitted, he was under considerable pressure from "the front office" to have Dr. Borden transferred.[18]

By War Department Special Orders No. 75, April 1, 1907, William Cline Borden was relieved from duty at Washington Barracks, scheduled, on expiration of his leave, to sail on the first available transport for the Philippines.[19] The *Washington Evening Star* paid tribute to his activity in the movement which resulted in Congressional appropriations for erection of a model military hospital "on a tract of land on the Brightwood Road due west from the Battle Cemetery. The officer of the Medical Department detailed to relieve Major Borden will have charge of the hospital when it is completed."[20]

The peace-loving Surgeon General O'Reilly, who respected Major Borden's "shrewdness and good judgment" and used his special abilities without stint, avoided unpleasant situations whenever possible. On the morning following public announcement of Borden's military transfer, the Surgeon General, who anticipated an explosive outburst from the forthright doctor, was, according to Mrs. O'Reilly, unable to attend to his official duties.[21] However, after due persuasion by some of his younger friends he appeared at the office as usual, offering to Major Borden, when he called, any other assignment than the Philippines.[22] Such consideration may have been due to friendship or perhaps to the fact that the doctor required expert dental attention[23] which may not have been available at a foreign station. With dignity and in the spirit of the true soldier, however, he refused a change of orders, sailing in the early autumn for the new station.[24]

Although not embittered over the circumstances which prevented him from actually commanding the new hospital, Major Borden was disheartened. He had served his Corps long and well under the peculiar requirements of the day. In the late summer of 1908 he was required to make the long return trip from Manila to Washington to meet the Examining Board for promotion to Lieutenant Colonel. During this ordeal he suffered a coronary attack and was immediately retired from the Army. He became, in May 1909, the month his brain-child, the Walter Reed U.S. Army Hospital, opened to patients, dean of the George Washington (Columbian College) Medical School.[25]

The Occupation

When Company "B" of the Hospital Corps returned from Cuba, the already crowded quarters at Washington Barracks proved inadequate to house both complements of men. As a means of meeting the overflow, in April 1909 Company "C" was temporarily sent into camp on the high ridge of the western extremity of the new hospital grounds.[26]

The permanent buildings then on the reservation included Building No. 2, a double set of sergeant's quarters, completed in April 1908, and the unoccupied Building No. 1, the Main or Administration building, completed in December of the same year. Both structures were of brick built on concrete foundations, with Georgia pine flooring with fireproof roofs, electric lighting, central heat and water and sewer connections.[27] Building No. 3, a second double set of sergeant's quarters was completed in March 1909, but to the tent-sheltered Company "C" roughing it on the ridge, these were domiciles of unknown luxury.

The standardization of medical supplies, usually an uninteresting subject to doctors until some defective product jeopardizes their techniques, first gained recognition through the efforts of the chemist, Major Carl R. Darnall (then professor of Chemistry and secretary of the new Army Medical School). Thus much of the early investigative program concerned laboratory experimentation and credit for the development

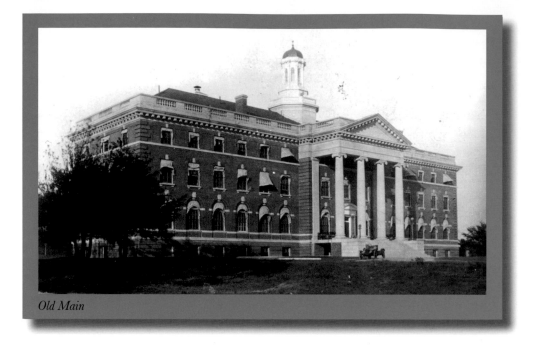

Old Main

of one of the Army's most efficient supply programs is rarely accorded the faculty of the Army Medical School. There were other things of importance besides drugs and hospital equipment, and rapid evacuation of the wounded was, like ready provisions of field supplies and equipment, a grave problem under combat conditions. Commercial development of steam-driven motors caused the Surgeon General to propose, in 1902, without subsequent favorable action by the Quartermaster, construction of a motor ambulance. Undiscouraged, in 1906, he recommended purchase of a steam-driven motor ambulance for experimental and testing purposes at Washington Barracks. Built by R. H. White of the White Sewing Machine Company, without expense to the government, the motor ambulance was used to supplement the escort wagons[28] in shifting equipment and supplies from the old hospital to the new in May 1909.

Building No. 4, the combined Storehouse, Quartermaster and Commissary; Building No. 5, a stable with capacity for thirty-two animals, and Building No. 6, a wagon shed and garage, with capacity for twelve horse-drawn vehicles and three automobiles, were completed in January 1910.[29] Lack of storage space resulted in the use of part of the old Lay Mansion, or Norway, at the southern end of the reservation, as a supply depot.[30] The remaining part of the building was occupied by Charley Anderson, a "handy" civilian employee and his family.

Building No. 7, the Hospital Corps barracks, with capacity for 200 men, was completed in March 1910. The plan of assigning a field hospital company to the station for training purposes and demonstration of field equipment for the Army Medical School students resulted in a shortage of housing fully as unsatisfactory as conditions at Washington Barracks had been. Within two years Building No. 7 was entirely inadequate, and the Surgeon General was complaining officially because part of the detachment was quartered in the attic of the hospital proper which "was not originally intended to be used as quarters and is but a makeshift." It was, he said, "excessively hot in summer and illy ventilated in winter,"[31] a circumstance personally subscribed to by later occupants, especially historians.

Buildings eight and nine, officers' quarters, built to accommodate "one captain and his household," were completed during the spring of 1910, and finally in August 1910, Building No. 10, a seventy-five foot iron flagstaff with concrete foundation, was erected in front of the Main Building.[32] This last addition gave to the small group of colonial buildings the distinctive air of a military reservation, and it provided fun for pranksters who took an especial delight in sending bemused new recruits in search of a presumably formal architectural structure.

The main building, originally planned with bed capacity for only sixty-five patients,[33] consisted of three floors. The first floor accommodated the Commanding Officer, the Adjutant, the Officer of the Day,[34] the Resident physician, Eye, Ear, and Throat, with no record of a "department for noses," space for a future Dental Surgeon, clerks, a laboratory, waiting room, dining room, reception room, a dark room for X-ray work, the Library, which consisted of a small collection of professional books in the custody of the First Sergeant, and the various laboratories. The second floor provided space for a women's ward, linen room, dining room, wards and convalescent wards and a nurse's office, although there was no nurse (prison ward was located in basement). The third floor was given over largely to the operating room, instrument, sterilizing and recovery rooms, wards and other rooms with the specialized nomenclature characteristic of a modern hospital.[35]

When the Reorganization Bill, with authority for the Medical Reserve Corps, finally passed on April 23, 1908, and Army pay was increased as of the pay bill, Act of May 11, 1908, a number of officers acknowledged the signs of prosperity by purchasing automobiles. The mysteries of the gasoline motor absorbed the thoughts of more than one Washingtonian, including the temperamental Lt. Colonel Arthur, whom the Surgeon General had detailed as Major Borden's successor at President Theodore Roosevelt's request.[36] One member of the Ambulance Company was an especially proficient driver and gave lessons to some of the doctors. When Colonel Arthur complained bitterly over his ineptness in managing his run-about, the supply officer proposed having the ambulance driver assist in securing his license. With his usual unpredictability, Colonel Arthur assumed that he had been asked to have a soldier impersonate an officer when applying for the license. Roaring and rumbling, he personally reported the circumstance to the Surgeon General, demanding that his supply officer be court-martialed for his attempt to defraud the Government.[37] Imperturbably, the Surgeon General sent him home to attend to more important professional affairs.

Colonel Arthur secured the license and learned to drive the run-about, which in those days he could park in front of Building No. 1 without fear of molestation from meddlesome military policemen. His sturdy little vehicle soon showed as much recalcitrant individuality as its owner. For on more than one occasion, as he cranked it vigorously, the little car got out of hand, and before being brought under control pursued the doctor as he fled down the slope toward Cameron's Creek.[38] Station assignment at the Walter Reed U.S. Army General Hospital was especially pleasant during the first two years. Opened in April 1909, there were then on duty five officers, sixty-two enlisted men of the Hospital Corps and four civilian employees. Of the four civilians one was the "handy" carpenter residing in the Lay House, one was the Post engineer, one a cook and the fourth was the hospital matron. Company "C" of the Hospital Corps, which occupied the barracks, had one officer and eighty-two enlisted men and constituted a "Field Hospital Unit." Although Company "C" was attached to the station primarily for the field medical training of Army Medical School students, it was fiscally supported from the hospital budget.[39]

Only five officers, eleven enlisted men, two retired enlisted men and one civilian had received treatment at the end of the first thirty-day accounting period. It was not a fixed policy of the Medical Department to send patients long distances for hospitalization, nor were travel funds available had the Surgeon General believed this a necessity. Medical officers assigned to station or Post hospitals had general training, were self-reliant and not only wanted but were expected to treat the sick. Under the circumstances, professional activities at Walter Reed were not too strenuous, and during the humid summer months the customary halfday tropical schedule was maintained. Some of the officers used the additional leisure time to good advantage, for the ravine crest made an excellent location for teeing-off golf balls; the ensuing scramble for recovery amidst the underbush of the ravine provided exercise of a special sort.[40]

Many of Washington's principal avenues were being named for the states, and by 1909 an irate Senator from Georgia, successful in his plea for "states' rights," suc-ceeded in having the historic Seventh Street Road, otherwise Brightwood Avenue, appropriately renamed. In spite of the transportation afforded by the direct streetcar line to the city, and Colonel Arthur's run-about, the Walter Reed reservation was still an isolated rural post.

Public officials in Washington were governed by rigid protocol. Leaving cards at the White House and at the home of the Secretary of War was a "must." These were the days when high-ranking Army officers were a curiosity; when Colonels were important, when good manners and good breeding were the characteristic rather than the afterthought. If medical officers in these early days of the century were selected for their cultural as well as professional background, their wives were no less important to their military careers. "At homes" were held on specified days, and white-gloved, parasol-equipped ladies arrived by carriage for afternoon tea and visiting. Mrs. Arthur was talented, agreeable and sociable, and she met her responsibilities to younger officers' wives with charm.[41]

How Times Have Changed!

There is some difference in the recorded statements concerning the bed-size of the new hospital. The original history, written in 1921, listed the number at sixty-five in 1909. The Surgeon General's Annual Report, based on the fiscal year, listed eighty beds, noting that places were available for women requiring hospital treatment or surgical operation.[42] As a professional institution Walter Reed was immediately successful and the building was hardly occupied before the Surgeon General, or possibly Colonel Arthur, proposed securing an additional eighteen acres of land to the west, thus providing an entrance on the-soon-to-be-extended Fourteenth Street. Purchase of additional acreage would not only provide high ground but would prevent the crowding of buildings in the northeast corner of the plot, making "it possible to keep out of sight from the main street the necessary administrative buildings such as stables, storehouses, power houses etc., and... allow spaces for a hospital garden, dairy and laundry."[43]

Concealing the presence of Building No. 5, a stable with accommodation for thirty-two animals was doubtless more than an aesthetic problem. Interestingly, by the fiscal accounting of 1911, there were 565 patients with the total expenditure listed at $27,381.79. Moreover, the animals were undoubtedly costlier in some respects than the patients, for even two years later the amount of monies expended for the purchase of non-issuable Medical Supplies totaled only $1,156.66, while Dr. Paul Halloran, the Post Quartermaster, paid out $3,875.04 to provide bran, hay, oats and straw[44] for the four-footed "beasties."

Sergeant Newport had moved from the Barracks to the hospital, occupying one of the double sets of stewards' quarters, enveloped nearly forty years later by the Eye Clinic. A sensitive as well as a forward-looking man, Sergeant Newport planted a catalpa tree outside his door in celebration of the birth of his son, Georgie. No doubt he deplored the proximity of the stables, and perhaps even the barracks. With all the spartan qualities of the responsible non-commissioned officer, pride in the conduct of the men of his organization caused him to regret extension of the streetcar line from Brightwood Village, for the one-mile walk to the Post tended to sober inebriated soldiers before they reached the Post[45] — and fell into Sergeant Newport's unsympathetic hands. This was, of course, a less strenuous way of sobering drunks than Arthur had employed at Vancouver Barracks in 1896, but there is no record to prove that the Colonel had mellowed to the point of evaluating a brisk walk in the fresh air as more effective than the stomach pump and cayenne pepper.

Sergeant Newport was not the only member of the command with homesteading instincts, and the hospital reservation was undergoing its first real landscaping. One hundred thirty-five Norway maples were planted; hedges were set along the entire length of Georgia Avenue and around the officers' and non-commissioned officers' quarters. Lawns were made, graded and drained; bushes and flowering shrubs were planted; roads were repaired and maintained; and five arc lights were replaced by fifteen incandescent street lamps. "Practically all of these improvements were effected by the labor of troops,"[46] reported the hospital commander. It is a small wonder, therefore, that the animals foraged more heavily or that the Troop Command may have tippled more lustily than usual, for both were working with unaccustomed vigor.

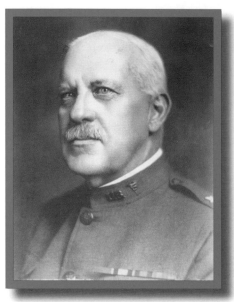

William H. Arthur, Commanding Officer, June 1, 1908–July 11, 1911

Enter: The Women!

Col. Arthur, like the other physicians of his day, took seriously the Florence Nightingale mandate on nurses: "Nurses are not 'medical men'," she wrote to Dr. W.G. Wylie in 1872. "On the contrary, the nurses are there, and solely there, to carry out the orders of the medical and surgical staff.... "[47] But wherever else they were, nurses were not at Walter Reed in 1909. Col. Arthur's mighty wrath over the 1902 strike in the Philippines had cooled somewhat, but he was still reluctant to accept female nurses, for, being women, they were not subject to the rough and ready military discipline.

Such was the intrepid doctor's influence on younger officers that many of them shared his skepticism and dislike, and even the nurses believed that he flatly refused to accept the distaff branch. According to the possibly embellished legend, Col. Arthur was standing by the elevator cage on the second floor of the hospital when the ten-dollar-a-month matron reported off duty. Fortunately or unfortunately, depending on the viewpoint, her suitcase fell open at his feet, disclosing an Army blanket, government property, being removed from the military reservation.[48] The horrible fact that civilian employees could or would purloin his supplies presumably brought a complete change of heart in regard to quasi-military female personnel. According to the Surgeon General's less colorful but doubtless more factual record, failure to have female nurses at Walter Reed was a simple case of logistics. A great deal of essential construction was necessary; funds were limited; quarters for nurses were not built until 1911.

Prior to the opening of the nurses' residence, on the main drive and facing the Commanding Officer's quarters, all newly appointed nurses in the Army Nurse Corps received preliminary orientation at the Presidio.[49] This was a costly arrangement, for some nurses made the long trip from the East only to be found unsuitable for military service. Others were disappointed and wanted to return home. The Superintendent of the Army Nurse Corps, aware of the uncertain military position of her charges, favored establishing an orientation course at Walter Reed, where all new appointees would come under her watchful eye for screening.[50] This was an important concession, and the preparation for receiving nurses at Walter Reed moved the conservative *American Journal of Nursing* to report:

The location is most attractive, with ample grounds and wooded hills in the distance, but easily accessible, being directly on a car line. The house is commodious, admiral in architecture, with open fire places and wide verandas.... It is hoped that all newly appointed nurses may spend a few months at Walter Reed Hospital, receiving there special instruction in the organization and discipline of military hospitals and the duties peculiar to the service of the Army Nurse Corps.[51]

Innocent of any irony, the Surgeon General's Annual Report for 1911 merely noted that "a building for quarters for nurses (Building No. 12) of the Army Nurse Corps to accommodate 20 nurses had been constructed and was ready for occupancy June 1, 1911."[52]

The stately Jane A. Delano was Superintendent of the Army Nurse Corps at the time. Of powerful influence in the young but rapidly enlarging national nursing organizations, Miss Delano was likewise a personal friend of Kean's and secured through his support many concessions favorable to the nurses.[53] Selecting the first Chief Nurse for so exacting a commander was not an easy matter, and the legend that surrounds Jane Molloy's assignment to Walter Reed is as ripe with colorful interpretation as Colonel Arthur's own story. A petite little person who, like many of her generation, studied nursing in order to be of service to humanity, Jane Molloy was in her quiet way an even match for the fiery Colonel. "I was chosen," she said emphatically, "because I could handle him." Reserved, dignified, well educated and cultured, Jane Molloy kept tight rein on the thirteen nurses remaining on duty at Walter Reed at the end of the year 1911, a number then adequate to meet institutional needs.

Acceptance of the women nurses marked a forward stride in the doctor-training program as the admission of female patients insured broader clinical resources. In spite of her special qualifications for managing recalcitrant Colonels, Jane Molloy had other problems to meet. It was still the era in nursing when many directors combined the characteristics of supervisor, Mother Superior and warden in the discharge of their obligations. And at Walter Reed more than one young nurse who too long lingered on the ward at the noon hour found the double doors to the nurses' dining room closed in her face [54] — or Miss Molloy grimly rocking on the front porch. Exacting in her requirements and particular of small details, some not only believed she was eccentric but that she failed to fight aggressively for the nurses. Detached and objective, she was refined, scholarly and progressive.[55] She preferred, therefore, woman's usual weapon — oblique strategy rather than outright defiance.

Marketing for the nurses' food service, or mess as it was called in those days, was a real problem, for the women found the heavy standardized military ration distasteful, preferring salads and other delicacies which the troops disdained. The Army ration had a cash value, raised from thirty to forty cents for the Army Nurse Corps of 1911, but even this increase did not ease the budgetary problem. It was some months before Miss Molloy learned to her chagrin that in exchanging surplus ration commodities with the Commissary Sergeant she invariably got the short end of the financial arrangement, the wily Sergeant crediting her with the cost of lower priced items and charging for the higher, the profit to be applied to improving the meals served his own personnel. Green groceries and delicacies were procured in the city, and with market basket on her arm the Chief Nurse made the long trip by street car several times each week. Afternoon tea and dainty cakes were provided for her tired charges whenever funds were available, but this was not a standing arrangement, for the "tea fund" accumulated only from ten cent fines imposed on young ladies reporting on duty with their petticoats hanging below their uniform skirt.[56]

The Army Nurse Corps uniform of the period consisted of a waist, belt and skirt of suitable white material, a bishop collar and white cap made to the Surgeon General's specifications. Their insignia consisted of a gold or gilt caduceus superimposed on the white enameled letters ANC. A government issue of women's clothing was unheard of, and the nurses considered themselves lucky to have their hospital uniforms laundered at government expense.

Miss Molloy had an insatiable taste, which she called an addiction, for *Blackstone's Commentaries* and foreign travel. The first she satisfied by reading and the

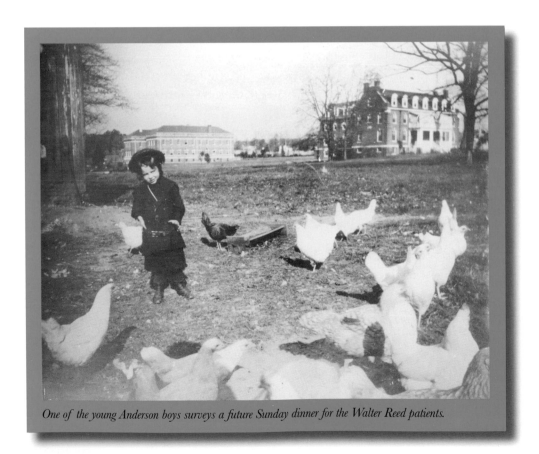

One of the young Anderson boys surveys a future Sunday dinner for the Walter Reed patients.

second by "long and frequent vacations." As individualistic as Colonel Arthur, a legendary story credits her with meeting inclement weather with fortitude. For, as the story goes, she negotiated the muddy path between the nurses' residence and the hospital wearing high-buttoned yellow shoes and a soldier's campaign hat.[57] It is more probably, however, that to this frail, detached,[58] blue-eyed little woman who "early came under Mohammedan influence"[59] has been credited the flash of gaily stockinged leg as some young charge climbed aboard the escort wagon which called for the nurses in bad weather. Without doubt the long trailing skirts of the day concealed many physical defects and the Medical Department established no regulations on either bootery or calf. Sedate and decorous as to outward appearances, the distaff branch compensated for their sober professional mien by wearing a garden-variety of pastel stockings.[60]

Ironically, the preparations for psychological warfare between the commanding officer and the first Chief Nurse were wasted. Like Doctor Borden, Walter Reed's second commander had served his day in the sacred shadow of the Capitol. The first nurses arrived on June 21, 1911; on July 11, Colonel Arthur began his final leave before reassignment in the Philippines. During the two-month interim prior to the arrival of his quiet and unimpressive successor,[61] Colonel Charles Richard, administrative affairs at the little hospital were apparently managed by the executive officer.

Any successor to the stentorian, irascible Arthur would seem colorless in comparison, for of the nineteen men who by accident or design commanded the U.S. Army General Hospital after 1898, Arthur was recalled with the greatest affection and uniformity of opinion as the one indomitable individualist. Richards was then fifty-seven years old and although his professional background was impeccable,[62] he had commanded nothing more spectacular than a hospital train during the brief war with Spain. Called a pleasant "old duffer" by some of his contemporaries[63] and irascible and cantankerous by others,[64] on the whole he was considered a good administrator and if not progressive he was at least not destructive. Small, quiet-appearing,[65] even "mousey,"[66] he was apparently an unexceptional surgeon but an able administrator as some considered him the "wheelhorse" of the Surgeon General's Office during World War I. As is often the case with quiet people, some mistakenly believed that he lacked interest in other people.[67]

His wife was inclined to be shy;[68] thus the combination of two quiet personalities resulted in criticism of the retiring[69] Richardses who "did not hold their end up."[70] Some of his associates considered the little doctor's unchanging manner a tribute to the solid standards of respectability characteristic of the medical officers of the "old school" type.[71] Small, neat and of unusual "military bearing" for a doctor, Colonel Richard was, surprisingly, a bit on the "saucy" side of good manners.[72] He not only swore energetically on occasion, but through the years he had acquired the reputation for having the best "vocabulary" of any doctor in the Corps,[73] a definition of *vocabulary* which students of semantics might deplore.

On Seventh Street South

The work of the Yellow Fever Board brought prestige as well as increased responsibilities to Army medical officers. By 1903, when Walter Reed hospital was opened to patients, Colonel W.C. Gorgas had been five years in Panama as sanitary officer for the canal project. Among his assistants, three, Lt. Colonel John L. Phillips, Major Charles F. Mason and Captain Robert E. Noble are of interest in the hospital story. Major J.R. Kean was again in Cuba as sanitary officer but exercising his usual judicious influence over corps affairs.[74]

Colonel Valery Havard was then completing his third year as president of the Army Medical School faculty. In 1904 he had prepared a paper for the *Military Surgeon* on venereal disease,[75] the ever-present plague of Army commanders. By 1909 he had written a textbook which applied "in a practical manner for military use the latest advances in preventive medicine and the results of the author's wide experience during thirty-eight years of service."[76] The photographic-minded Walter Drew McCaw had succeeded the more military Colonel Calvin DeWitt as librarian of the Army Medical Library in 1908, and would remain in that capacity for nine years. An intellectual and humorous man, he was an omnivorous reader but produced less original writing than might have been expected of one of his capabilities.[77]

Concurrently, Percy M. Ashburn was achieving modest recognition for preparing a manual in "an attractive style for nonprofessional readers." Charles F. Mason's revised edition of the *Handbook for the Hospital Corps* was off the press, and Charles Lynch, by then detailed as liaison to the American National Red Cross, was writing brochures on first-aid and relief work. Of two men destined to bring great professional distinction to the Army Medical School, little was said. Charles F. Craig, interested in Malta Fevers as early as 1904, was in 1909–1910 writing energetically on mosquito-borne fevers. Captain F.F. Russell, interested in anti-malarial work in 1904, was listed only as the School's professor of clinical microscopy and bacteriology, having succeeded the recently deceased James Carroll. He was, however, junior member of a Board of officers which recommended voluntary vaccination against typhoid fever.[78]

Captain Russell's scientific star was in the ascendancy, for in 1908 he was the Surgeon General's emissary in Europe to investigate the bacterial prophylaxis against typhoid fever in European services. The method proposed for the United States was primarily a modification of the earlier work of an English doctor, Sir Almroth E. Wright. Capt. Russell not only returned home with some of the European bacterial cultures, for the laboratory staff at the School to study, but the School began the manufacture of vaccine which "by February 1909, ...was ready for issue.... "[79] As in the case of many other untried therapeutic measures, there was no sudden stampede by applicants anxious for inoculation.[80]

H.P. Birmingham had a short tour of duty as Post Surgeon at Washington Barracks during these early years. Conscientious, determined and subscribing to high professional standards for his Corps, he let nothing interfere with the proper discharge of his "duty."[81]

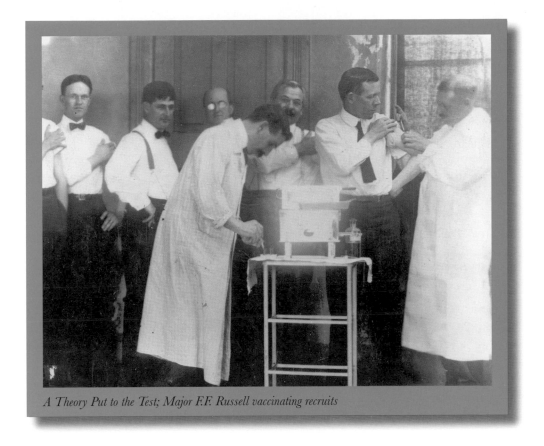

A Theory Put to the Test; Major F.F. Russell vaccinating recruits

In March and September, therefore, Russell not only immunized Majors Ireland and Kean but also the Ireland, Kean, and Birmingham wives and children,[82] for it seemed necessary to encourage the recruits with examples of innocent martyrdom. The entire class of the Army Medical School likewise faced the ordeal bravely, and by the end of the year the Surgeon General was able to report that 830 immunizations had been given.[83] Such is the effect of noble example that the director of the French Army Medical Service cited the fortitude of the American women and children as a stimulus to his officers.[84]

In 1910, the Army Medical School moved from its cramped quarters in the Library-Museum building to the six-storied building at 721 Thirteenth Street, known as the Builder's Exchange and later occupied by the Sloan auctioneers. The fourth floor was given over almost entirely to the bacteriological department, comfortably arranged so that sixty students could be instructed simultaneously rather than in sections as formerly. Captains Charles F. Craig and Henry J. Nichols assisted Major Russell with his work on the bacteriological and serum diagnosis of diseases, typhoid fever, dysentery, cholera and diphtheria receiving special attention.[85]

Russell's work with typhoid fever vaccine had placed the United States far ahead of other countries, and the Surgeon General was naturally anxious to apply the principle of immunization in order to reduce the non-effective rate from this cause. Major General Frederick C. Ainsworth was still the Adjutant General[86] and though usually rather sympathetic to Medical Department problems he considered it within his administrative province to oppose compulsory vaccination of the troops. He not only demanded a precedent from continental armies but withheld his consent on the grounds of expediency. As if to clinch the argument he voiced his own personal opinion that the anti-vivisectionists "would make a great row over it and the War Department would back down."[87] Under the approved general staff organization, the Adjutant General was the record keeper of the Army, not, as the Ainsworth interpretation would have it, the final voice of authority. A brother medical officer, Leonard Wood, was made Chief of Staff in 1910. When General Ainsworth attempted to usurp General Wood's military prerogatives, the resulting personal feud between the doctor-administrators reached proportions unparalleled in Medical Department history.[88]

In March 1911, at about the time the mortuary, Building No. 11, was being completed at Walter Reed, the War Department ordered mobilized at Fort Sam Houston, Texas, an Infantry Division and a brigade of Calvary. The Surgeon General was directed to assemble medical units to support this reinforced organization, called a "maneuver camp," but obviously intended for ready action against Mexico. Colonel Birmingham became the Division Surgeon,[89] and the forty-nine qualified Army Medical School students were graduated on March 20, two months earlier than usual, as the field work was considered of more value than the remaining weeks of formal instruction.[90] The Chief of Staff consented to vaccination of the entire military command, apparently prior to a request from the field commander, General Carter, for this measure. "In this way," said Kean, "the maneuver Division became a test on a large scale of typhoid vaccinations with only one unvaccinated teamster succumbing to typhoid."[91]

Colonel Arthur was still at Walter Reed during the early part of the year and mourning the fact that he could neither quarter all of his officers and men on the reservation nor provide a suitable recreation room for "an organization like the Field Hospital, which is largely composed of recruits." He found, however, that part of his problem melted away on March 9, when Company "C" of the Hospital Corps, three officers and ninety-nine enlisted men, with the impediments of Field Hospital Number 3 and Ambulance Company Number 3, departed for the south. The mobilization was short-lived and on April 17, 1911, the Secretary of War declared the emergency over. Company "C" was therefore reassigned, but not at Walter Reed.[92]

Some eight months after the Surgeon General proposed routine vaccination of all troops, as a part of the mobilization plan, and the Adjutant General aborted the decision, the matter was reopened. General Wood was known for his lack of partiality to the Medical Department,[93] but on October 7, 1911, all officers and men under forty-five were required by War Department order to be vaccinated.[94]

Studies on the epidemiology of typhoid fever had aroused interest in water purification, and in 1910 Major Darnall devised apparatus for purifying drinking water with chlorine gas, later improved for the use of liquid chlorine.[95] This was a public health measure of the greatest importance and like vaccinations and venereal disease control, of national rather than purely military significance.

Epidemics, alcohol and venereal disease were the medical officers' time-resistant and historic enemies. Troop education was practically the only means of controlling the non-effective rate for the latter causes, and these man-made problems created incalculable medical, military and social costs. Captain Henry Nichols is especially deserving of recognition, for through his work with yaws-infected rabbits brought from the Philippines he was the first physician in the United States to try a specific treatment for syphilis. While he was on a later trip to Europe, Erhlich not only encouraged him to go ahead with this work but presented him with the first "606" or salvarsan ever brought to the United States, thus enabling the laboratory instructors of the Army Medical School to proceed with this monumental research problem.[96]

The clinical investigation of syphilis was limited for lack of time in 1909, but in 1910, the Surgeon General issued a circular letter on the use of "606." The venereal disease studies were again pursued vigorously in 1911, with the cases for study secured from nearby garrisons and treated at Walter Reed.[97] Serology was receiving more careful attention, and because of the increased interest in tropical diseases, protozoology. An increasing amount of time was devoted to X-ray work,[98] and courses in ophthalmology and optometry were changed from the didactic to the practical.[99]

Subjoining the School and Hospital

Among the permanent commissioned personnel assigned to Walter Reed in 1912, there were: one Colonel; two Majors; two Captains and one First Lieutenant, with an additional Major carried on a detached service status. The small staff of School and hospital, and the limited amount of operating funds for each, encouraged continuation of the interchangeable professional assignments which had permitted the School to survive lean budgetary years. While hospital administrative problems were essentially local, and the School program was departmental, the two were complementary. Functionally, both involved the Hospital Corps, without which the Medical Service could not operate in peace or war. The caliber of the corpsmen then enlisting was believed to be no better and rarely as good as the average line recruit; the authorized manpower strength was insufficient; attrition was heavy. The Army had always attempted to find satisfactory psychological excuses to justify the citizens' basic dislike for regimented military service. Thus the Medical Department had felt justified in encouraging proportionately higher pay for corpsmen as compensation for performing unattractive hospital tasks. Nevertheless, the Surgeon General was still finding in 1912 that even monetary inducements could not keep manpower availability and effective strength apace of the requirements of a growing medical service.

The local situation at Walter Reed was a telling example. A peacetime detachment was necessary for maintenance of the buildings grounds and performance of minor admin-

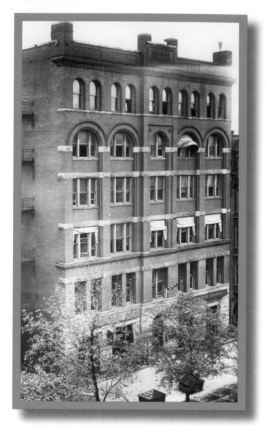

The Army Medical School, 721 Thirteenth Street, N.W., 1910

istrative duties. The plant was growing rapidly, and the inpatient census was increasing, with 687 patients admitted to the two services of medicine and surgery during the year.[100] Corpsmen were performing fewer nursing duties than at any time since the general hospital opened in 1898, for by the end of the calendar year seventeen graduate female nurses were on duty. Of this number one nurse served as chief and housekeeper; six each were assigned to the officers' ward and enlisted wards; three to the operating room and one as dietitian.[101] Still, the assignment of female nurses encouraged the admission of female patients and dependents, so by and large there was more to do. Whereas 122 more patients were admitted in 1912 than in 1911, the laboratory examinations increased by 6,271 procedures. The most noticeable increases concerned urinalyses, malaria, sputum and feces examinations, and all of these reflected the line of investigation being pursued so vigorously at the School.

In spite of the increase in patients, only two enlisted men were assigned to day ward nursing duty; three to night duty; four as Wardmaster; one to the operating room and one to the laboratory. When the Hospital Company moved from the unsuitable attic, over the operating room, to the modern new barracks formerly occupied by Field Hospital No. 3, all other possible conveniences and inducements were provided for the corpsmen. In spite of the physical comforts, the Hospital Company continued to be so depleted of men due to expiration of term of service, discharge by purchase etc.,

> *... as to make it difficult to properly care for the public animals, police and care for the grounds and attend to the various duties necessary for the proper up keep of a military post which this hospital, aside from the primary one for caring for the sick, essentially is.*

Metropolitan area patients were transferred to the hospital by automobile ambulances, whose general usage was then increasing, but there were few other signs that a mechanized era was dawning. Horse-drawn vehicles were used for post service functions — commissary deliveries, ice, the custodial work of buildings and grounds. As a result, animal maintenance was costly and the Post Quartermaster expended more for forage than for nonstandard medical supplies procurable by purchase.[102]

By Special Orders No. 156, War Department, July 3, 1912, Colonel Richard relieved Colonel Louis A. La Garde as instructor in military surgery at the Army Medical School. By Special Order No. 12, August 26, he succeeded him as Commandant. According to the official hospital record, the quiet little Doctor Richards, whom his contemporaries recall as a man of military bearing and colorful vocabulary, served at Walter Reed for a year and a day,[103] long enough to be the probable proponent of a recommendation regarding

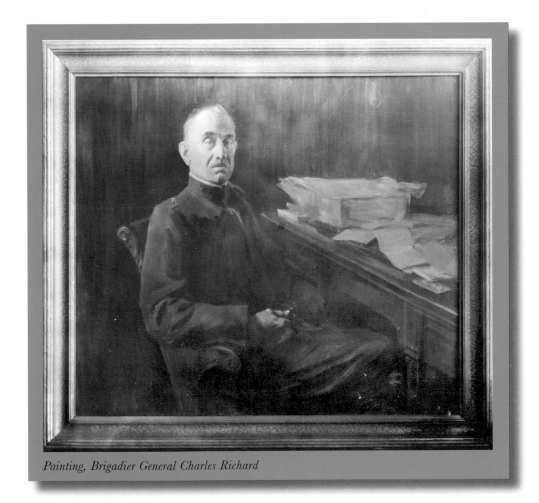

Painting, Brigadier General Charles Richard

> *... the desirability of building quarters at (the) hospital for the student officers in attendance at the Army Medical School, whereby they could be placed in a proper military environment at the beginning or formative period in their military careers at which time the inculcation of discipline and the forming of proper military habits is so essential. In addition they would have the advantage afforded in a medical and administrative way by this large hospital and all this could be done with a decided pecuniary saving to the government.[104]*

A quiet, thoughtful man, Colonel Richards undoubtedly figured the $8,680.00 annual rent expended for housing the Army Medical School could as well be applied to a capital investment.[105] He was three years at the Army Medical School, after which assignment he followed the course of so many of his predecessors, becoming commanding officer of the Division Hospital in Manila. With the versatility expected of the medical officers of his day, he subsequently served at the Medical Supply Depot, New York Port of Embarkation, and, as noted, during World War I, in the Surgeon General's Office, from which he retired November 10, 1918. In writing his obituary, following his death at the age of 86, *The Military Surgeon* noted that Charles Richards was "a gentle and courteous man of retiring disposition, who brought industry and high intelligence to every duty he was called upon to perform." [106]

References

1.   Editorial, *Military Surgeon*, February 1910, pg 375.

2.   Annual Rpt TSG... 1906, pg 120.

3.   *Ibid*, pg 38.

4.   *Ibid*, pg 21.

5.   *Ibid*, pg 116.

6.   *Ibid*, pg 118.

7.   *Ibid*, 1907, pg 125.

8.   *Ibid*, 1908, pg 62.

9.   *Ibid*, 1907, pg 119.

10. *Ibid*.

11. *Ibid*, pg 122.

12. *Ibid*, pg 121-123.

13. Ltr from Col. James D. Fife, M.C., Ret., to the writer, Jan. 11, 1951.

14. Scrapbook of Wm. Cline Borden, containing papers and records of his military service. Jan. 2, 1903 to NY; Aug. 19, 1903 to Ft. Bayard, N.M., & Presidio etc.

15. MSS of Brig. Gen. Jefferson R. Kean, pg 97; Ltr from acting AG, W.P. Hall, to Col. Clarence Edwards (cc) named Bd. of Officers, Oct. 12, 1903, composed of Edwards, Chf. Bureau of Insular Affairs; Borden for TSG; and Capt. Chancey B. Baker, QM, to ascertain a suitable location within DC but without committing U.S. either for final purchase or for any expense of option. Copy in Borden's Scrapbook.

16. *The Washington Evening Star*, April 4, 1907.

17. Interview with Col. Herbert N. Dean, MAC, Ret., April 12, 1950.

18. Interview with Daniel L. Borden, M.D., Jan. 7, 1951.

19. WD SO #75, Borden's Scrapbook. ("A True Copy").

20. *The Washington Evening Star*, *op cit*.

21. Interview with Brig. Gen. Albert G. Love, Ret., April 5, 1950.

22. Interview with Daniel L. Borden, Jan. 7, 1951.

23. Ltr Wm. Cline Borden, Maj. Surgeon to TSG, April 20, 1907. Copy in Borden's Scrapbook.

24. WD Spec. Orders #75, April 1, 1907. Copy in Borden's Scrapbook.

25. "Phillips Ousted as Medical Dean... Succeeded by Borden," *Washington Star*, Wednesday, May 19, 1909.

26. Annual Rpt... 1909, pg 130; interview with Maj. Gen. Robert U. Patterson, Ret., Aug. 24, 29, 1950, who accompanied the group as a Lieutenant.

27. *Med. Dept. of the U.S. Army in the World War*, Military Hospitals in the United States, Vol. V, pg 274; original manuscript, Hist. of WRGH, prep. In 1921, on file Library, WRAH.

28. SGO 3501 — Ambulance (Washington Barracks, D.C.) Correspondence 21 March 1902 (quoted) War Rec. Div., Nat'l Archives; See also 1904-1915.

29. WR MSS, *op cit*, pg 8, 9.

30. Interview with Col. John Huggins, MC., Ret., April 20, 1950.

31. Annual Rpt TSG... 1912, pg 156.

32. WR MSS, *op cit*, pg 13.

33. *Ibid*, pg 7.

34. The small room immediately to the right of the main entrance, presently used as a telegraph office.

35. *Ibid.*

36. Interview with Brig. Gen. Jefferson R. Kean, M.C., Ret., April 17, 1950.

37. Interview with Colonel John Huggins, M.C., Ret., April 20, 1950.

38. *Ibid.*

39. Med. Dept..., Vol. V, pg 277, 278.

40. Interview with Colonel James F. Hall, M.C., Ret., April 17, 1950; August 8, 1951.

41. Interviews with Miss Anne Halloran, April 19, 1950; Mrs. Mathew Reasoner, April 17, 1950; Mrs. M.W. Ireland, April 14, 1950.

42. Annual Rpt TSG... 1909, pg 140.

43. *Ibid.*

44. Annual Rpt WRGH, 1911, (cc).

45. Dean interview, *op cit.*

46. Annual Rpt TSG... 1912, pg 156.

47. Ltr frm Florence Nightingale to Dr. W.G. Wylie, representing the founders of Bellevue (School of Nursing) in 1872, and originally presented in the report of the committee on Hospitals of the NY State Charities Aid Association, Dec. 23, 1872.

48. Interviews with Col. James F. Hall, MC Ret., April 17, 1950; Col. John Huggins, M.C., Ret., April 20, 1950; Maj. Gen. Morrison C. Stayer, M.C., Ret., June 10, 1950. All of these officers were assigned to Walter Reed within the first year of operation; WR MSS, pg 20. Interview with Miss Jane Molloy, first CN,WRGH, June 30, 1950; Interview with Miss Dora Thompson, former Supt. ANC, June 26, 1950.

49. *American Jrn. of Nursing*, Vol. 12, 1911/12, pg 240.

50. Annual Rpt TSG... 1911, pg 172.

51. *American Jrn. of Nursing*, Vol. 11, 1910/11, pg 654.

52. Annual Rpt TSG... 1911.

53. See *Organized Nursing and the Army in Three Wars*, MSS on file HD, SGO.

54. Interview with Lt. Col. Jessie M. Braden, ANC Ret., June 26, 1950; Interview with Lt. Col. Ida W. Danielson, Chf. Nurse, WRAH, June 7, 1950.

55. Interview with First Lt. Florence Baily, ANC, Ret., June 25, 1950.

56. Braden interview, *op cit*; Molloy interview *op cit*.

57. Telephone conversation with Lt. Col. Nellie Close, ANC, Ret., June 1950.

58. Interview with Major Sara M. Schoenberger, ANC, Ret., June 26, 1950.

59. Molloy interview, *op cit*.

60. Interview with Lt. Col. Lydia M. Keener, ANC, Ret., former Chief Nurse, WRGH, June 28, 1950.

61. Halloran interview, *op cit*.

62. Obituary, "Charles Richard," *Military Surgeon*, Vol. 86, June 1940, pg 617.

63. Kean interview, April 17, 1950.

64. Conversation with Brig. Gen. George C. Callander, M.C., Ret., Feb. 22, 1951.

65. Interview with Maj. Gen. Morrison C. Stayer, M.C., Ret., June 10, 1950.

66. Interview with Colonel Mathew W. Phalen, M.C., Ret., April 19, 1950.

67. Interview with Brig. Gen. Frank Keefer, M.C., Ret., April 20, 1950.

68. Reasoner interview, *op cit*.

69. Interview with Colonel James D. Fife, M.C., Ret., May 26, 1950.

70. Reasoner interview, *op cit*.

71. Stayer interview, *op cit*.

72. Keefer interview, *op cit*.

73. Stayer intervier, *op cit*.

74. Biography of General J.R. Kean, MSS on file AML, Washington, D.C.

75. "The Value of Statistics in Connection with Venereal Diseases in the Army and Navy," (quoted) Edgar Erskine Hume, *A History of Our First Half Century*, 1891–1941, pub. by Ass. Military Surgeon, 1941, pg 39.

76. Annual Rpt TSG... 1909, pg 136; *Manual of Military Hygiene For the Military Services of the United States*.

77. Ltr H.W. Jones, M.C., Ret. to writer, Aug. 2, 1951.

78. S.O. #279, W.D. 1 Dec. 1908; G.O. #10, W.D. 21 Jan. 1909.

79. Ahsburn, *op cit*, pg 273.

80. Dean interview, *op cit*.

81. Based on interviews, see later chapter.

82. Kean, *op cit*, pg 124; Interview with Mrs. J.R. Kean.

83. Ashburn, *loc cit.*

84. Kean, *loc cit.*

85. Minutes... Fifteenth Session, AMS on file AMS, AMC; Annual Report... TSG, 1910, pg 132.

86. Known as Mil. Secy. from April 23, 1904 – March 2, 1907.

87. Kean, *op cit*, pg. 137.

88. Otto L. Nelson... Chp. IV, pg 73–184.

89. Kean, *op cit*, pg 140.

90. Minutes... Fifteenth Session, *op cit*.

91. Kean, *loc cit*.

92. Annual Rpt. WRGH, 1911.

93. Kean, *op cit*, pg 139; Ashburn, *op cit*, pg 249, 250.

94. Kean, *op cit*, pg 143.

95. Army Medical Bulletin No. 46, October 1938, pg 1, et seq.

96. Love interview, *op cit*.

97. Annual Rpt TSG... 1911, pg 160.

98. *Ibid*, 1912, pg 174.

99. *Ibid*, pg 184.

100. Annual Rpt WRGH, 1912.

101. Annual Rpt WRGH, 1912.

102. $2,688.42 for forage, oats and straw and $858.08 for nonstandard medicine; Annual Rpt WRGH, 1912.

103. Records of service dates provided by Historical Division, SGO.

104. Annual Rpt. WRGH, 1912.

105. Annual Rpt.... TSG, 1914, pg 177.

106. *Military Surgeon*, Vol. 86, June 1940, pg 617.

Normal Growth

1913–1916

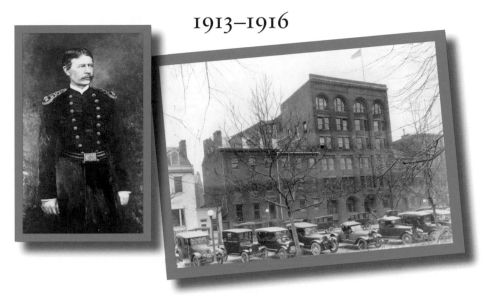

"It seems to me that too much time is given up to laboratory work in the School and not enough attention is paid to sanitary tactics." [1]

"The Old Soldier"

The years immediately prior to World War I were more significant for the number of commanding officers at Walter Reed than for additions to the physical plant. Colonel H.P. Birmingham returned from his southwestern assignment with the maneuver division to replace Colonel Richard, transferred to the Army Medical School. A fine figure of a man, veteran of the Indian Wars, he was called "The Old Soldier" by his friends.[2] Nervous, capable and exacting,[3] he was quick-tempered; like Colonel Richards, he punctuated his speech with sharp and colorful expletives.[4] An able administrator,[5] he tempered his military efficiency[6] with kindness, his discipline with wit.[7] Slender, of distinctive military bearing, well groomed to a dandified neatness, the pince-nez-equipped Birmingham could stare "the best of them" into an uncomfortable state of confusion, and few of the men called before him for infractions of discipline forgot his piercing blue eyes.

Sixteenth Street was as yet unopened, and within a few yards of Building No. 10, the flagpole, the hospital grounds were wooded and uncultivated as during the days of Jubal Early's encampment. As he was an enthusiastic horseman, the neat Colonel rode with his children in the surrounding areas of Silver Spring and Takoma Park. The Birmingham children were the only juvenile members of the command, and their year at Walter Reed was an all-too-short idyll. Cameron's Creek provided hideaways for book-loving youngsters escaping household chores. And in spite of fatherly admonitions, unavoidable homework was always postponed for the hour-long trip in the "glass wagon," the enclosed escort wagon which carried the little girls across town to the convent school. Happy and carefree, they had long since forgiven their stern parent for using them, somewhat unwillingly, as Major Russell's laboratory subjects. Conditioned as they were to his moods, "Father," in the seclusion of the home, was not an awesome figure, and they took especial delight in undermining his regal manners.

If his friends and contemporaries called Colonel Birmingham "The Old Soldier," with mixed affection and respect, the hospital corpsmen at Walter Reed, as subordinates invariably do, called him "the old man." One of the Birmingham children, unexpectedly hospitalized for appendicitis, overheard two of the corpsmen talking in the hall.

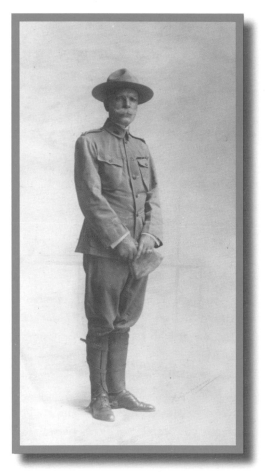

"Who you got in there?" said the first.

*"The old man's kid,"
said the other laconically.*

*"God pity them poor children,"
said the other piously, to
the later delight of all the
Birmingham clan.*[8]

Thus Colonel Birmingham, like Colonel Arthur, was a colorful character, and like his later successor, James D. Glennan, he was called a martinet.[9] To these three, one-time members of Army Examining Boards, perhaps more than to any other medical officers of their generation, is due credit for upholding the high admission standards of the

"The Old Soldier;" Col. H.P. Birmingham, 1914

Corps. Stony-hearted, Walter Reed had called some of the examineers on the 1902 Board,[10] for without hesitation or compunction they failed unlikely candidates for commission on the preliminary admission examinations. Because of his long experience, sound military background and excellent judgment, Colonel Birmingham was frequently used as a trouble-shooter for the Medical Department. And as a complete antithesis to this spartan and outspoken man, Sophy Burns, who succeeded Jane Molloy as Chief Nurse, was best known for her devotion to small details and to her church work.[11]

As early as 1778, venereally diseased officers were fined $10.00 and enlisted men $4.00, and *War Department Rules and Regulations*, published May 2, 1814 not only stopped their pay but deducted the price of all medicine used during treatment. As social concepts as well as therapy began to change, more responsibility for venereal disease instruction was placed on Army Commanders, as they were directly concerned with maintaining an effective troop strength. Consequently the Army Medical School investigative program, and the use of "606," were especially important to the health of the Army. In 1909 the Surgeon General issued a memorandum on the control of venereal disease,[12] and as a preventive medicine factor, the prophylactic "K" packet was first sold in the Post Exchanges.

Under the provisions of General Order No. 17, WD 1912, military pay was still mulcted[13] for known cases, a policy which may have contributed to its spread, for the average soldier could ill afford the deduction, and so many failed to report infections. In the Eastern Department, at least, the "K" packet was unpopular and the Surgeon General soon recommended distribution without cost — or that passes be restricted.[14] As the venereal disease investigative program was pursued vigorously during this period, after publication of SGO Circular No. 10, *Salversan*, some Army hospital staffs began control studies; the first such work was actually done at Walter Reed on a group of twenty carefully selected patients, with a report made in the "Boston Medical and Surgical Journal" in 1911.

There was little new construction at Walter Reed during 1913, except a Post Exchange opened on August 1, in the basement of the barracks; the Quartermaster's landscaping project[15] was one of the highlights of the year, for twenty-six Norway maples, twenty-eight American elms, nine white pines, twenty-eight

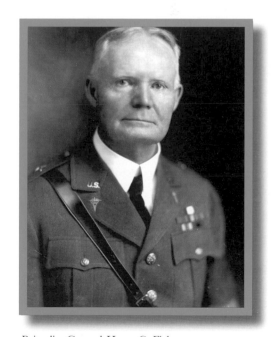

Brigadier General Henry C. Fisher

evergreens, two dogwood and one Japanese maple tree were planted. In addition to the gardener, the small Quartermaster Detachment included three teamsters, all Privates 1st Class; a boiler fireman and an overseer in charge of the stables. The Hospital Corps detachment was quite as representative of skills, for it included a printer, gardener, painter, trumpeter, elevator attendants, kitchen police, special dietitians and a night watchman. Moreover, there were, during 1913, only five of its members assigned to day and two to night nursing duty, one to the operating room, one to the laboratory and five as wardmasters.[16]

The Walter Reed detachment seemingly provided the necessary number of men for all the institutional requirements. Still, times were changing and by 1914 the Surgeon General was proposing a reorganization of the Corps in order to draw into it the men of intelligence necessary to perform the specialized duties of "anesthetists, pharmacists, surgical, laboratory and sanitary assistants." Discouraged over the general manpower situation, he expressed the opinion that men nurses and cooks could get better pay and hours outside the Army.[17]

Business As Usual

The slow physical growth of the institution was neither accelerated nor retarded during Colonel Birmingham's short tenure. Building No. 13, a twelve-bed isolation hospital, familiarly called *The Pest House*,[18] was opened November 13, 1913, only three months after Colonel Henry C. ("Pinky") Fisher assumed command. The new hospital commander made no change in the organization of the professional services, still divided into the broad classes of medicine and surgery, nor did the fact that eighty-one, or approximately ten per cent, of the 817 admissions during 1913 were for injuries stir him to comment. In preparing the *Annual Report* for that year, the need for proper Post housing for the Army Medical School students was reaffirmed, and he noted that "a satisfactory start has been made toward the establishment of a general hospital that shall be a credit to the Army. The work should be continued along the plans already made." [19]

"Pinky" Fisher was a quiet and ultra-conservative man, as a result of which some of his associates considered him indecisive as well as unimpressive. He rarely antagonized anyone, which was certainly to his credit, seldom refused a reasonable request and since these characteristics were contrary to the traditional concept of a military man as a fire-breathing grenadier, some believed he made many of his decisions by default.[20] As he was shy and withdrawn, others among his contemporaries credited him with a meager knowledge of medicine.[21] In contrast, some who knew him well objected violently[22] to allegations that he was "mousey" and unspectacular.[23] Nor would they concede that because he was hard-working, although apparently without imagination or haste, he lacked leadership.[24] Perhaps the very fact that he worked without unseemly haste, adhered strictly to Army regulations[25] and made no demands for a prima donna role retained him in the good graces of some of the most influential men in the corps.[26] At any rate, regardless of varying appraisals of his personality, his service record was excellent, he was held in high esteem and appears to have led an exemplary life as soldier. In May 1914 he was transferred from Walter Reed for a three-year tour of duty in the Surgeon General's Office.

Enigmatic and self-contained, "Pinky" Fisher had married late in life, choosing a congenial companion of similar type. Socially, little was seen of the Fisher family, for they did not encourage the trivial social activities so necessary for entertainment at the isolated military stations.[27] Further, the Colonel refused to attend formal dances, allegedly because he objected to having other men's arms around his wife.[28] Regardless of their temperamental preference for seclusion, the Fishers always had satisfactory military medical assignments, especially the coveted, and in "Pinky's" case prolonged, detail as Chief Health office in Panama. Later, from July 1, 1925 until October 5, 1929, as a Brigadier General, he served as Commandant of the Army Medical Center, the third officer in the institutional lineage to fill the role of both hospital commander and dominie.[29] Again, he progressed to the Surgeon General's Office, where he served with distinction as Assistant Surgeon General in the closing years of the Ireland administration.

Old-timers delight in recounting an episode from the Fishers' post-military life. As the General was born in Montgomery County, Maryland, graduated with the class of '86, Central High School, Washington, D.C.,[30] and having received in turn the AM and MD degrees from George Washington University, it was only natural that he choose to retire in the familiar surroundings. Thus he selected for his homesite a high lot in Arlington Heights, Virginia, a plot owned by the congregation of a Negro church. No other location was acceptable. Strong in his determined isolation, he finally succeeded in purchasing the location, in spite of protests from the noisy church-goers. There he retired in splendor in a two-story house which, although it was none of their business, his friends believed too large and too pretentious for elderly unsociable people. Unfortunately the land venture did not include an option on the surrounding lots in this then unrestricted and nearly rural area. Without difficulty, it seems, the congregation relocated in close proximity to the Fisher mansion, where its hearty hymn-singing plagued the remaining years of this "...quiet, Christian gentleman (who was) very efficient." [31]

Additions and Subtractions

Ward "A," the west wing of Building No. 1, consisting of a basement recreation room and a first floor ward, was ready for occupancy by April 6, 1914.[32] Completed on December 14, 1914, the kitchen and mess, added to the north side of the Main Building, not only provided much-needed additional space but eliminated some of the odors of cookery from the hospital proper. A year later, when the new concrete roadway was completed in this area, the servicing of wagons was both easier and cleaner. Moreover, the roadway diverted much surface drainage that formerly washed directly toward and partly through the basement.[33] A hydrotherapeutic plant was opened in 1914, with the treatments given by Hospital Corpsmen receiving extra duty pay from the Hospital Fund rather than the government. The term insanity was becoming less popular as a specific diagnosis than heretofore, and on January 1, the Surgeon General invoked a change in medical nomenclature. Mental alienation[34] was a sufficiently broad diagnosis to cover such conditions as mental defectiveness, constitutional psychopathic state, hypochondriasis and nostalgia. When Ward "B," counterpart of Ward "A," was opened May 8, 1915 and attached to the eastern end of the Main Building, it provided two rooms for housing insane patients and two rooms for cooks, not that there was any correlation between affliction and occupation. The insane wards were much needed, for of the 1175 patients admitted to Walter Reed in 1915, 44.7 per cent of the enlisted men and 24 per cent of the officers were diagnosed as mental cases.[35]

An enlargement to the nurses' residence was completed in April 1915, providing space for six additional nurses. The attendance of female nurses was becoming increasingly important, for "…In keeping with modern tendencies, specialization (had) developed…."[36] This tendency was viewed with considerable alarm by Dr. Fielding H. Garrison, successor to Dr. Robert Fletcher as editor of the Surgeon General's great Index-Catalogue. Dr. Garrison, with his ready purview of the world, was concerned because *The Journal of the American Medical Association*, whose editor had once told him it was designed to meet the needs of the country practitioner, had become so "splendidly scientific" that this group was becoming estranged.[37] The Medical Department, Dr. Garrison included, viewed the trend toward specialization in terms of physicians' services, but it was destined to affect the collateral branch fully as much. Of the total inpatient census, 15 per cent were women requiring medical care and 15 per cent were women requiring surgical care. No females were then admitted to Walter Reed for mental or venereal disease, recognized afflictions of the troops, nor did this hospital's "nearness and convenience to a metropolis and the monotony of sickness make for derelictions in the way of drink (as) by too many Hospital Corpsmen and (male) patients." Although female patients showed marked sobriety, forty-eight required professional attention of a type peculiar to women, for the surgical staff performed forty-four gynecological operations and delivered four infants.[38]

The aggregate cost of general administration per diem, per patient, in 1915, exclusive of subsistence, was $4.06, with a total cost of $138,243.77 for the year. There were other unaccounted costs, however, such as the extra pay for the hydrotherapist met from the Detachment fund, and the pay of maids working on the women's wards. Such costs troubled the commanding officer, for he objected to subsidizing the incumbents in these positions from the special welfare fund.[39]

There appears to have been no general shortage of trained nurses at this time, for the Surgeon General reported more applications for Army Nurse Corps assignments than vacancies.[40] The hospital was still so small at this time that nursing duties could hardly have been as arduous as described. Still, in times of stress, there was an insufficient general allotment of nurses to provide for their own sickness and for their leaves of absence. Moreover, as the units mobilizing on the Mexican Border required nurses with military experience, five of the Regular Army nurses at Walter Reed were replaced by five contract nurses, the first non-military or strictly civilian nurses to be assigned since the "matron" was dropped from the personnel roles.[41]

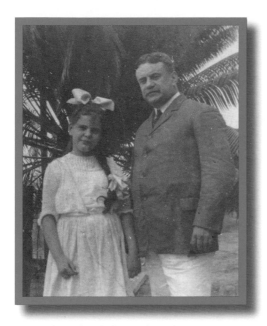

Colonel John L. Phillips and daughter, Frances; Panama, about 1912

"Go West, Young Man"

William Crawford Gorgas, by then an international expert on sanitation because of his position as Chief Sanitary Office of the Panama Canal project, became Surgeon General on January 16, 1914. On April 24, he telegraphed his former Assistant Chief Sanitary Officer,[42] and one-time manager of Ancon Hospital, Colonel John L. Phillips, and offered him the detail as Chief Surgeon, base line of communications,[43] an excellent position in case of war. This potentially excellent position was refused as Phillips preferred to command Walter Reed, where he reported as "Pinky" Fisher's relief on May 12.

Born in Chapel Hill, North Carolina on April 1, 1859, Colonel Phillips attended the University of North Carolina for two years and the University of Virginia for one year. In 1882 he received his medical diploma from the College of Physicians and Surgeons, New York. The chairman of his faculty had attested to the fact that young Phillips was diligent, studious and made the best use of his time.[44] Son of the Solicitor General of the United States, on October 29, 1883, he applied to Robert Todd Lincoln, Secretary of War, for appointment as Assistant Surgeon in the U.S. Army, stating both his family and academic credentials. The preliminary appointment procedures were apparently handled without undue bureaucratic delay, and by November 19, 1883, the young doctor was subscribing to the usual oath whereby prospective officers declared themselves to be mentally and physically sound.[45] In accordance with established Medical Department policy he was sent west for his first station, the detail to include two four-year assignments followed by a two-year assignment in the East.[46]

Six years later rather than eight, his father requested the Secretary of War, Redfield Proctor, to have his son reassigned to Governor's Island, New York, stating that the President had given his permission.[47] The letter followed the customary course through the interested divisions and to the Surgeon General's Office. On January 15, 1890, Surgeon General John Moore declined to make any reassignments which would penalize other officers.[48] Nevertheless, young Phillips was relocated from Camp Crawford, Colorado, to the Oklahoma Territory in November 1890, and although he requested service at the front during the Spanish-American War, he was first ordered from Walla Walla, Washington, to Alcatraz Island, California, for post duty, before the order was amended and he was sent east to Camp Alger, Falls Church, Virginia, and thence to Greenville, North Carolina, as Chief Surgeon of the 2nd Division, 2nd Army Corps.[49]

While John L. Phillips was apparently not one of the small group of Ireland intimates, nor had he earned a distinguished place[50] among the pioneer scientists of the Army Medical School, he filled one of the most useful and probably satisfactory roles permitted the peacetime Army doctor — that of post surgeon and thereby the family physician. By November 1902, less than a year before Lt. General A.R. Chaffee was sent to Washington as understudy for the position of Chief of Staff,[51] he requested that Captain Phillips be assigned as attending Surgeon at Governor's Island, New York, as he had charge of Mrs. Chaffee's case.[52]

A large rather heavy-set man,[53] strangers thought the quiet-appearing Army doctor shy and[54] somewhat melancholy.[55] Intimates, and especially some friends of his young daughter, recalled him as kindly, gentle and humorous but a lonely man.[56] He reported for duty at Walter Reed on May 12, 1914, but on January 15, 1915 he suffered a severe attack of gout, accompanied by renal complications. By February 2, 1915, he was undergoing treatment at the Army and Navy General Hospital, the Medical Department's special hospital for rheumatic diseases. His prognosis for a permanent cure was considered unfavorable.[57] He did, however, return to duty at Walter Reed on April 7, 1915, although far from well. During the evening of September 18, Colonel Phillips fell from the second floor elevator shaft at Walter Reed,[58] incurring several fractured ribs, severe contusions on the right side of the trunk and pelvis and, more serious, a fractured kidney. As an interim measure, the Chief of the Medical Service and Executive Officer, Major Percy M. Ashburn, assumed command of the hospital. The renal complications undoubtedly retarded the general recovery, and as he was still unwell after a four-month sick leave, Colonel Phillips was carried as sick in quarters for an additional six weeks.

All of the officers who served on the Panama Canal project were presumed to have undergone grueling experiences, and so in order to compensate them properly for their sacrifices, the Congress passed a law permitting voluntary and discretionary retirement in a grade higher than their Regular Army grade.[59] This privilege could have been Colonel Phillips' had he so desired. Instead he died unexpectedly on May 22, 1916, during a solitary walk along Cameron's Creek.

The chain of command now took a sudden dip toward youth, for Ashburn, the interim commander, became commanding officer in fact, the first and only time in the history of the hospital that a major held the post on permanent assignment. Quiet, introverted and scholarly,[60] he was especially interested in tropical diseases. However able in his own field, he was not acknowledged by Army men as the "command" type. A versatile and prolific writer on military medical topics, he became, by some strange anomaly[61] of circumstance, the first commandant of the Medical Field Service School, opened at Carlisle, Pennsylvania, in 1920, when the field training program was separated from the clinical.[62]

The hospital, including the new basement wards, had a capacity of approximately 180 beds by 1916, with an additional seventeen beds in the isolation building. Moreover, in case of emergency, at least one hundred patients could be housed temporarily in the detachment barracks. The number of patient days increased by twenty-three per cent during the year, making the accommodations for officers, women and others on officer status inadequate. As a result of the frequent shifting of patients, the hospital commander noted both discomfort and dissatisfaction.

There were other causes for complaint, for of the eleven Medical Officers and two Dental Officers then on duty two families had quarters on the Post. Among the utilitarian services the stables needed concrete flooring for easier cleaning and to prevent fly breeding. The unsightly coal sheds, a source of complaint for many years, were in need of repair or replacement. A proper entrance was needed on Georgia Avenue with a waiting pavilion for streetcar passengers. The hospital grounds needed grading, draining and the roads surfacing. In spite of minor administrative inadequacies listed by the commanding officer of the hospital, Army personnel were becoming increasingly confident that the professional staff was one of the best in the East. Consequently the hospital was becoming something of a popular resort, and military patients spoke with pride of having been "out to Walter Reed."

Perhaps the strain of urban life or the prospect of a war began to tell on Army wives about this time, or the pleasant prospect of having a safe place to restrain them encouraged busy husbands, but whatever the cause, 19.2 per cent of the fifty mental cases admitted in 1916 were women. Of the remaining members, 22.4 per cent were officers; 32.5 per cent were enlisted men and 32.2 were male civilians.[63] Wards "A" and "B" were already too small and two-storied additions were being considered.

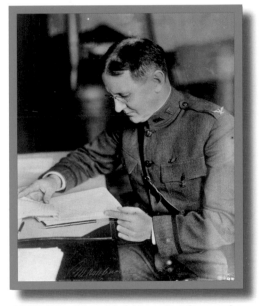

1915, Colonel Percy M. Ashburn; Post Commander, September 19, 1915 – October 5, 1916

There had been, since August 1913, commanding officers, and among the nurses changes were more frequent than otherwise, for many stayed at Walter Reed only long enough to receive a general sort of orientation training. Miss Estelle Hine, one of the first three nurses reporting to Walter Reed on June 21, 1911, returned on May 23, 1914 as Chief Nurse. Tall, angular and a strict disciplinarian, she managed the nurses' mess economically by reducing the food servings. According to her hungry charges even the mantel clock protested the sparse meals and instead of striking, pled in a tired and hungry voice for "coffee-coffee-coffee."[64] Handsome, quiet and meticulous, Miss Hine was considered a superior nurse. She was quite artistic; as she had some knowledge of interior decorating she was frequently sent to new Posts to open quarters for the nurses.[65] Like others, her stay at Walter Reed was short. Elizabeth Reid, her successor, was a large, stern and unimaginative woman.[66] The complete antithesis of Miss Hine, she had a taste for delicate cuisine and was herself an excellent cook. A splendid executive and strict disciplinarian, she held her subordinates accountable for any infractions of the rules.[67] Fortunately she held no grudges and attempted no reprisals.[68]

The Surgeon General sent military medical observers to Europe as early as 1914, for the Balkan Wars were exciting new interest in mobilization planning. Under authority of the National Defense Act of 1916, Colonel Kean was assigned as Director General of Military Relief for the American National Red Cross and began at once to assemble mobile hospital units for overseas shipment, as assistance to beleaguered countries. In the event of American participation the units would be on hand, ready for use. As the War Department was not in an active state of preparedness, this was the best effort which some military medical planners could devise for meeting an unexpected emergency. Miss Delano had resigned from the Army Nurse Corps in 1912 to devote her life to Red Cross work. As part of her nursing she had listed a roster of reserve nurses willing to serve with the Armed Forces in time of war. And so, as during her assignment as the Superintendent of the Army Nurse Corps, she was again associated with her old friend, Colonel Kean. She was interested in principles rather than politics, but these two were in complete agreement on health and medical policies, and together they made a formidable team in upholding standards for Medical Department nursing personnel.

While international events were accumulating with the rapidity of storm clouds, personnel problems were besetting Major Ashburn, who had begun to feel the administrative pinch of trying to maintain business as usual, but with a fluid staff. As if it were not trial enough to have the doctors and nurses changing rapidly, he encountered personnel problems in the enlisted detachment for "the character of recruits received during the year was below normal; many are very young and irresponsible, others are hard drinkers, and still others (seemed) incorrigible."[69]

There were few permanent changes or additions to the institution during this last pre-war period. The controversy over credit for the work of the Yellow Fever Commission had subsided, but the Congress had not yet authorized a suitable memorial.

General Gorgas had ordered a posthumous portrait of the scientist Reed, to grace the foyer of the hospital,[70] for which the artist, selected by Mrs. Reed, was charging $550.00, including the frame.[71] A Major Crosby P. Miller of the Quartermaster Corps served as stand-in, and the features were painted from old photographs. The artist believed Mrs. Reed, her daughter and "others" approved the work and informed the Surgeon General that she was "proud and highly pleased to have been able to succeed in obtaining such a perfect likeness...."[72]

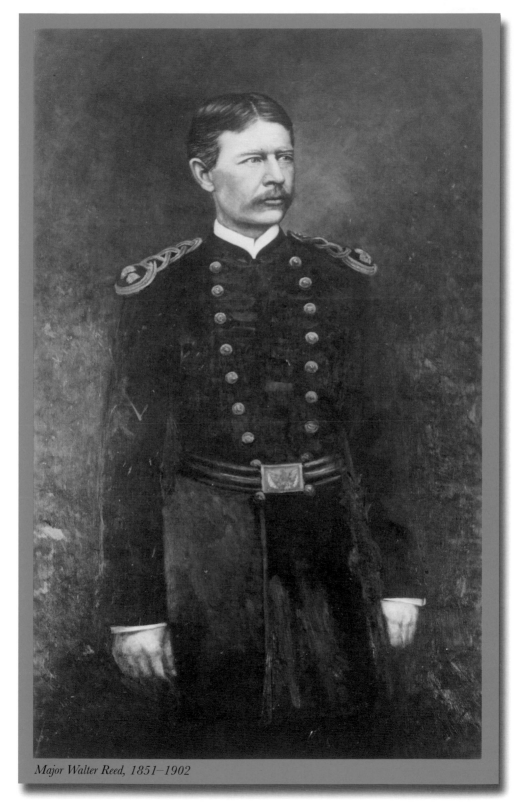

Major Walter Reed, 1851–1902

Arthur, who was something of an artist himself, exploded forcefully to the young Charles R. Reynolds, one of the original staff members at the hospital "...for God's sake, have you seen this oil painting of Reed? A drunken cow could paint a better picture with her tail." (Ltr, Maj Gen C. R. Reynolds, M.C., ret., to writer, 21 March 1952.)

The picture was hung in due time, but Colonel Kean, busy man that he was, had other ideas regarding the likeness and noted thoughtfully:

> *I went with the Surgeon General to see the full length portrait of Walter Reed at the Walter Reed Hospital, which the Surgeon General had... painted by a woman recommended by Mrs. Reed.... We agreed that it was a <u>bum</u> job. He suggested that it might be improved by cutting off the legs and making a half length of it!* [73]

And so it was altered, in military parlance — according to directives.

The Academic Emphasis

Administration of the Army Medical School, like that of the hospital, changed little during Charles Richard's assignment. Considerably more class time was spent on clinical microscopy and bacteriology and sanitary chemistry than on other subjects. The classes continued to have clinics at the hospital, but medicine and surgery were presented on alternate weeks. Actually, the course in military surgery was didactic rather than practical, with the lectures on gunshot, sword, saber and bayonet wounds well illustrated by "...lantern slides, skiagraphs, and experimental gunshot wounds on the cadaver." [74] First Lieutenant George R. Callander of the Medical Reserve Corps earned the Sternberg Medal in 1913, but a quarter of a century later he was better known as the Medical Department's only wound ballistics expert than a bacteriologist.

Some lectures and demonstrations on "psychiatrics" were given at St. Elizabeth's, *The Government Hospital For the Insane*, but the series of special lectures delivered by distinguished members of the Medical Reserve Corps showed a decided trend toward surgical interests. As more in keeping with the professional reputation of its lecturers, effective January 25, 1913, the Secretary of War authorized a change in faculty titles from instructor and assistant instructor to professor and assistant professor. [75]

This was a period of expanding opportunities for medical officers, and in 1912–1913 they were engaged in various extra-curricular activities such as flood relief work in the Ohio and Mississippi Valleys and as observers in the Balkan Wars. Major Russell, of the Army Medical School faculty, had a temporary assignment in Porto Rico with Lt. Colonel Kean to investigate an outbreak of bubonic plague, and Captain J.F. "Dusty" Siler began his life-time research work with an investigation of pellagra. Of approximately eighty-one articles prepared by medical officers and approved for publication by the Surgeon General's Office, only twenty-four were on military medical rather than clinical subjects. Of the twenty-four, eight were by Captain Louis C. Duncan, the budding military medical historian.[76]

Too few para-typhoid cases were reported during the year to justify preparation of a mixed strain of vaccine for special use or to necessitate any change in the highly acceptable typhoid vaccine which the Army Medical School prepared for distribution to other government agencies.[77] The Wasserman reaction was then as satisfactory as could be achieved in that laboratory and the faculty believed the time had come for a general survey on the prevalence and distribution of syphilis in the Army. By 1915, when Vedder's work on syphilis was published as SGO Bulletin No. 8, some 10,000 Wasserman reactions had been recorded.

Colonel Richard wanted to increase the number of students at the School, as well as to erect buildings at Walter Reed in order to use the clinical advantages of the hospital while training students in the practical aspects of hospital administration.[78] Inasmuch as the School served as the central laboratory for the Department of the East, thereby performing all of the more complicated laboratory procedures for the hospital, the Commandant's proposals had definite substance. Further, the Builder's Exchange Building, occupied so joyously only four years previously, was now deemed unsatisfactory because of high rent, noise and the poor state of repair.

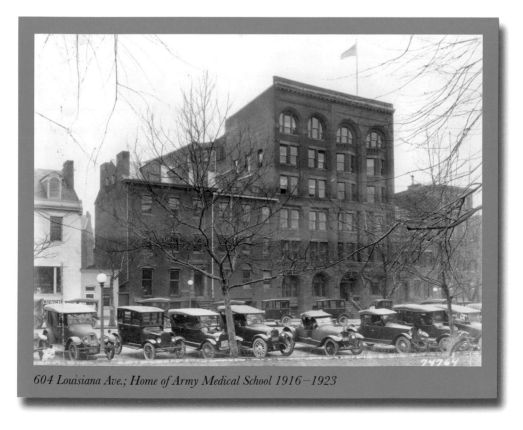

604 Louisiana Ave.; Home of Army Medical School 1916–1923

Improved X-ray procedures, which became more apparent as the need for clinical care of the peacetime Army personnel gained importance, came into the limelight during the eighteenth session, October 1, 1913–June 1, 1914, when Captain Arthur C. Christie published *A Manual of X-ray Technique*. This was an especially significant test, for in addition to the officers, a few carefully selected non-commissioned officers of the Hospital Corps were being trained each year.[79] Dentistry, still a technical rather than a professional ally, received a boost when *First Aid Dentistry* was prepared by Dental Surgeon E.P.R. Ryan and published by P. Blackstone's Sons; for good measure, the War Department purchased 122 copies.

The change in nomenclature from the stark term *insanity* to *mental alienation* was probably more significant to the faculty and students of the School than to the maintenance of exact clinical records in the hospitals, for it signified the beginning of a changing perspective in the treatment of mental disease, for which there was then too little in the way of specific therapy. Although on occasion the Surgeon General detailed medical officers for special study of mental disease, this later popular specialty was not especially interesting to the Army doctors of the period, and was considered an incidental subsection of medicine and as part and parcel of the total clinical evaluation. There may have been less disease per population ratio at this time, or less self exploitation in the discussion of maladjustments, for personnel counselling and psychoanalysis were not encouraged. Patients either lived with their fantasies or were "put away." A diagnosis of mental disease carried a social stigma and alienists were shunned, for this was before the days when the psychoanalysts had become a popular human crutch and personal maladjustments were accepted parlor topics.

Dr. William A. White of the *Government Hospital For the Insane* lectured to the Army Medical School students, some of whom may have pursued independent investigations of their own. In 1914, for instance, with war just around the corner, the class was stimulated to new thought by clinical demonstrations on the various symptoms of mental disease; lectures on dementia praecox and syphilitic diseases of the brain and cord; the usual mental diseases found in the military service, including those most frequently observed during war… "and the general effect of war in producing mental disease."[80] Perhaps as a consequence, the Surgeon General appointed a board to investigate the reclassification of general military prisoners… "with special reference to mental alienation."[81]

While not of immediate significance in the Army Medical School or Walter Reed Hospital, in August 1914, Major Joseph H. Ford was detached as a military observer in Europe, to study the hospital corps organization of the continental armies. Meanwhile, other Medical Department officers were studying and evaluating the increased use of motor ambulances in modern warfare. Moreover, a board was appointed to consider revision of the soldier's first aid packet, with the introduction of ampules of iodine.

In October 1915 Colonel Arthur replaced Colonel Richard as Commandant of the Army Medical School. In 1916 General Gorgas called attention to the School's unusually successful year under Arthur's management and the special emphasis on medico-military subjects. As no approval had been obtained for a new building at Walter Reed, and as the old one was outmoded as well as outgrown, 604 Louisiana Avenue was selected as the new home of the Army Medical School.

Evidence of Changes to Come

The School and hospital functions were spiritually if not physically identified, but the functional ties with the Army Medical Museum and Library,[82] included as an essential part of a medical center by both Surgeon General Hammond and Dr. Borden,[83] became more remote after the School moved to the Builders' Exchange Building on Thirteenth Street. The relocation left the Museum, which had long since outgrown the Hammond concept of its function as a collection de guerre as it had collected pathological items at an amazing rate, and the Surgeon General's Library in possession of the increasingly shabby building at Seventh and B Southwest. Both institutions were invaluable to the Medical Department blood and bone of its research and teaching program.

Dr. Billings' (Dr. John Shaw Billings) achievement in creating the Index-Catalogue had maintained him, in the period from 1870–1890, both at home and abroad, as the best-known American physician, and his personal reputation had brought considerable fame to the Library. In 1876 Billings alluded to the Army collection as a national medical library when publishing his *Fasciculus*, a name which the editor of *The Nation* warned might enable the Congress "to bring it under the control of politics," of which it then was entirely free.

In 1892 and again in 1901, Congress made the collection available to the civilian medical profession. It is especially interesting, therefore, that in the late nineties, during the real dawn of scientific medicine, that an unsuccessful attempt was made to annex the Army collection to the Library of Congress.[84] The American Medical Association began expanding its own publishing and indexing activities at about the same time. Dr. Fletcher had some difficulty in securing funds for publishing the Index Medicus and from 1900 to 1902 suspended the activity. By 1914 an insurgent movement had developed to assign the Army collection to the Library of Congress, largely defeated by Congressman Lloyd, of Missouri, with the open support of the AMA. Dr. Garrison had a well established academic feud under way with Dr. Simmons, editor of the *Journal of the American Medical Association*, with whom he had disagreed[85] over the kind and number of journals that should be indexed and to whom he voiced objection to the AMA's lack of encouragement to smaller medical journals then struggling for existence. It is more than probable that the movement to attach the Surgeon General's Library to the Library of Congress stems from the competition between the two organizations in regard to indexing and publications, for the Surgeon General's Library had, for over thirty years, performed under military direction and with the support of military funds, a function properly chargeable to the medical profession-at-large. There was, however, definite competition between the AMA-sponsored "Guide to Current Medical Literature," designed as a ready reference for busy physicians, and the Army-created-Army-sponsored Index

Medicus. Later, after the AMA absorbed the Index-Medicus, the great Index-Catalogue became the professional bone of contention which deprived the Army Medical Center, outgrowth of the Walter Reed General Hospital, of the Library.

The political hiatus gained the attention of the Secretary of War, Lindley Garrison, who at first supported the transfer to the Library of Congress, for, when the Army Appropriations Bill for the fiscal year 1915 was under discussion, the Senate Military Affairs Committee proposed an amendment, outgrowth of an extemporary suggestion made during the hearings, to which he assented, that is, that on or before January 1, 1915 the transfer be effected. In the meantime Army protagonists secured enough support to defeat the proposed action. On April 6, 1914, while the bill was still in conference, both the Secretary of War and the Senate and House Committees withdrew their proposals. Thus amendment 148 480 did not become law in the Act of April 27, 1914 (Army Bill for 1915). The affair was minimized, and probably as an attempt to establish in the eyes of American medicine the fact that the Library served the public as well as the military interests, the Surgeon General's great collection of scientific and professional books was more frequently referred to as the *National Medical Library*, in spite of *The Nation's* earlier warning.

Victory was conceded to the Missourians, but like the Battle of Fort Stevens, the 1914 attempt to strip the Medical Department of its most famous possession was only a skirmish.[86] The plans for a complete Army Medical Center were still so nebulous, however, that the lobbying activities of acquisitive groups were of little or no concern to the small professional staff at Walter Reed General Hospital, still thought of as out in the country rather than in the city proper.

Under the National Defense Act of 1916, the Dental Corps, an integral part of the Army since March 3, 1911, was reorganized and the three-year probationary contract required for eligibility as dental surgeons was abandoned. The Veterinary Corps functions were separated from the Quartermaster Corps, with the Corps established as an integral part of the Medical Department. Among other changes and authorizations, the government was allowed to provide storage space for Red Cross medical supplies and to permit erection of Red Cross storehouses and buildings on military reservations.[87] Each of these provisions in some way later affected military hospital management.

Because of the increased use of motor vehicles the commanding officer at Walter Reed advocated an additional Hospital Corps grade for chauffeur-sergeant and blamed the poor quality of the recruits on the inadequate military pay. The nine medical officers and nurses on duty during 1916 cared for 1175 patients, apparently without overexertion. While the interchangeable duties of clinician and professor were not allowed to interfere with the proper care of the sick, the hospital commander believed the detail of officers to work outside the institution interfered with their administrative duties such as "officers-of-the-day duty, instruction of the Hospital Corps, (assignment as members of) disability boards, consultation boards and committees and attendance at Journal Club and clinical meetings," all of which were necessary administrative functions.[88]

Officers at the Army Medical School made the long streetcar ride out to Walter Reed to perform professional and officer-of-the-day duties, that is, as a resident on call during the night hours. On the other hand, Colonel Arthur complained because his students did not spend at least two weeks in a military camp, which *could* be at Walter Reed. He agreed that laboratory work was important, but he seemed especially apprehensive because medical officers were not learning to care for themselves in camp, the details of camp sanitation or their general duties in the field.[89] Arthur, the old campaigner, believed it time to prepare for a war!

References

1. William H. Arthur, Report of the Commandant, Army Med. Sch; Annual Rpt TSG...1916, pg 200.

2. Interview with Brig. Gen. J.R. Kean, MC, Ret., April 17, 1950; Major Gen. Morrison C. Stayer, MC. Ret., June 10, 1950.

3. Interview with Brig. Gen. Frank Keefer, MC, Ret., April 20, 1950.

4. Interview with Maj. Gen. S.U. Marietta, MC, Ret., April 25, 1950.

5. Interview with Col. James F. Hall, MC, Ret., April 17, 1950; Marietta interview, *op cit*.

6. Interview with Col. James M. Phalen, MC, Ret., April 19, 1950; Hall interview, *op cit*; Keefer interview, *op cit*.

7. Kean interview, *op cit*.

8. Interview with Miss Clara Birmingham and sister, Mrs. Everett Harman, Jan. 24, 1951.

9. Phalen interview, *op cit*.

10. Ltr Walter Reed to W.C. Gorgas, Feb. 4, 1902 (quoted) W.C. Gorgas, *Sanitation in Panama*, NY & London, D. Appleton & Company, 1915, pg 105.

11. Interview Lt. Col. Jessie M. Braden, ANC, Ret., June 26, 1950.

12. Memorandum by TSG Torney, 25 Jan. 1909.

13. Became a law by Act of 27 April 1914 (38 Stat 353).

14. Annual Rpt TSG...1914, pg 56, 57.

15. Annual Rpt WRGH, 1913.

16. Annual Rpt WRGH, 1913.

17. Annual Rpt TSG...1914, pg 12, 13.

18. Birmingham interview, *op cit*.

19.   Annual Rpt WRGH, 1913.

20.   Stayer Interview, *op cit*.

21.   Keefer, Huggins, Stayer interviews, *op cit*.

22.   Interview Brig. Gen. Albert G. Love, MC, Ret., Feb. 13, 1951.

23.   Phalen interview, *op cit*.

24.   Love interview, *op cit*.

25.   Marietta interview, *op cit*.

26.   Keefer, Huggins, Stayer, Marietta interviews, *op cit*.

27.   Interview with Mrs. Mathew Reasoner, April 17, 1950.

28.   Interview with Mrs. M.W. Ireland, April 14, 1950.

29.   Henry C. Fisher (obt) *Military Surgeon*, Vol. 80, 1937, pg 87–89.

30.   Keefer interview, *op cit*.

31.   Ireland interview, *op cit*.

32.   Annual Rpt, WRGH, 1914.

33.   Annual Rpt, WRGH, 1915.

34.   Annual Rpt, TSG...1914, pg 69.

35.   Annual Rpt, WRGH, 1915.

36.   Annual Rpt TSG...1914, pg 13.

37.   Ltr F.H. Garrison to Dr. George H. Simmons, Ed., J.A.M.A., Aug. 5, 1914. Collection of the Institute of History of Medicine, Welch Med. Lib., Baltimore, MD.

38.   Annual Rpt WRGH, 1915.

39.   Annual Rpt WRGH, 1915.

40.   Annual Rpt TSG...1915, pg 161.

41.   John Babson Soule, Article in the Terre Haute Ind. *Express*, 1851.

42.   Ltr from Frances Phillips to writer, Jan. 23, 1951; Wm. Crawford Gorgas, *Sanitation in Panama*, *op cit*, pg 243.

43.   Tlgm Gorgas to Phillips, Apr. 24, 1914, SGO folder 1430, War Rec. Div. Nat'l Archives.

44. Endorsement signed by James F. Harrison, M.D., Oct. 2, 1883, *Ibid.*

45. SGO Folder 1430, *op cit.*

46. Ltr to S.F. Phillips, signed "JM" (John Moore) Surgeon General U.S. Army, Jan. 10, 1890, Folder 1403, *op cit.*

47. Ltr from S.F. Phillips, Senate Bldg. Wash., D.C., to TSW, Jan. 10, 1890, Folder 1430, *op cit.*

48. *Ibid.*

49. AGO SO 121, par 31, 24 May 1898; AGO SO 138; 14 June 1898; AGO SO 166, 13 October 1898.

50. Interview with Col. Herbert N. Dean, MAC, Ret., April 12, 1950.

51. Otto L. Nelson, *op cit*, pg 82.

52. Folder 1430, *op cit.*

53. Hall interview, *op cit.*

54. Ireland interview, *op cit.*

55. Kean interview, *op cit.*

56. Interview Mrs. Aileen Gorgas Wrightson, July 18, 1950.

57. Folder 1430, *op cit*, Rpt signed by F.A. Winker, CO, A&NH, Feb. 2, 1915.

58. Answer to questions submitted by Lt. Col. Andre W. Brewster, I.G., No. 88..."One officer opened elevator door at night and stepped off into space, the elevator not being at that floor. The fault was not in the elevator." Annual Inspection, WRGH, Dec. 1916, signed P.M. Ashburn, Maj., M.C. and Chf of Medical Service. Incident mentioned in all interviews on Phillips.

59. Hall interview, *op cit.*

60. Marietta interview, *op cit*; Stayer interview, *op cit.*

61. Stayer interview, *op cit.*

62. Edgar Erskine Hume, *History of the Military Surgeon...op cit*, pg 87.

63. Annual Rpt., WRGH, 1916.

64. Braden April 1945; June 26, 1950.

65. Danielson interview, *op cit.*

66. Danielson, Thompson, Braden interviews, *op cit*; Miss Bernice Hansen, ANC, Ret., July 18, 1950. (Telephone)

67. *Ibid.*

68. Braden, *op cit*; Ltr from Lt. Col. Elvira Helgren, ANC, Ret. to writer, June 6, 1950.

69. Annual Rpt WRGH, 1916.

70. Kean MSS, pg 133.

71. Ltr from N.M. Miller 631 Penna Ave., N.W. to TSG, W.C. Gorgas, War Dept. Nov. 23, 1951, SGO file 19928, War Rec. Div. Nat'l Archives.

72. *Ibid.*

73. Kean, *op cit.*

74. Annual Rpt TSG...1913, pg 171.

75. *Ibid*, pg 172.

76. *Ibid*, pg 180–182.

77. *Ibid*, 1914, pg 146–149.

78. *Ibid*, 1914, pg 149.

79. *Ibid*, 1915, pg 162–163.

80. *Ibid*, 1914, pg 163.

81. *Ibid*, 1915, pg 164.

82. Division of the Surgeon General's Office.

83. Memo frm Robert W. Patterson, TSG to TAG, Sept. 14, 1931. Subject, The Surgeon General's Library and The Army Medical Museum. SGO 631.-1 (Judge Thompson's files).

84. Conversation with Dr. Caludius Mayer, Chf. Index-Catalogue Division, AMI, as proposed by the Director Lt. Col. Frank B. Rogers.

85. Ltr Garrison to Simmons, Ap. 26, 1911; Ap. 5 and 8, 1914. Collection... *op cit.*

86. SGO 631.1 (The Army Medical Library), CG, (Judge Thompson's files).

87. Annual Rpt TSG...1916, pg 16.

88. *Ibid*, pg 163.

89. *Ibid*, pg 200.

The War Years
1917–1918

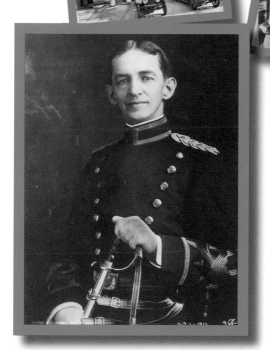

*1916, Colonel Charles F. Mason, Post Commander;
October 6, 1916 – November 27, 1917*

*"Modern wars are so short and
decisive that it would
be criminal to delay preparation
until the moment of rupture."[1]*

The Line of Succession

Colonel Charles M. Mason succeeded Major Ashburn as commander at Walter Reed on October 6, 1916. Although his first and most continuing professional interest was in surgery, he was, as noted, author of a handbook which *The Military Surgeon* called the medical soldier's "Bible."[2]

He was quiet,[3] refined, scholarly, cultured[4] and had charming manners.[5] Like Colonel Richard he was small of stature, with little inclination for any athletic exercise except walking. He was somewhat solitary in his habits and derived more enjoyment from playing classical records on his gramophone than from hilarious parties. The Mason family had moved to Panama in 1909, where they remained for seven interesting and exciting years. Although Colonel Mason was in charge of the Ancon Hospital, where the records of that period show he had a flair for economic management,[6] he did not confine his activities entirely to administration. Gorgas' mosquito prevention work had caught the imagination of the entire world by this time, and as the Army medical laboratory was across the street from the Mason's quarters, the children were encouraged to breed mosquitoes from larvae in order to facilitate their father's research. It was, therefore, with real regret that the family returned to North America and a more routinized military life, in spite of the advantages of advanced schools for the children.

The geographical change from the tropical climate of Panama to the unpredictable one of Washington was at first accepted reluctantly, for city life had little appeal. Family visits to the adjoining Shepherd estate were delightful events, and like the Birmingham children, the young Masons found life on the military reservation of the U.S. Army General Hospital a pleasant adventure. The slope above Cameron's Creek provided an excellent sled-run in winter, and in the spring the surrounding violet-filled woods afforded the same sort of hide-away from household chores that had protected the young Birminghams from the all-seeing eyes of chore-minded parents. Domestic chores may have been avoidable, but Colonel Mason's scholarly instincts encouraged no procrastination with school work. The Takoma School kept the younger members of the family occupied, and Charles Mason assured his older daughter a proper skill on the typewriter,[7] for he set her to copying the manuscript for the fourth edition of the handbook, published by W. Wood and Company of New York in 1917.

General Gorgas was more interested in international public health work than in administration, and in January 1917, he informed the Secretary of War that he wished to retire. Colonel Birmingham had organized the *Division of Sanitation* in the Surgeon General's Office. He was not only efficient but also a senior officer,

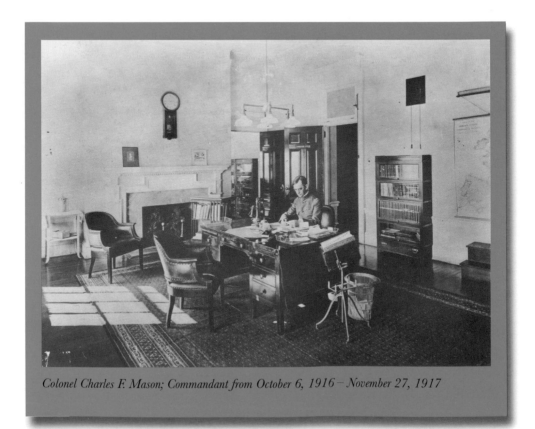

Colonel Charles F. Mason; Commandant from October 6, 1916 – November 27, 1917

and General Gorgas proposed him for the Surgeon Generalcy.[8] However, the critical military situation in Europe, with the probability of American intervention, caused him to remain in office. After Birmingham's detail as Assistant Surgeon General terminated, Lieutenant Colonel Robert E. Noble,[9] one of General Gorgas' former assistants in Panama, gradually became more influential in Medical Department policies. When Noble was promoted to a temporary Brigadier Generalcy in the National Army and "jumped" not only his contemporaries but many of his seniors in rank, the situation had an adverse effect on Medical Corps morale.[10]

Insofar as Walter Reed Hospital was concerned, the "Panama Influence" seemingly governed the appointment of the next two commanding officers. Colonel Williard F. Truby, also a former assistant of General Gorgas,[11] was appointed as Mason's replacement on November 28, 1917. Of German extraction,[12] the Colonel was a quiet, phlegmatic bachelor.

Shy, but with a great deal of personality,[13] his humorously cynical thoughts sometimes found outlet in verse,[14] apparently his preferred means of self-expression as he was notably a poor correspondent.[15] He had entered the Medical Corps in 1898, more from patriotic duty than because of a preference for military life.[16] More interested in the clinical than in the administrative functions of his Corps,

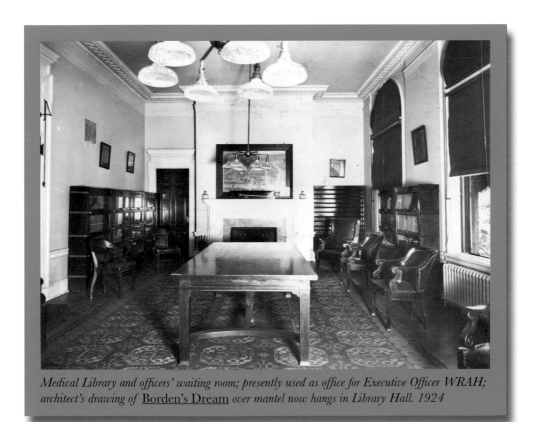

Medical Library and officers' waiting room; presently used as office for Executive Officer WRAH; architect's drawing of <u>Borden's Dream</u> *over mantel now hangs in Library Hall. 1924*

he well deserved his reputation for being an excellent internist.[17] Therefore when the opportunity for retirement with physical disability came on November 28, 1918, Colonel Truby accepted it with alacrity,[18] returning to his native New York State to practice medicine successfully for more than thirty years.

In contrast to the usual civilian opinion of Army officers as raging bloodthirsty autocrats, Walter Reed Hospital either had a surprising number of small quiet men as managers or, with the adjudication of philosophers, those contemporaries who recalled the early commanders frame their recollections entirely with kindness. For of the conscientious, serious, somewhat humorless[19] Colonel Edward R. Schreiner, commanding officer from August 27, 1918 until March 15, 1919, very little is known.[20]

Expanding the Bed Capacity

Construction of temporary war-model frame buildings began in June 1917, with preparations made for expanding the facilities to accept some 2,500 to 3,000 patients. A one-story frame building for housing fifty additional nurses and a two-story frame barracks for 250 enlisted men were erected on the Georgia Avenue side of the reservation. A mess hall capable of seating 250 men; a storehouse for medical supplies; a one-story frame guardhouse for fifteen prisoners and four guards, built near to Ward "B" and almost in front of the hospital; a Receiving Ward for storage of personal effects and accommodation of eight patients prior to assignment to wards; a "linen" building and ten single one-story forty-five-bed wards; three double one-story eighty-five-bed wards and one thirty-two-bed officers' ward were all built during the remainder of the year. Further, to increase the bed capacity an overflow of thirty patients could be accommodated on each of the ward porches. Amazingly, in 1917, as the pressure of war activities mounted and accumulated fatigue should have placed greater strain on all military personnel, the average number of patient days spent in the hospital decreased by twenty-eight per cent.[21]

The expansion of the physical plant created requirements for a larger staff and ultimately some fifty-three medical officers and eight dentists were on duty at Walter Reed. A modern fully equipped X-ray laboratory was installed on the third floor of the Main Building, where 1,498 patients were examined during the year, with 160 of the examinations requested by the dental service. In September, a Quartermaster detachment of one officer and one hundred men undertook the receipt and shipment of all medical and Quartermaster property not handled by the separate Property Division, responsible for the medical supplies necessary for the proper operation of the hospital and for procuring from outside sources and as required immediately, "such articles as are urgently needed to prevent suffering and save life."[22] The Quartermaster had charge of all animal-drawn vehicles, but the ambulance service was under the direction of the Property Division, and from four ambulances (and two chauffeurs) on January 1, 1917, this service increased to ten ambulances a year later.

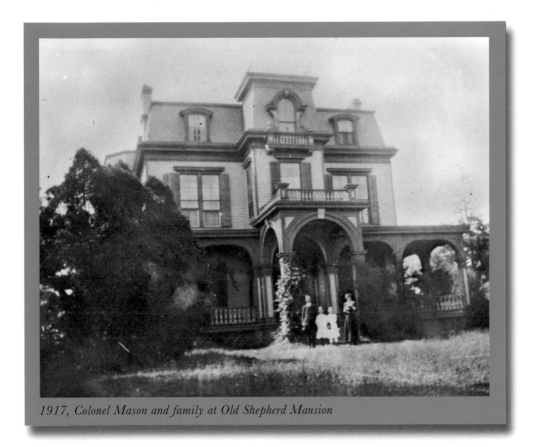

1917, Colonel Mason and family at Old Shepherd Mansion

In fact all of the former hospital services were outgrown before the end of the year. The laboratory, two rooms in the Main Building, was too small and had insufficient apparatus; kitchen floor space and equipment were needed to provide food service for the anticipated 2,500 persons; a new incinerator was a necessity, and a complete disinfecting plant. Dentistry, with the case load steadily increasing, required an entire wing in one of the new buildings; the surgeons wanted a separate building, leaving Old Main for administration, or at least separate operating pavilions for clean and infected cases; a cystoscopy room; etherizing room; cast room and, in anticipation of war casualties, special

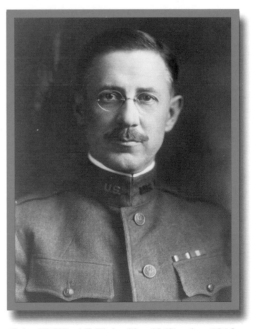

Colonel Williard F. Truby; Nov. 1917 – Aug 1918

orthopedic rooms. Similarly, the Eye, Ear, Nose and Throat work increased so rapidly that an entire new clinic building was discussed, complete with recovery room and a preparatory room for sterile dressings and water. Buildings were needed for physical therapy and hobby work, such as a therapeutic workshop, so necessary in the physical rehabilitation of the maimed soldiers.

Inpatient admissions were classified as to status in the Regular Army and the National Army, and including civilians, 4,256 patients were admitted during the year, of whom only 174 were classed as insane. Interestingly, in comparing the statistics for hospital admissions for the two groups, a noticeably higher proportion of both officers and enlisted men of the Regular Army were admitted for treatment of venereal disease and mental disturbances than of the National Army. The Post census for April 1917, the month war was declared, showed that fifteen officers, 145 Medical Department enlisted men and thirteen men of the Quartermaster Detachment were on duty. There was one Commanding Officer; one Chief of the Service who also served as a summary court officer; one Chief of EENT who also served as recruiting officer and as Assistant Professor of Ophthalmology at the Army Medical School; one officer who served as Quartermaster, Ordnance Officer and Commanding Officer of both the Quartermaster and Medical Detachments; one officer who served as adjutant, registrar and mess officer; one officer who served as pathologist and roentgenologist, and one dental officer.

The remaining officers were departmental assistants and served as board members, post exchange officer, athletic officer, librarian etc. The permanent buildings then included, as listed previously, the Main Building; mortuary; coal shed; isolation hospital; Quartermaster office; stables; garage; wagon shed; barracks; nurses' residence; quarters one and two for officers and the "Old Frame House" occupied by the Charley Andersons. Temporary buildings No. 200-208, as cited, were built during the year. Commodity prices had not increased appreciably at this time, for the average aggregate cost of general administration, exclusive of subsistence per inpatient, was less than in 1915. Strangely, the Surgeon General's Annual Report for 1917 noted the Walter Reed statistics for 1916. Whereas the hospital reported a bed capacity of 950 during this year of expansion,[23] the Surgeon General listed only 297,[24] one hundred of which would be temporary in the barracks.

A permanent power house structure was begun in May 1917 and completed the following year. Other permanent buildings included an incinerator, a brick morgue, and a garage addition with a connection to the old stables,[25] still in general use as the hospital reports carried expenditures for forage and the shoeing of horses. By the end of 1918, the reservation presented a hybrid appearance, for several other similar structures had been added to the 1917 group of temporary buildings. The few dignified red brick colonial buildings seemed out of place in the mass of barracks-like structures so familiar in cantonments throughout the United States.[26]

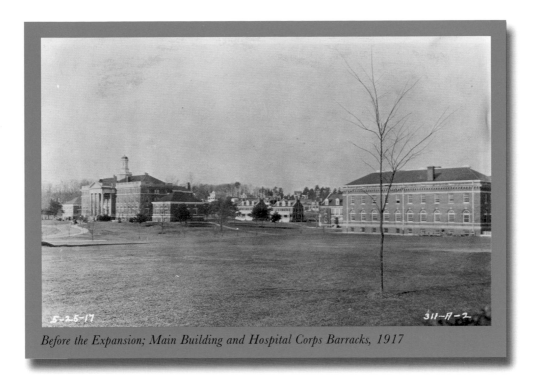

Before the Expansion; Main Building and Hospital Corps Barracks, 1917

No doubt Dr. Borden, who returned to active duty on June 6, 1917 as chief of the surgical service, found his creation, *Borden's Dream*, an architectural nightmare. Sprawled about the hillocks, connected by ramps and covered corridors, the low rambling wards clung to the wooded slopes of Cameron's Creek like the tentacles of an octopus. Even a bridge had been built across this feeble trickle in order to protect the long dragging skirts of the nurses from ground soil. It is more than possible that had the war continued longer the expansion would have developed as Dr. Borden predicted ten years earlier, for to "the west of Sixteenth Street (was) Rock Creek Park with its high ridges where temporary camps (could) be placed if such (were) required."[27]

As a consequence of the war, the surgical service had its most significant growth during the eighteen months that Dr. Borden served as chief. By January 7, 1919, however, "the greatest war in history" was past tense for all but students of military strategy and historians. Regular Army personnel was again available for domestic assignment, and Dr. Borden returned to his duty as Dean of the George Washington Medical School. He had, at last, served in the institution he created, but not as its chief executive. In the following years he had little association with the Medical Corps, and soon he was all but forgotten. That is, by all but Kean, who with his unfailing care, steadfastly gave credit where credit was due:

Dec. 20, 1927

My dear Colonel Borden

    I had occasion to go to Walter Reed Hospital…
and was much interested to see the group of fine
buildings there that are approaching completion
— The original main building with the two new
great wings make a noble façade —

    I thought how Borden's baby had grown and how
proud it should make him to see what a great
and beautiful as well as useful creation has
grown up from the foundation which he laid —

    The thought also came to me, and saddened me
to think how few of the younger men who work
there know about how entirely its inception
and the acquisition of the original site and
building were due to your initiative….[20]

Dr. Borden died in 1934, after a long illness. An editorial in the October issue of the *Military Surgeon*, apparently prepared by Kean, stated that "Walter Reed Hospital, the greatest of American military hospitals, originated in his foresight and was built as a result of his personal efforts and unwearied persistence."

In time the Medical Department fostered a custom of commemorating the services of distinguished medical officers with bronze plaques, mounted in the halls of the new Army Medical School. The money was supplied by "outside" sources; the applications for recognition were made by descendants of the deceased; a board appointed by the Surgeon General approved the proposals.

In the early forties some unused monies permitted erection of several plaques for which no applications had been made. Because of its size, or perhaps because

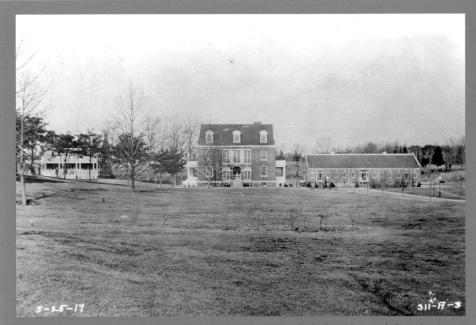

1917 – Prior to erection of East Wing, Main Building; Left: Double set of Qtrs, later replaced by Isolation Wards; Center: "The Pest House", later ward for Interne's Quarters; Extreme Right: Quartermaster Building.

few people know what it actually was, the original painting of *Borden's Dream* had been in the Army Medical School building but unhung for some years previously. Now, however, it served a useful purpose, for the "artists drawing of a proposed medical center which was made during his administration" was the convincing credential that secured a plaque for William Cline Borden. His family was apparently unaware of this belated and somewhat insignificant honor,[29] until after the Borden General Hospital, a temporary war service structure, was named for him in late 1942.[30]

Organization

The mushroom growth of the hospital plant was matched by the complicated organizational structure of the hospital services. Gone were the days when the institution was an "uncrowded, unhurried sanitarium for the care of (a) small quota."[31]

The usual carefully prescribed Medical Department regulations governed the tight organizational structure, divided for convenience into six principal operating divisions.

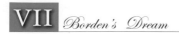

Hospital Organization.
THE COMMANDING OFFICER.
Department of Administration.

1. The Executive Officer.
    (a). Officer of the Day.
    (b). Night Administrative Officer.

2. Correspondence and Records
    (a). Adjutant.
    (b). Personnel Adjutant.
        (1). Insurance Officer.
    (c). Supervisor of Clinical Records.
        (1). Registrar.
        (2). Curator, Department of Illustration.
        (3). Medical Examining Board for Officers.
        (4). Disability Board for Enlisted Men.
        (5). Demobilization Board.

3. Inspection.
    (a). Hospital Inspector (inspection of administration and service departments).
    (b). Sanitary Inspector (inspection of grounds and buildings for sanitation and maintenance).
    (c). Post Surgeon (inspection of dairies, food supplies, etc.)
    (d). Adjutant (inspection of public funds).
    (e). Survey Officer (inspection of unserviceable property).

4. Detachment Administration.
    (a). Detachment Commander, Patients.
        (1). Receiving Officer.
        (2). Disposition Officer.
    (b). Detachment Commander, Medical Detachment.
    (c). Detachment Commander, Quartermaster Detachment.
    (d). Detachment Commander of Nurses.
    (e). Detachment Commander of Aides.

5. Police and Fire Protection.
    (a). Intelligence Officer.
    (b). Prison Officer.
    (c). Fire Marshals.
    (d). Police Officer.
    (e). Courts Martial.

Department of Service and Supply.

1. Service of Supply.
      (a). Supply Officer.
      (b). Ordnance Officer.
      (c). Finance Officer.
      (d). Transportation Officer.
      (e). Salvage Officer.
      (f). Medical Supply Officer.

2. Constructing and Utilities Service.
      (a). Constructing Quartermaster.
      (b). Utilities Officer.

3. Mess Service.
      (a). Mess Officer.
      (b). Dietitians.

4. Motor Transport Service.
      (a). Motor Transport Officer.

5. Telephone and Telegraph Service.
      (a). Signal Officer.

6. Post Exchange.
      (a). Exchange Officer.

7. Recruiting Service.
      (a). Recruiting Officer.

8. Morale, Education and Recreation Service.
      (a). Chaplains.
      (b). Morale Officer.
      (c). Education and Recreation Officer.
      (d). Service Club Hostess.
      (e). Librarian.

Department of Professional Services.

1. Surgical Service.
      Chief of Service.
      (a). Administrative Officers.
            (1). Assistant to Chief of Service.

(2). Chiefs of Sections.

(3). Ward Surgeons.

(4). Surgical Emergency Officers.

(b). Professional Sections.

(1). General Surgery.

(2). Septic Surgery.

(3). Empyema.

(4). Maxillo-Facial.

(5). Neuro-Surgical.

(6). Eye, Ear, Nose and Throat. (In July 1918, subdivided into Eye Section and ENT Section.)

(7). Orthopaedic. (Separate from General Surgery in July 1918; Central Dressing Station opened for all ambulatory orthopedic cases, Dec. 17, 1918.)

(8). Amputation.

(9). Dermatology and Syphilis.

(10). Urology.

(11). Obstetric and Gynecologic.

(c). Professional Departments.

(1). Dental.

(2). X-ray.

(3). Orthopaedic Appliance Shop.

(4). Anesthesia.

2. Medical Service.

Chief of Service.

(a). Assistant to the Chief of Service.

(b). Chiefs of Section.

(1). General Medicine Section.

(2). Neuro-Psychiatric Section. (Early in 1918, hospital became one of six centers for care of nervous and mental cases. Five 150-bed wards were assigned.)

(3). Contagious Disease Section.

(c). Receiving Officer.

(d). Post Surgeon.

(e). Ward Surgeons.

(f). Medical Emergency Officer.

Laboratory Department.

(a). Bacteriological Section.

(b). Chemical Section.

(c). Pathological Section — (Mortuary).

Reconstruction and Education Departments.

1. Ward Handicrafts.

   For patients unable to leave their wards.

2. Curative Shop Work.

   For patients whose primary requirement is curative; occupational therapy.

   (a). Wood working.

   (b). Rug weaving.

   (c). Clay modeling.

   (d). Gardening.

   (e). Typewriting.

3. Educational and Vocational Training.

   (a). Academic: English, reading, writing, arithmetic, etc.

   (b). Commercial: Shorthand, typewriting, bookkeeping, accounting, office appliances.

   (c). Trade and vocational training:

      (1). Auto mechanics.

      (2). Garden and greenhouse management.

      (3). Electrical wiring and dynamo tending.

      (4). Drafting.

      (5). Jewelry making and repairing.

      (6). Machine shop practice.

      (7). Motion picture operating.

      (8). Photography.

      (9). Rug weaving and repairing.

      (10). Wireless telegraphy.

      (11). Oxy-acetylene welding.

      (12). Vulcanizing and tire repairing.

      (13). General printing.

      (14). Linotype operating.

      (15). Wood shop practice.

Physio-Therapy Department.

1. Measurement and Record Section.

2. Hydro-therapy.

3. Electro-therapy.

4. Massage.

5. Medical Gymnastics.

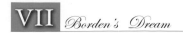

Nursing Department.

1. Army Nurse Corps – Principal Chief Nurse.
      (a). Assistant Chief Nurse (Records and Correspondence).
      (b). Day Supervisor for Graduate Nurses.
      (c). Night Supervisor for Graduate Nurses.

2. Army School of Nursing.
      (a). Superintendent.
         (1). Theoretical Instructor.
         (2). Practical Instructor.
         (3). Circulating Supervisors for Student Nurses. [32]

Whereas a mean average of 22.8 medical officers, 223.197 Medical Department and Quartermaster personnel and 44.7 Army Nurses were on duty in 1917, a year later the mean average strength had increased to 86.3 officers, 689.1 Medical Department enlisted men, 136.7 Quartermaster enlisted men, 147.8 Army nurses, 33.6 Reconstruction Aides and 18.9 civilian employees;[33] there were, during 1918, some 13,752 patients treated.

New Functions

Occupational therapy and rehabilitation was a new function in therapeutic care of patients and required considerable space and equipment. In February 1918, "a single room was secured in what was originally the Lay Homestead, dating from Civil War Days, and tenanted by the Post carpenter and his family."[34] In spite of limitation to simple carpentry with Charley Anderson's discarded tools, the work was from the first successful as a morale builder.

The first aides, arriving on February 15, began their work on an orthopedic ward, teaching men to weave colored wool squares for blankets. From this small beginning the activities broadened to include both remedial and palliative courses. By April 1918, when the Division of Physical Reconstruction of the Surgeon General's Office authorized funds for shop equipment and the payment of expert educational directors, the value of this new function was already evident. By the latter part of the summer the Department of Occupational Therapy was not only stimulating patient interest through weekly staff meetings, but it was serving as a training and demonstration school for other hospitals. Like many other "firsts" in military medicine, Walter Reed was the first American military hospital to have a professional psychologist on its staff.[35]

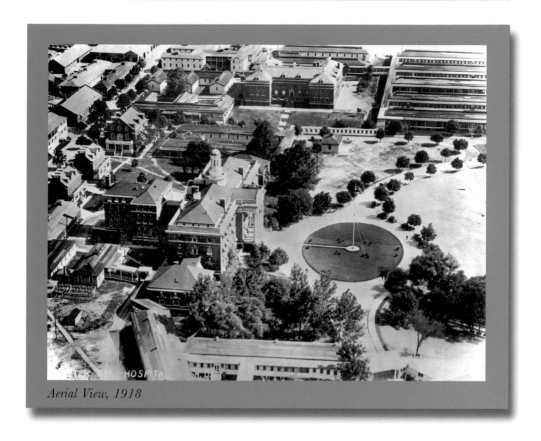

Aerial View, 1918

This department was divided into five sections: Administrative, Psychological and Statistical, General and Academic, Technical, and Recreational. By the end of the year the usual academic and technical courses were being offered. These included *Agriculture*, with outdoor truck farming, forced growth under glass; flowers and textbook studies; *Printing*, hand, linotype and press; *Mechanical and Electrical* work such as automobile repairing, oxyacetylene welding; wiring, telegraphy and radio operation; *Machine Shop Practice*, with electrical and mechanical studies; *Drafting*; *Woodworking*; *Display Painting*; *Arts and Crafts*; *Leather Work*; *Rug Weaving*, and *Physical Education*.[36] The program eventually became so popular that five occupational therapy buildings were required. The hydrotherapy, electrotherapy, gymnasium and physical therapy sections expanded in proportion to their respective needs.

In September 1918, the Lane Convalescent Home, with capacity for ten enlisted men, was opened in Takoma Park; in November, Mrs. Evelyn Walsh McLean released "Friendship House" as a convalescent home for fifty officers. A hospital newspaper, *The Come Back*, made its first appearance on December 4, 1918. All of the work was performed by volunteers, and the profits were presented to the Donation Fund in the Surgeon General's Office.[37]

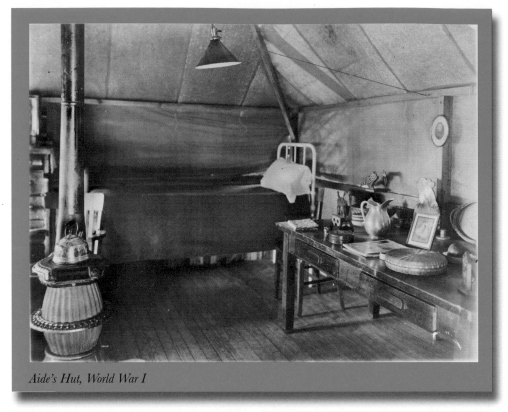

Aide's Hut, World War I

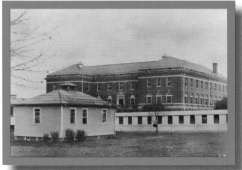
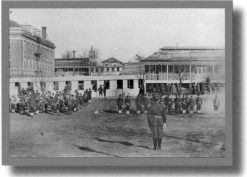

1919; Left: Main Barracks showing Old Guard House; Right: Post Band and Grand Inspection

In accordance with its prescribed mission to the Medical Department, the American Red Cross was erecting convalescent houses at the base and general hospitals in the United States, including Walter Reed. As one of its special service projects, in February 1918, the American National Red Cross authorities asked Mrs. Edith Oliver Rea, a wealthy Pittsburgh philanthropist residing temporarily in Washington, to interest a group of volunteer ladies in welfare work at Walter Reed. Mrs. Rea became Field Director of the Red Cross project and Miss Margaret Lower the Assistant Field Director, as approximately 75 ladies signed up for ward service on certain days.

The hospital was divided into three sections, each with a volunteer supervisor and four helpers. Thus only fifteen carefully selected women did the first ward visiting. Their first activities included recreation, games, group singing, oral reading, letter writing and a shopping service for the benefit of the patients. When the Convalescent House was completed on May 11, the volunteer socialites arrived with brooms, mops, buckets and soap to clean the building for presentation to the commanding officer on June 11. This proved to be a greater undertaking than visualized, but the indomitable ladies placed a GI[38] trash can in the fireplace, heated their own water, and with the assistance of some ambulatory patients, set the place in order.

The first "uniforms" were light blue aprons, similar to the uniforms used by volunteer workers in the District of Columbia Chapter. In July 1918 the National Headquarters directed that all volunteer lay workers in the Convalescent Houses wear a drab shade of gray gingham. This proposal met with opposition from Mrs. Rea and her group, and as a result of their protests the soft pearl gray uniform-dress selected by Mrs. Rea was used. As the casualties began arriving from overseas in large numbers, and responded to the well meaning kindness of their benefactors, such terms as "My Gray Lady of the Red Cross" or "My Monday Gray Lady" etc., became familiar terms. The title, which the "Gray Ladies" accepted as a term of endearment, was thus bestowed by the doughboys themselves.[39]

In December, the American Library Association used part of the Red Cross building for a central recreation library of some 6,500 books. Ward service was provided for all bed patients, and the library collection of technical books was adequate to supplement the academic courses sponsored by the reconstruction program.[40]

Various welfare organizations contributed generously in both equipment and personnel. The YMCA "hut" first located in the basement of the Main Building, later had its own headquarters on Dogwood Street, across from the Post. The Knights of Columbus opened a "hut" in November 1918, and the Jewish Welfare Board maintained quarters in a nearby residence on Butternut Street. The principal Service Club, No. I, provided by the National Catholic War Council, was opened on December 15, 1919. Equipped with a cafeteria and dining room, lounge and a number of bedrooms for rent to transient visitors, it featured entertainments and socials all during the active emergency. In addition to the Red Cross, the various clubs sponsored recreational activities for patients such as celebrity shows, musicals, movies, dances, classes in dancing, lectures, sight-seeing trips, corn roasts, picnics, theater parties, athletic teams, dramatics, masquerades etc. The special personnel such as aides, recreation workers and nurses likewise had their own entertainments.[41]

Organized athletics played an important part in rehabilitation, and playing fields and tennis courts were built, and during the early postwar period Mrs. Rea provided funds for a swimming pool. Enclosed on each side by occupational therapy wards, this prized recreation spot was eventually used as an all-purpose swimming pool for the entire command.

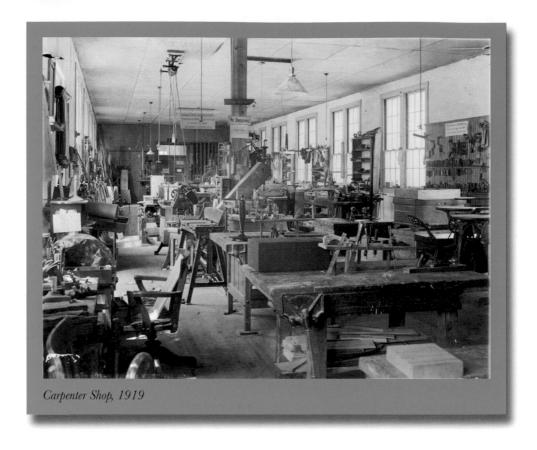

Carpenter Shop, 1919

The Post Exchange grew in proportion to other installation support activities and sponsored a barber shop, soda fountain, restaurant, laundry, tailor shop and cobbler.

The medical post was like a busy little city, and its transient population was united in a common attempt to rehabilitate and return to civilian life as useful citizens, the injured doughboys from France. The war was officially over, but the Quartermaster at Walter Reed had endless trouble with the records and equipment of soldier-patients transferred from the rapidly closing cantonments, from which they were made to take all the possessions on their descriptive list. In many cases the clothing was not invoiced at the last Quartermaster station, an omission which caused extensive correspondence and misunderstanding between the Quartermaster and the patients. At the Walter Reed U.S. Army General Hospital it was disconcerting, to say the least, to have patients reporting in at the hospital's receiving ward equipped with rifles and one hundred fifty rounds of ammunition.[42]

Nursing

There were a number of Chief Nurses at Walter Reed during 1917-1918, and providing an accurate biographical list has defied even the Nursing Division of the Surgeon General's Office. Some of them apparently stayed for a month or two and then moved on to open new stations or to go overseas with mobile units. The annual reports carry few references to personnel, and the sections prepared by the Nursing Service are mere recitals of skeleton facts — an average of so many nurses were on duty at a given time. The writer has had singularly satisfactory experiences with the nursing service at Walter Reed, and so the 147.8 mean average of nurses reported as on duty during 1918, leaves a bewildering sense of frustration as to who composed the .8 per cent, unless that figure can be assigned to the elusive Chief Nurses who came and went about their duties but left no record of their activities. Miss Bessie S. Bell, the principal Chief Nurse, was released from Walter Reed in October 1917, to become director of the Army Nursing Service of the American Expeditionary Forces.[43] Frail-looking, modest, retiring and unaggressive,[44] she was as pleasant, lady-like and gentle as her euphonious name suggests.[45] Though efficient with records, she was not an aggressive personality, and her reputation for being an accomplished pianist did little to mollify contemporaries who judged her lack of positive leadership by the feminist patterns of the day. Like her chief, Miss Dora E. Thompson, Superintendent of the Corps, she was quietly efficient but not spectacular. In fact, the Medical Officers apparently believed that their "quiet efficiency was such that both women so blended with the team that (they) have to be grabbed, as it were, and dragged into view."[46]

These were turbulent days in nursing circles, for the Army increased its demands for personnel with predictable certainty. More, more, more was the constant plea, as nurse leaders and teachers planned frantically to reconcile demand and supply. As a former Superintendent of the Army Nurse Corps, Miss Delano was not only Army-minded, but she had taken seriously the Red Cross mandate to provide reserve nurses for the Army in time of war, for civilian communities in time of disaster.

The three-year training period was an insurmountable obstacle in keeping a ready supply of nurses flowing to the Armed Forces, and so the Red Cross had long planned to use health aides as assistants in case of a national emergency. A carefully prescribed program limited their duties and placed them under the jurisdiction of graduate nurses. Academically, nurse training was not out of the "dark ages" of being a service rather than a profession, and many of the prominent leaders feared acceptance of aides would undermine their economic security.[47] War or no war, this was a social problem of grave significance to an emergent group.

Miss Thompson appreciated more fully than her civilian contemporaries the transitory nature of military expansions. Knowing that evacuated casualties must have immediate nursing care, she supported Miss Delano in the Red Cross proposal for immediate and temporary use of aides.

As director of the Hospital Division, Office of the Surgeon General,[48] created in July 1917, General Noble held an extremely influential position, and regardless of the fact that Gorgas was the Surgeon General, he essentially held the balance of power when the Amazonian dispute between the national nursing groups began in the spring of 1918. Several of the doctors from Johns Hopkins, including Dr. William Henry Welch, friend of the Surgeon General since the days of Major Walter Reed, exerted considerable influence on national medical policies, including the Medical Department of the Army. Some of these men freely voiced their opinion of Regular Army administrative methods and personnel management, and they apparently persuaded Generals Gorgas and Noble to disregard the advice of experienced Regular Army personnel, including Miss Thompson, and accept the civilian interpretation of Army needs. Such was the situation in regard to the plans for using "trained" nurses rather than nurses' aides to provide immediate nursing care for men in the cantonment hospitals.

Nurse leaders from the Department of Nursing Education, Teachers College, Columbia University, adopted an intransigent stand for the training of additional nurses. They found fault with the nursing service as rendered by the corpsmen in Army hospitals and under the supervision of an all-graduate even if quickly expanded Nurse Corps. Inconsistently, therefore, they insisted on using the Army hospitals as training schools, with accredited supplementary work in the specialties given in civilian hospitals. The ensuing dispute between the two factions, the Army Nurse Corps and the Red Cross Nursing Service interested in providing immediate care, and the national nursing organizations determined to raise the academic standards of nursing education and train nurses at government expense, is basic to the history of nursing in these United States. Between politics and wiles, organized nursing won its greatest academic battle in the half-century.

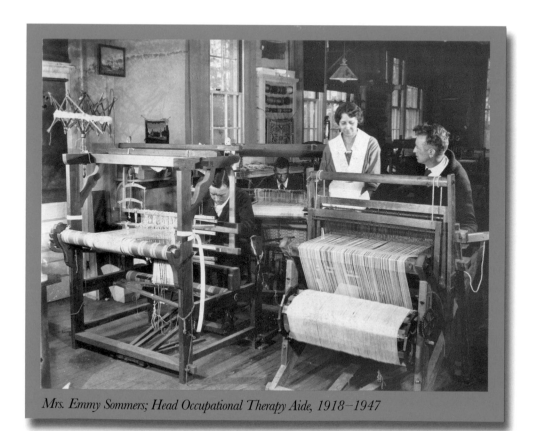

Mrs. Emmy Sommers; Head Occupational Therapy Aide, 1918–1947

In spite of the consistent and determined efforts of the Red Cross Nursing Service to provide an adequate number of nurses for the Army, recruitment was difficult all during the war. This was a period of turmoil and confusion, and not all conflicts in ideology were restricted to international events; cleavages between civilian and military medical health groups may have been more apparent than inter-agency disagreements, but the Army and the Red Cross likewise had some misunderstanding over priority of function. In regard to nurse procurement, it was the usually discreet "Pinky" Fisher who became so incensed at the proprietary attitude of Red Cross officials that he asked the Superintendent of the Army Nurse Corps caustically if the dog wagged the tail or the tail wagged the dog.[49]

The Army School of Nursing, proposed in March and authorized in May 1918, was a turning point not only in the history of the Army Nurse Corps but of the Medical Department itself. Whereas in 1908 medical officers had used civilian influence to further departmental plans for improving the status and benefits of Army doctors,[50] parenthetically the shoe was on the other foot, and a program dear to the hearts of civilian advisers was foisted on the Army. Dr. Welch and Dr. Franklin Martin were powerful allies of the non-military nurse protagonists. To the dismay of the Red Cross Nursing Service, which was thereby unable to make firm plans for assisting the Army, General Gorgas vacillated on the question of using aides, giving at least three different decisions. The controversial question was finally settled by the Armistice rather than by an acceptable policy.[51]

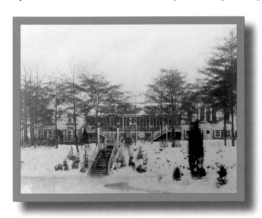

Red Cross "Hut," 1920

On August 5, 1918 Walter Reed General Hospital opened one of the first units of the Army School of Nursing and by September had a class of some forty-five students. Before the close of the year the class totaled fifty-one.[52] The influenza epidemic which swept the nation in the autumn of 1918, crippled the training program severely, and Army students were released from class work to render nursing care on the wards.[53]

In retrospect it seems obvious that cessation of war should have brought termination of the Army School of Nursing.[54] However, in March and April 1919, release was offered those students who entered the school primarily because of public pleas to render patriotic service; although begun as an emergency program, the school was continued as a civil or non-militarized activity of the Medical Department. The daily nursing duty consisted of eight hours on the wards, one hour of class and one of study, with an eight-week rotating service in the various professional services. Moreover, it required essentially two professional staffs, for the school, under the general direction of the Principal Chief Nurse, had its own director, teachers and floor supervisors, while patient care was provided by the hospital's regular nursing staff. As the program closed in the approved cantonment hospitals, the students were con-centrated at the Letterman General Hospital at the old Presidio of San Francisco and Walter Reed. Eventually, Walter Reed became the last outpost of the Army School of Nursing, the Mother House for the training of student nurses.

The professional activities carried on at Walter Reed during 1917-1918 were so greatly magnified by the expansion and departmentalization that the tranquil life of the pre-war days was unrecognizable. The expansion in the service of medicine, surgery, dentistry and nursing was no greater than that made by the laboratory service. Lieutenant Colonel[55] Henry J. Nichols became Chief of this service April 9, 1918, in time to participate in the general development of the new laboratory, storeroom, animal house and addition to the morgue. The need for the latter was made apparent during the influenza epidemic when it was necessary to erect a tent near the morgue in order to find room for the caskets and bodies. The hospital was now performing many of the Laboratory procedures formerly sent to the Army Medical School, which, likewise under expansion, was feeling the increased tempo of the times.

As in his pioneer work at the Army Medical School, Henry J. Nichols made a lasting impression on the laboratory service of Walter Reed Hospital. Here he began an intensive study of the *Streptococcus hemolytica*, culturing from the unusual number of empyema cases, from tonsils and from throats. He emphasized the importance

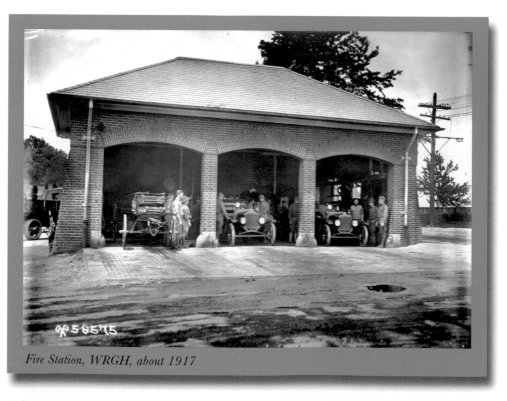

Fire Station, WRGH, about 1917

of post-mortem examinations in substantiating clinical findings, and he sponsored the detailed study of the influenza cases, both through laboratory techniques and X-ray. Of perhaps greater significance to the other professional services, he instituted the practice of joint staff meetings, rotating the responsibility and presentation of clinical material between the three major services of Laboratory, Medicine and Surgery, or one of their sub-sections.[56]

Collateral Activities

Mobilization of "practically the entire National Guard, the increase in the Regular Army and Navy" and plans for mobilizing the National Army taxed the Army Medical School facilities to the fullest. An increase in the size of the physical plant was therefore necessary if enormous quantities of vaccine were to be prepared for ready shipment to the various medical supply depots and thence for direct issue to post and camp surgeons.[57] Arthur, a Brigadier General in the National Army after October 9, 1917,[58] estimated that in that year alone the $240,000.00 net cost of vaccine manufactured at the School would have grossed $1,200,000.00 in the civilian market. Further, the 6,701 Wasserman reactions performed at slightly less than one dollar each would have cost some $33,505 if performed in a civilian laboratory.[59] The Army Medical School was therefore a profitable health investment for the Medical Department.

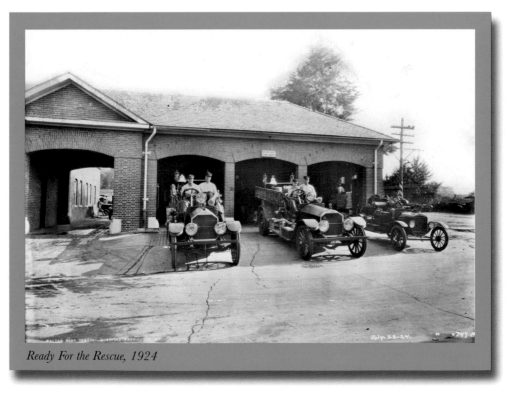

Ready For the Rescue, 1924

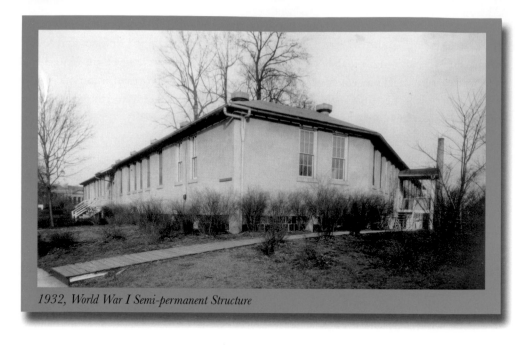

1932, World War I Semi-permanent Structure

As a War Department General Order of May 14, 1908 prescribed an annual physical test for officers, as well as examination before promotion to higher grades, the School faculty had performed this service for officer candidates in and around Washington. With expansion of the various sections of the Reserve Corps, the physical examination became a burdensome part of the School's administrative activities. Ultimately, as the records of large contingents of Reserve Officers were processed for overseas assignment, the School became essentially a small induction station, and an appropriate section called *The Foreign Service Bureau* was established.

A new responsibility was added to the academic activities during 1917, for medical officers assigned to lecture tours required moving pictures, lantern slides, charts, graphs and other addenda for illustration.[60] These were supernumerary activities and affected, primarily, the services of the younger or junior faculty members.

Many of the older and more experienced Army doctors, heads of departments and separate laboratories, were frequently engaged in teaching and writing, usually on professional subjects. In spite of being Commandant of the School, General Arthur was at heart a field officer rather than a clinician, laboratory technician or research worker. For this current literary endeavor, he chose, therefore, a subject in harmony with his own interests, and the *Military Surgeon* for January 1917, published his article on "The Advantages of Military Training for Young Men," which a later editor noted was "written with his characteristic wit and genius."[61] He spent a great part of his time during this period reviewing many Medical Department items prior to standardization, for as in the case of the Walter Reed professional facilities, these organizations were logical proving grounds and natural testing laboratories for the

Surgeon General's Office proper. This was a natural function within the organizational structure, and General Arthur participated intimately in Medical Department activities at the national level. Thus it is not surprising that in the two-year period from July 3, 1915 to June 25, 1917, he served on fourteen important Army boards.

The usual eight-month course at the Army Medical School had been shortened to accommodate the increased number of students, and the faculty substituted three four-month sessions. On November 12, 1917, an elaborate course in orthopedic surgery was opened which included sections on mechanical prostheses, research, development and repair of orthopedic appliances. This represented a distinct departure from former policies as the Medical Department usually procured, under the law of June 17, 1870, prostheses from civilian sources.[62] The required expansion in the physical plant was finally met in 1918, by leasing and adjoining a neighboring building.

Some idea of Medical Department prestige of the World War I period is reflected in the assignment, from the Rockefeller Institute for Medical Research, of one hundred fifty Medical Reserve Corps and Sanitary Corps Officers for a one-month course of laboratory instruction. Further, some thirty-six enlisted men were trained in the orthopedic workshops, and four hundred thirteen enlisted men were instructed in laboratory and X-ray procedures. In the latter case the didactic instruction was supplemented by practical on-the-job experience in nearby hospitals, military and civilian, including Walter Reed.

General Arthur estimated that the accrued savings for 1918, in School-sponsored tests and vaccines, equaled $92,189.00 on Wasserman reactions and $3,600,000.00 on the 18,000,000 doses of vaccine.[63] Moreover, the laboratory staff was actively experimenting with oil suspension rather than saline suspension of vaccines, while other qualified personnel advised the Surgeon General's Office regarding a suitable design for and manufacture of an X-ray ambulance for the portable X-ray unit, and other pieces of new equipment. Further, in addition to the numerous curricula activities, the Army Medical School staff did extensive photographic and printing work for the Surgeon General's Office, and X-ray work for the Government Hospital for the Insane.

The policy of accepting a small "advanced" class of Regular Army officers for an intensive course was abandoned as the Regular Army personnel was needed to staff new installations and overseas units. Neither the experience of the war period nor General Arthur's thirty-seven years of service with the Medical Department[64] had convinced him that bestowal of the degree of Doctor of Medicine necessarily equipped its possessor to meet the varied requirements of a medical officer in the United States Army. Thus in contemplating the phenomenal growth of the Army Medical School and possibly the prospect of a return to peacetime standards, he viewed its academic mission in terms of "a post graduate institution, with all the... equipment, and facilities for teaching everything necessary including field work to make Army Medical Officers out of selected graduates of medical schools."[65] Clearly, the Commandant viewed the School's

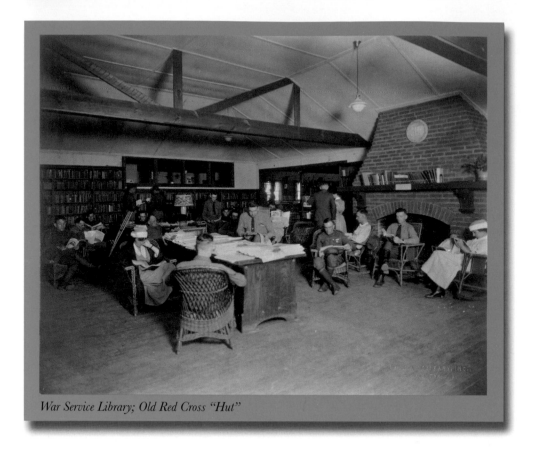

War Service Library; Old Red Cross "Hut"

future in terms of its magnificent past: a return to the eight-month course, increased physical accommodations, and a good drill and camping ground for the furtherance of field training. For if the experience of the World War I mobilization period had taught medical planners any lesson, it was in relation to adequate field medical training for the Corps and proper means of evacuating the wounded.

General Arthur had, until the autumn of 1918, a successful and distinguished career in the Medical Department. As the senior of sixty-three Regular Army Colonels[66] and temporarily a Brigadier General in the National Army, he not only considered himself an eligible successor to General Gorgas, but, with the latter's permission and endorsement, stated his credentials for the Secretary of War. In spite of his tendency to be a bit critical, even hasty in his judgment of people, in many respects he represented the ideal medical officer by the standards of the day: a positive but charming personality; courtly manners; wit; technical proficiency in his preferred field of medicine — anatomy and surgery; a cultural background which included the ability to read and speak French fluently and translate Portuguese and Italian. Moreover, he had an articulate philosophy on the Medical Department's first responsibility — support of the fighting forces of the Army. Some of his associates believed him irascible and that his facility with pen and pencil was merely an outlet for an erratic personality.[67] In any case, this latter accomplishment was his undoing.

There was considerable competition between Regular Army and Reserve officers during World War I, with the latter group compelled to wear identifying insignia. Many of the doctors believed they were unsatisfactorily placed, their services were unappreciated and that the prize assignments invariably went to members of the Regular Army Medical Corps. Once in uniform, military mores, rank and precedence, assumed dimensional importance. If as civilians they had dismissed the Army doctors as of negligible importance to medicine itself, their perspective changed rapidly as seniority became an operative factor in their own lives. Age and experience, training and assignment, were command sequelae to the regulars; to the reserve they represented a new-found prestige as well as compensation. Many reserve officers, particularly the specialist groups, alleged that the Regular Army not only failed to use their particular qualifications, but they were bitter that prescribed War Department regulations stymied reserve promotions. Unavoidably, a schism developed between the two groups.

As noted before, General Noble, through his association with General Gorgas in the Canal project, held an enviable position near the "throne." He was apparently popular and well-liked by the several distinguished and politically influential Reserve and National Guard officers stationed in the Surgeon General's Office, including Dr. Welch, who likewise held a commission and energetically inspected military camps,[68] and the civilian nurses.[69] As thirty-sixth on the list of permanent Lieutenant Colonels, he was many years the junior of some of the men then under his jurisdiction. Arthur had no assurance of being selected as Surgeon General, but it was rumored in the late summer and early fall of 1918 that General Noble might succeed to this position when General Gorgas retired for age on October 3.

Many of the most experienced and certainly the most influential men in the Corps were in responsible overseas positions at this time. Some of them undoubtedly believed, as did many officers during World War II, that the men who stayed safely at home in office positions received more rapid promotions and better rewards than those who served in the field. To them the prospect of having the civilian group of consultants and/or National Army officers control the appointment of the Surgeon General was demoralizing.

Almost as a brotherhood the Ireland faction united. Colonel Kean was elected spokesman. An appeal was presented to General Pershing to have Ireland, his Chief Surgeon during the punitive expedition in Texas, and Chief Surgeon in France, appointed Surgeon General. Pershing cabled the Secretary of War, who referred the matter to the President.[70] Again there are indications of the far-reaching Welch influence, for by July he had written the President and, more intimately, Secretary of War Baker, saying that Ireland seemed to be just the man.[71] Of more importance, perhaps, was the influence of the distinguished reserve officer, Colonel J.M.T. Finney, likewise of Baltimore, personal physician of the President and present at the European meeting where, "the Ireland gang" surrendered their individual claims to the Medical Department's highest office. (Ltr M.W. Jones, Col., M.C. ret., to writer, 10 June 1952). On October 4, 1918,

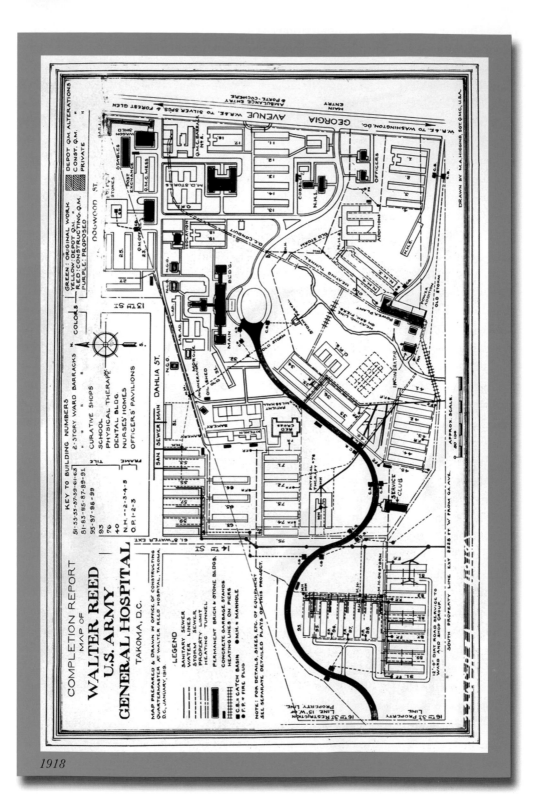

1918

Merritte W. Ireland was appointed Surgeon General. He had come a long way since his assignment as Company Commander of the First Company of Instruction to be organized at Ft. Riley, Kansas.[72]

General Nobel was rotated to overseas assignment, on his own understanding that he was General Ireland's replacement in the AEF. He was therefore both surprised and disappointed on hearing that the key assignment had gone to Colonel Walter D. McCaw and that he was to be assigned as Surgeon of the Port of Bordeaux.[73] Brigadier General Charles Richard filled the position of acting Surgeon General during October and early November 1918, in the brief interim prior to General Ireland's arrival in the United States.

Temporary promotion, or in fact any irregularity of promotion which disregards age and experience in a group structure built on seniority, seems to affect morale adversely. Thus General Noble's rapid advance over such men as Arthur, Kean, McCaw, Glennan, Keefer, Fisher, Darnall and others of the "old-timers" group rankled.[74] Ireland had disposed of the psychological aspect of the "command" problem by having Noble assigned to a minor position, but Arthur, perhaps without ready knowledge of affairs in Europe, with haste rather than foresight, penned a scathing letter to General Noble, attributing his rapid rise in rank on his ability to infatuate "a weak and misguided old man."[75]

It is useless to conjecture on "what might have been" had General Noble not been embittered, but like the Chaucerian tales, his participation in the Arthur fiasco has been preserved through many repetitions. He forwarded the Arthur letter to the already retired General Gorgas, suggesting disciplinary action. Perhaps as a result of his recent experiences with other health and medical politics, Newton D. Baker, Secretary of War, made short work of the complaint. General Arthur was reduced to his Regular Army grade of Colonel, and being sixty-two years of age he was directed to retire by order of the President.[76]

All stories must have an end, even those from real life. General Arthur's summary retirement from the Medical Corps has a pathetic side. The Noble letter was written in confidence, and although about a man for thirty years his friend,[77] his rapier-like thrusts were doubtless no more caustic than usual. Well known for his wit, his caricatures and his inclination for letter-writing, he apparently expressed the viewpoint of other more timorous officers. There is little doubt that General Gorgas had many times enjoyed the barbs directed at others, and under other circumstances he might have been more indulgent.[78]

Following his retirement, General Arthur lived for many years in Washington, visiting the Walter Reed General Hospital regularly and using the Post Library facilities with great enthusiasm. Never, even in his old age, did he lose the dignity, distinction and charming manners[79] which set him apart as the hospital's most individualistic commander. On April 19, 1936, at the age of eighty years and eighteen days, the corpulent old campaigner, veteran of the Indian Wars, commander of a hospital ship in the Spanish-American War, member of the China Relief Expedition in 1901, one-time Chief

Surgeon of the Philippine Division, Commandant of the Army Medical School, anatomist, artist and wit died at Walter Reed General Hospital, the institution he opened for the Medical Department in 1909.[80]

References

1. Elihu Root, Annual Rpt TSW, Nov. 27, 1901, quoted from Otto L. Nelson, pg 49.

2. *History of Association of Military Surgeons in U.S., 1891–1941*; Washington, The Ass. of Mil. Surgeon, 1941, pg 17.

3. Interview with Maj. Gen. Morrison C. Stayer, M.C., Ret., June 10, 1950.

4. Interview with Brig. Gen. Jefferson R. Kean, M.C., Ret., April 17, 1950.

5. Telephone conversation with Lt. Col. Nellie Close, ANC, Ret., June 1950.

6. William C. Gorgas, *Sanitation in Panama*, NY & London, D. Appleton & Company, 1915, pg 243.

7. Interview with Mrs. Montgomery Blair (Virginia Mason) and Mrs. William Blair (Mary-Eula Mason) May 29, 1951.

8. James M. Phalen (comp) *Chfs. of the Med. Dept. U.S. Army 1775–1940* (published by Army Medical Bulletin) pg 92.

9. Permanent Lieutenant Colonel, Regular Army, 15 May 1917. Colonel National Army, 26 January 1918. Brig. General National Army, 9 May 1918. Maj. Gen., USA, Asst. SG AEF, 30 October 1918.

10. Kean interview, *op cit.*

11. Interview with Col. Herbert N. Dean, MAC, Ret., April 12, 1950.

12. SGO Folder 50135, War Rec., Nat'l Archives.

13. Interview with Brig. Gen. Albert E. Truby, M.C., Ret., June 27–28, 1950.

14. Stayer interview, *op cit.*

15. Truby interview, *op cit.*

16. *Ibid.*

17. Interview with Brig. Gen. J.E. Bastion, Sept. 14, 1950; A.E. Truby interview, *op cit.*

18. A.E. Truby interview, *op cit.*

19. Ltr frm H.W. Jones, Col., M.C., Ret. to writer Aug. 12, 1951.

20. Bastion, Close, Dean interviews, *op cit*.

21. Annual Rpt WRGH, 1917.

22. *Ibid*.

23. Hist. of WRGH, prep. in 1921, on file Library, WRAH, pg 22.

24. Annual Rpt TSG, 1917, pg 230 (based on F.Y.)

25. Hist. of WRGH, *op cit*, pg 26.

26. See Annual Rpt WRGH 1918 for detailed listing.

27. Maj. Wm. C. Borden, *The Walter Reed General Hospital*, Mil. Surg., Vol. XX, 1907, pgs 20–35.

28. Ltr. Jefferson Randolf Kean to W.C. Borden, Dec. 20, 1927 (hand written) filed in Borden scrapbook.

29. Ltr. Harold W. Jones, Col. U.S. Army, Librarian AML to Colonel Daniel L. Borden, Commanding, Station Hospital, Fort Eustis, Virginia, Dec. 28, 1942 (SPMCL). Original in Borden Scrapbook; GO 64, 24 Nov. 1942.

30. Activated Nov. 1, 1942 and declared surplus in the general reduction of force, 30 June 1946.

31. Hist. of WRGH, *op cit*, pg 56.

32. Hist. of WRGH, *op cit*, pgs 57–61.

33. Hist. of WRGH, *op cit*, pg 33.

34. *Ibid*, pg 48.

35. *Ibid*, pg 55.

36. *Ibid*, pg 51.

37. *Ibid*, pg 110.

38. Government Issue.

39. Annual Rpt TSG...1918, pg 446; Ext. from ARC Nat'l Convention San Francisco, California, Hospital and Recreation Service Round Table, May 3, 1938 (Miss Margaret Lower's statement). On file Archives, ANRC.

40. Med. Dept. Hist....Vol. 5, pg 319, 320.

41. *Ibid*, pg 314.

42. Annual Rpt WRGH, 1918.

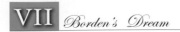

43. P.M. Ashburn, *A History of the Medical Department of the United States Army*, Boston & New York, Houghton-Mifflin, 1929, pg 329.

44. Interview Ida W. Danielson, June 7, 1950; Lt. Col. Elida Raffensperger ANC, Ret., 26 June 1950.

45. Interview Jessie M. Braden, June 26, 1950; Miss Dora Thompson, former Supt. ANC; Miss Bernice Hansen, ANC Ret., July 18, 1950 (tel.).

46. Ashburn, *op cit*, pg 369.

47. Florence A. Blanchfield, *Organized Nursing and the Army in Three Wars*, MSS on file HD SGO, pg 48–150.

48. Surgeon General's Office.

49. Interview with Miss Dora Thompson, former Supt. ANC, March 18, 1947.

50. Biography of General J.R. Kean, *op cit*.

51. Blanchfield, *op cit*.

52. Hist. Med. Dept....Vol. 5, pg 302, 303.

53. Interview Miss Anne W. Goodrich, First Dean ASN, June 21, 1947.

54. Interview with Miss Dora Thompson, Supt., ANC, *op cit*; Miss Anne Williamson, director ASN during this period; Col. Florence A. Blanchfield, Supt., ANC, and approximately 8 Army Chief Nurses familiar with the Corps history.

55. Temporary promotion.

56. Annual Rpt WRGH, 1918.

57. Annual Rpt TSG... 1917, pg 323.

58. Army Register, 1918, pg 29.

59. Annual Rpt TSG... 1917, pg 300.

60. *Ibid*, pg 301.

61. Hume, *op cit*, pg 69.

62. Annual Rpt TSG... 1917, pg 324.

63. Annual Rpt TSG... 1918, pg 440.

64. App. Ass't. Surgeon March 1881.

65. Annual Rpt TSG... 1918, pg 443.

66. Charles Richard, one file ahead of Arthur, retired about five weeks after General Gorgas.

67. Interview with Brig. Gen. Albert G. Love, MC, Ret., Feb. 13, 1951.

68. Ltr Welch to Garrison, Sept. 13, 1919, Collection... *op cit*.

69. Thompson interview, *op cit*.

70. Interview with Brig. Gen. Jefferson R. Kean, August 17, 1950.

71. Ltr Welch to Pres. Wilson, July 15, 1918, hand-written. Also ltrs from Welch to Baker, collection... *op cit*.

72. Phalen, *Chiefs of the Medical Dept.... op cit*, pg 94.

73. Conversation, Col. James C. Kimbrough, MC, Ret., Feb. 5, 1951.

74. Kean interview, *op cit*.

75. Love interview, *op cit*; Interview with Col. John Huggins, MC, Ret., Apr. 20, 1950; Interview with Brig. Gen. Frank Keefer, MC, Ret., Apr. 20, 1950; Interview with Col. James D. Fife, MC, Ret., May 26, 1950; Interview with Col. James F. Hall, MC, Ret., Apr. 17, 1950, Aug. 8, 1951.

76. B.G. Nat'l Army vacated Nov. 29, 1918; Retired Dec. 2, 1918, by order of the President.

77. Interview with Mrs. Aileen Gorgas Wrightson, July 18, 1950.

78. Acc. to General A.E. Truby, Noble pursued the issue of Arthur's retirement; Gorgas was apparently unwell by this time. Two years later he died suddenly of apoplexy, Ashburn, *op cit*, pg 295.

79. Conversation, Miss Mary E. Schick, Librarian, WRAH, Feb. 5, 1951.

80. William Hemple Arthur, (obituary). *Washington Post*, April 20, 1936.

The Gardener

1919–1922

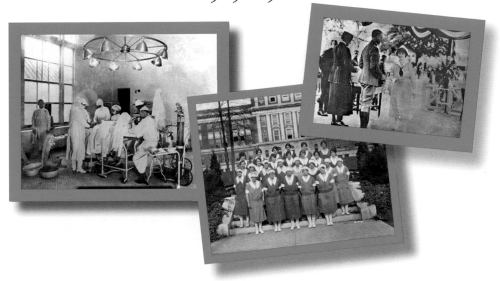

"To serve the art of medicine as it should be served one must love his fellow man."[1]

The 1914–1915 fright over the reassignment of the Army Medical Library to or near the Library of Congress apparently left key personnel in the Surgeon General's Office apprehensive lest the long-range plans for an ideal as well as complete medical post be thwarted by politicians. By the Act of May 19, 1917, the Congress appropriated $90,000 "to enlarge the Walter Reed Hospital," but to the Surgeon General's everlasting regret the exigencies of war required the erection of temporary rather than permanent buildings.

In the meantime, he was apparently able to interest some of the medical societies in the Army Medical Library's plight, and 150 letters and resolutions were on file in the Surgeon General's Office urging promotion of a new library structure.[2] The Public Building Commission proposal to develop the Mall area included razing the structure at 7th and B occupied by the Museum and Library, and the Fine Arts Commission proposed as a substitute site for the Library, the square at A and B and 4 1/2 and 6th Streets, S.W., which was assessed at $306,000.[3] Such a proposal was contrary to the long-standing Medical Department plans for a complete medical center, and in 1919 General Ireland secured the Chief of Staff's permission to add to Walter Reed certain activities such as the Army Medical School, the Army Veterinary School, the Army Dental School, and, among other buildings, an administrative and operating group, a ward group, a barracks group, power house, laundry, chapel, hospital library, nurses' residence, and officers' and non-commissioned officers' quarters at a total expenditure of $10,000,000.[4]

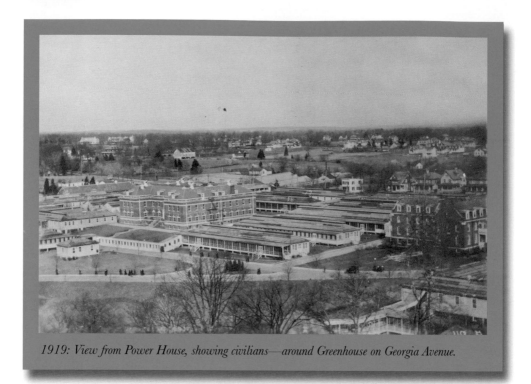

1919: View from Power House, showing civilians—around Greenhouse on Georgia Avenue.

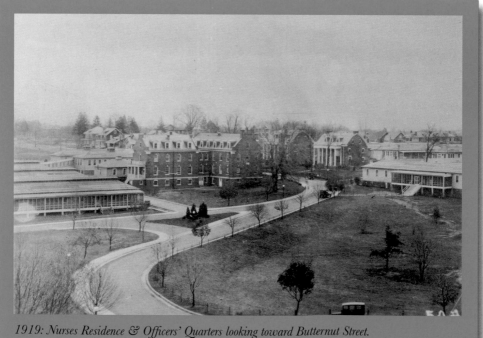

1919: Nurses Residence & Officers' Quarters looking toward Butternut Street.

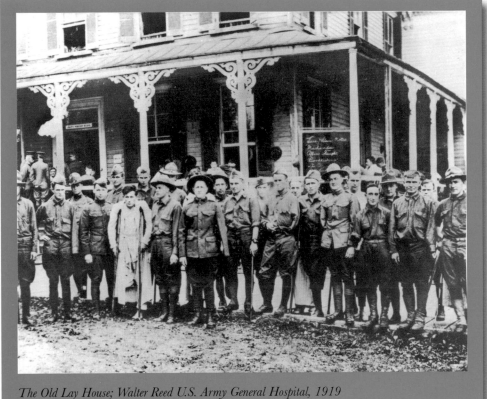

The Old Lay House; Walter Reed U.S. Army General Hospital, 1919

The Act of July 11, 1919 (41 Stat 122) provided $350,000 for the purchase of 26.9 acres of land for the *final location* of the Army Medical Museum and Library, a plan approved by the Bureau of the Budget and the President. Unless the Mall development was imminent, however, the President believed the Library project should be delayed because of a current fiscal deficit. The Director of the Budget countered with the proposal that Congress authorize the project in a special bill, with the actual monies appropriated at a later date.[5] Neither proposal resulted in action, and the principal handicap, which was to prevent indefinite development of the total plan on "Walter Reed Medical Center" now came into relief: the War Department was unwilling to support a costly technical service operation from its general appropriation, and the usual demands on the Medical Department budget prevented construction of the Library from its own current appropriation.

One section of the new 26.9 acre tract was bounded by Dogwood Street on the north, by 13th Street on the west, and to the southeast followed the line of the "original hospital reservation." This included part of the old Shepherd estate, with its stone gatehouse. A second section was bounded by Dahlia Street on the north, 14th Street on the west and on the southeast and followed the line of the "original hospital reservation." A third tract extended "the northern and southern boundary lines of the original reservation west of 16th Street." This addition increased the holdings to approximately 69.136 acres,[6] a number still insufficient for final realization of *Borden's Dream*, which, in any case, had neither appropriations for buildings nor a first priority over other Medical Department projects.

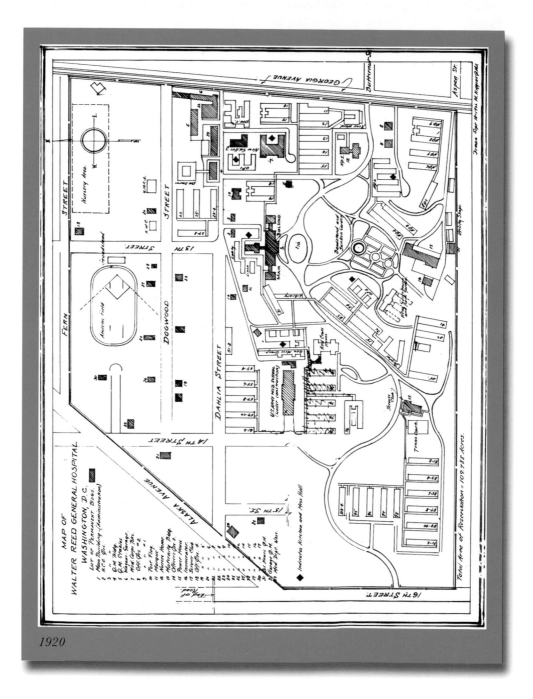

1920

As in 1915, the Library now came in for attention as a non-military activity, and although current publicity noted agreeably that the "three principal units in the contemplated medical center (were) the Walter Reed Hospital, the Medical Museum, and the Library," now widely separated, their assembly had the heartiest cooperation of "the entire medical fraternity of the United States and allied governments." The Library was compared to the great library in Petrograd, destroyed by fire and, said the *Washington Star* in a promotional spirit, it was "called Surgeon General's library but is in fact the library of the medical profession in the United States.[7]

In spite of now possessing land, the two more static institutions, the Library and Museum, represented no immediate housing problem, whereas the overgrown Army Medical School, with its expanding sub-service training programs, was in desperate need of shelter.

General Ireland was a man of strong likes and dislikes.[8] Well prepared for his position as Surgeon General both through training and temperament, he was extremely interested in developing the permanent general hospital to a new state of excellence, and he insistently exerted his not inconsiderable talents and charms for the general benefit of the Department.[9] Many of the Corps' most influential leaders agreed that the Army Medical School facilities were inadequate. Moreover, under the current plans for expanded field training at Carlisle Barracks, it seemed more important that the School activities, including the vitally needed vaccine laboratories, be housed at once.

Both the Surgeon General and General Kean were friendly to the General Staff,[10] and both were unusually successful in influencing both General Staff and Congressional support for Medical Department programs; the $500,000 appropriated under the Congressional Act of June 5, 1920, for the first portion of the Army Medical School was a tribute to this endeavor. The matter did not rest there, however, for the Acts of March 20 and July 1, 1922, provided $94,703.44 and $44,109.22 respectively to pay adjudicated awards for lands condemned by the War Department "for additions to the hospital and for the site of the Surgeon General's Library."[11] Therefore, for the time being, a medical center seemed assured.

"Noisy Jim"

James D. Glennan returned from Europe to become commandant of Walter Reed General Hospital on March 19, 1919. A long-time friend of the Surgeon General, who affectionately called him "Noisy Jim," this brilliant, quiet and almost abnormally reticent man was destined to leave an indelible mark on the buildings and grounds.[12] Long after his time, when only the composite beauty of the landscaping and a modest bronze plaque in the garden remained to identify him as God's servant in the great out-of-doors, James Glennan was still a topic for social conversation at Army dinner tables.[13]

The assignment at Walter Reed was ideal for one of his talents and interests, for little had been done in landscaping. Dr. David Lumsden, formerly of Cornell University, had been an enthusiastic member of the Plant and Agricultural part of the rehabilitation program during the war. Still in Washington, serving as horticulturist of the Department of Plant Immunization, U.S. Department of Agriculture,[14] he was a willing ally in the plans for landscaping the hospital grounds. James Holland, head gardener at Soldiers' Home during Colonel Glennan's incumbency prior to the war, joined this pair of nature-lovers in 1920.[15] And as the Colonel's interest in gardening became known, the hospital received many shrubs and trees as gifts, including the then rare weeping cherry tree transplanted from the disbanded Freeman Nursery to the sunken garden.

Between Colonel Glennan's enthusiasm, Professor Lumsden's technical knowledge and Mr. Holland's industry, all the trees, shrubs and plants on the grounds were identified, labeled and a cardex filing system was maintained in the Adjutant's office. Officers wore white shirts with their olive drab uniforms in those days, and it was not unusual for Colonel Glennan, when wandering about the hospital or grounds, to pencil his observations on his snow white cuffs. The ivy which grew profusely on the old stone gatehouse had been brought from England many years before, and it provided new growth on the walls of the permanent hospital buildings. The original start of mint, first transplanted around a small fountain in the sunken garden, but now growing wild around the reservation, was brought from England about 1600 and planted at Scuffletown Tavern,[16] in Orange County, Virginia. Like other horticultural contributions, it was given by interested friends.

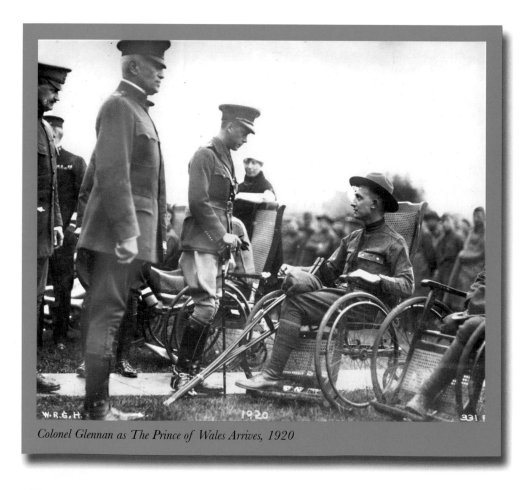

Colonel Glennan as The Prince of Wales Arrives, 1920

The colonial architecture of all of the permanent structures was approved by the Fine Arts Commission, and Colonel Glennan attempted to have the buildings erected in line with the Washington Monument. The Service Club, hastily built in 1920, did not comply with this surveying requirement, but the error was not discovered until four years later, after the Army Medical School building was erected and the dogwood trees were planted along the walk leading to the Rea swimming pool and the School. The day this irregularity was discovered was one long to be remembered, for the Colonel searched diligently for a scapegoat–and chose the unwary Adjutant as the object of his unpredictable wrath. He allegedly sulked for three days without so much as saying "Good Morning" to his office personnel.[17]

The Dominant Types

Colonel William L. Keller, a Regular Army doctor of exacting professional standards was allegedly passed by the Examining Board because of General Arthur's insistence that the early evidence of his professional acumen entitled him to special consideration. Having won his point, Arthur, as a later Division Surgeon in the Philippines, had an opportunity to see his protégé at work. For then the young Doctor Keller was using every opportunity to practice experimental surgery, and according to Arthur's lusty reminiscences, every time he saw the young surgeon he was trying frantically to dispose of "a bucket of dog guts."[18]

Quiet, conservative, reserved, and frugal,[19] the young surgeon blustered a good deal, probably in order to hide his extreme shyness[20] and to conceal his exceedingly deep sympathy for human suffering, especially in children.[21] Known for his gentleness, he was also known as a martinet.[22] Erect of posture, forbidding in appearance until one recognized the tenderly sympathetic expression in his tranquil blue eyes, the entourage of young surgeons who followed him on ward rounds did so in almost complete awe and silence. A hard worker, he established a rigid and inexorable custom of night visits, but he never imposed regulations or standards on others that he was unable or unwilling to meet. And to some who knew him well, his greatest contribution to military medicine was not in his brilliant pioneer work in empyema, performed at Walter Reed during the early twenties, but in the example set by his self-imposed and exceedingly high professional code, his sound and conservative surgical judgment, and the primary maxim used in training young surgeons – that the patients' interests always come first.[23] No hour was too late and no job was too difficult for him to undertake.[24] A non-Catholic, he nevertheless steadfastly refused to perform an abortion.

On one well-remembered occasion, the Chief of the Medical Service pled with him to surgically abort three seriously ill patients, all of whom had some morbid complication such as pulmonary tuberculosis. Flatly and unequivocally, the Chief of the Surgical Service refused. The Chief of Medical Service, equally obdurate in his quiet way, was indignant, for he expected the patients to die.

The situation came to a deadlock, with neither physician capitulating. It was well known that one of Colonel Keller's few self-indulgences was fishing, and that with great regularity he spent his thirty-day annual leave pursuing Colorado trout. It was not the fishing season, however, when quite unexpectedly the Chief of the Surgical Service announced that he wasn't feeling well, believed he was in need of a rest, and would be absent from Walter Reed for ten days or two weeks. He was noted for his rude good health; his staff was aghast at this break in his orderly routine. He had hardly departed for his "convalescence," however, when the Assistant Chief of the Surgical Service eased himself into the medical office to inquire if there were any cases for surgeons.[25]

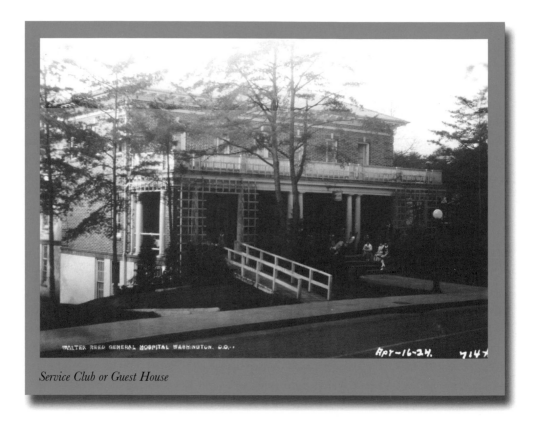

Service Club or Guest House

A second young surgeon, likewise assigned at Walter Reed in January 1919, was destined for distinction. The Army Medical School had started its special course in orthopedics in 1917, and as the overseas casualties began to arrive in considerable numbers, the hospital prepared for the overflow by separating orthopedics from general surgery. From January 1919 until May 1925, and again from June 1930 until March 1934, Norman T. Kirk was chief of this section at Walter Reed. From January 1941 until June 1942, he was Chief of the Surgical Service; from June 1943 until June 1947, he lived on the reservation, in the quarters formerly occupied by Colonel Keller but reassigned to the Surgeon General of the Army, the position he then filled with his usual energy and dispatch. In the "twice told tales" so familiar in Army social groups, an undocumented story is often repeated that as a young surgeon Kirk had no particular desire to specialize in orthopedics, and that Keller literally had to persuade him to undertake the necessary but not especially attractive role of becoming an "old sawbones," giving his personal word that he would never regret the decision. Although Colonel Keller refuted statements that through his tremendous prestige as "Surgeon Emeritus" of the Medical Department he tipped the political scales and influenced the appointment of Norman T. Kirk as Surgeon General, in 1943, this story, like others that people want to believe, gained wide circulation throughout the Medical Corps.

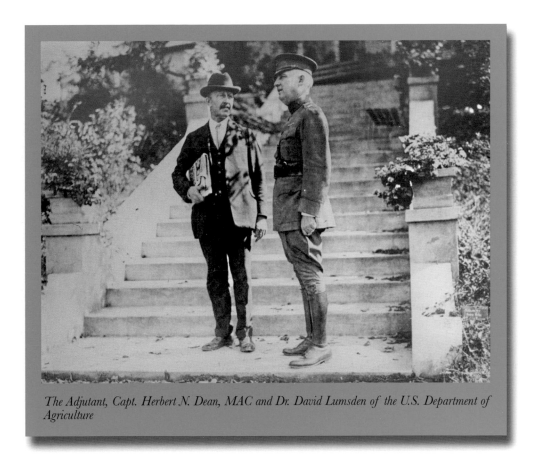

The Adjutant, Capt. Herbert N. Dean, MAC and Dr. David Lumsden of the U.S. Department of Agriculture

These two dynamic but compatible personalities worked together harmoniously through the years, and although entirely different in temperament they were constant friends. Where one was large, with leonine head and clear blue eyes, quiet, genteel, "Scotch" and unsociable the other was small, ruddy, brusque and with twinkling eyes as azure blue as the sea he loved so well. Like his preceptor, no hour was too late for him to return to the hospital to change a dressing or check the prognosis sheet; no patient was too humble to receive his expert best in surgical care. An ardent tuna fisherman, a successful amateur gardener and a satisfactory golfer, he was a man of lightning decisions and unstudied actions. No friend could ask too much of him; no enemy received quarter.[26] He was small, quick in his movement and with little that could be called "military bearing."

The soldiers swore by him; many nurses complained unnecessarily of his exacting professional standards.[27] Like many of the medical officers of his generation, one of his first Army assignments included a detail at the Barnes Hospital, U.S. Soldiers' Home. No purist, his vocabulary was a man's vocabulary. A rough and ready type, he appeared uncomfortable at the leisurely tea parties fashionable in that day. An old retainer at the Soldier's Home was apparently as omniscient of his future as Colonel Keller, for he predicted that the young lieutenant would sometime hold the Medical Department's highest office, and he promised that on the day of this appointment he would shine the little doctor's shoes. In 1943, when he was appointed Surgeon General of the Army, this loyal old man was one of the first to congratulate him, reminding his again of the long-ago promise and forgotten prediction.[28]

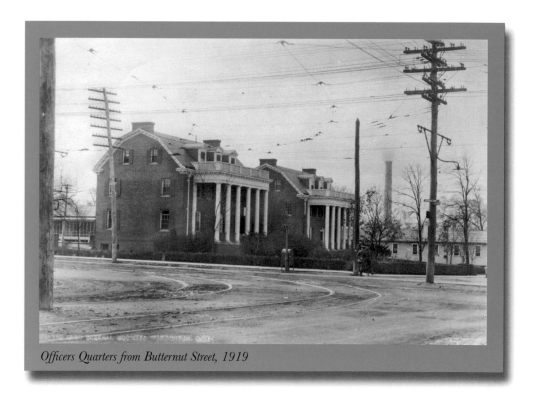

Officers Quarters from Butternut Street, 1919

Within These Walls

By 1920 the hospital had been reduced to a 1500-bed capacity, and Colonel Glennan was making strenuous attempts to restore both normal routine and a normal appearance. Some 7,923 cubic yards of earth were excavated from the area north of the stables, on Dogwood Street, and distributed in the re-graded sunken garden, which was created on top of the fourteen-foot causeway then encasing Cameron's Creek. Contracts were let for landscape supplies and nursery stocks, for painting of barracks, the non-commissioned officers' quarters and thirty-four hospital wards; a small nursery and greenhouse were erected.[29]

The professional activities were even more time-consuming than the administrative and some 5,407 patients were admitted to the principal services of medicine and surgery. No noteworthy new methods and treatments were devised during this year, but an electrocardiograph formerly used at the wartime General Hospital Number 9, Lakewood, New Jersey, was installed, and the first of 388 recordings for 1920 was made on April 26. Of further interest in the clinical care of patients, the Medical Service used the Tissot Gassometer and Russell-Sage modification of the Henderson Holdane Gas Analysis apparatus for recording basal metabolisms, for none of the newer, simpler and easier methods had proved entirely accurate and reliable.[30] In 1922, the laborious and time-consuming procedure of recording basal metabolisms was assigned to the Laboratory Service. Patients were transported from the various hospital wards by ambulance, and in accordance with accepted clinical practices, they were kept almost frighteningly inactive and quiet.

Walter Reed was by then a center for empyema work and many cases were transferred from home stations and abroad. It was in this special field that Colonel Keller earned his well-deserved reputation as a successful surgeon. Many acute cases resulted from the

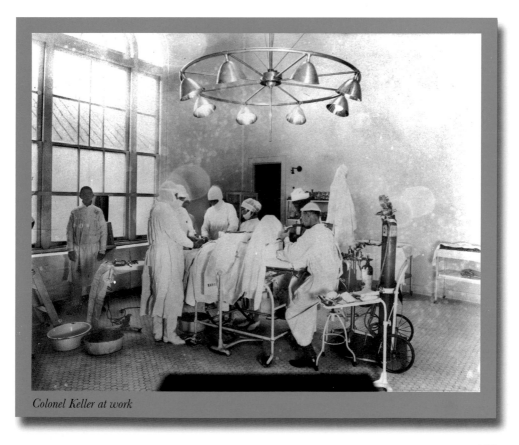

Colonel Keller at work

1918–1919 influenza epidemic, but they were treated so successfully that the mortality was less than five per cent. Further, none of the Keller-treated primary cases became chronic,[31] an unusual record for those antibioticless days, for the majority of the cases transferred to Walter Reed from other institutions had defied the usual treatment.[32]

The Neuro-Surgical Section was occupied chiefly with the remaining cases of war wounds, with approximately eighty per cent of the patients having gunshot wounds of the peripheral nerves. The Orthopedic Section discharged 367 cases that year as having been completely fitted and instructed in the use of prostheses. As the Troutman prostheses for thigh and leg stumps were highly satisfactory, permanent prosthesis for disarticulation of the hip was discontinued, and a light weight fiber thigh bucket with molded socket for hip, developed at the hospital, was substituted. As in the case of neuro-surgical disabilities, the majority of the cases treated on the Orthopedic Section resulted from gunshot wounds. Some had been unsuccessfully treated in other Army hospitals and some were transferred from hospitals that had closed. In general, however, the majority of cases required revision of the stump, and during 1920 alone, a total of 167 Orthopedic operations were performed.

Army surgeons may have been more pompous in those days, the Army regulations more strict, or pride in wearing the uniform more acute than in the generally civilian-minded Corps of a quarter of a century later. Sabres were worn for inspections, usually on Saturday morning, and at court martials; as a rule officers appeared in full dress uniform with slight encouragement. In the case of surgeons, it was the small gesture of exchanging sabre for scalpel that transformed the military medical officer into the king of all he surveyed–the operating room.[33]

Familiarly called "the grasshopper courses," the post-war surgical refresher courses for Regular Army officers, begun in June 1919, included assignment to the various surgical sub-sections where, regardless of the competence of his associates, Colonel Keller's rigid professional standards included a weekly inspection of all patients, and carefully supervised clinical instruction. It was probably during this period that he formed the habit of making ward rounds, flanked by the younger members of his staff. More than one patient quailed at the sound of tramping feet in the usually quiet halls of the surgical wards, where except for the courageous whispering of the laggards who composed "the rear echelon,"[34] there was no sound.

The hospital's dental staff was decreased from thirteen to nine officers during this year, but the reduced members managed, somehow, to meet the clinical load. The X-ray department, in spite of the decreasing number of war casualties, was obviously in more general clinical use, for 12,000 patients used some 30,000 plates and films. Dermatology and Urology were associated under one Section Chief, and in the latter specialty, 149 operations were performed, while a "large number" of venereal cases were treated. The Obstetrical and Gynecological section was proportionately busy, for 106 healthy infants were delivered, twenty-four of which were instrument cases; two mothers required caesarean operations.

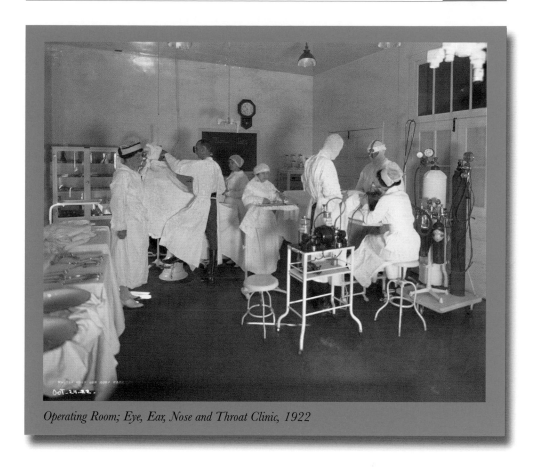

Operating Room; Eye, Ear, Nose and Throat Clinic, 1922

As the busy Surgical Service performed 2,439 operations during 1920, it is little wonder that the annual report carried a statement that "anesthesia is a developing field … and there is much to be investigated especially as to nitrous oxygen; it is the aim of this department to add its effort to the progress of this rather neglected branch of surgery." Two unnamed Army nurses and two civilian nurses from Providence Hospital, Washington, D.C., were trained in the use of gas oxygen anesthesia. Further, the Department of Anesthesia reported a detailed break-down on its cases: of the 1,305 general surgical cases exclusive of obstetrics, 649 received nitrous oxide; 123 nitrous oxide-oxygen-ether mixtures; 533 were nitrous oxide-ether sequences. Moreover, 797 local anesthetics were used in addition to the inhalation method. Of the 2,439 operations, the EENT Section led with 1,081; of the 1,358 remaining operations, 321 were in general surgery, with appendectomies and herniotomies leading the list.

Aloof and noncommittal "Noisy Jim" Glennan was sometimes misunderstood by some of his associates.[35] The Adjutant found it difficult to secure his official signature, and he held administrative officers accountable for routine and probably unavoidable administrative oversights. Occasionally he displayed a lusty temper, and he could be both contrary and cantankerous.[36] Withal he was beloved. Whatever his temperamental

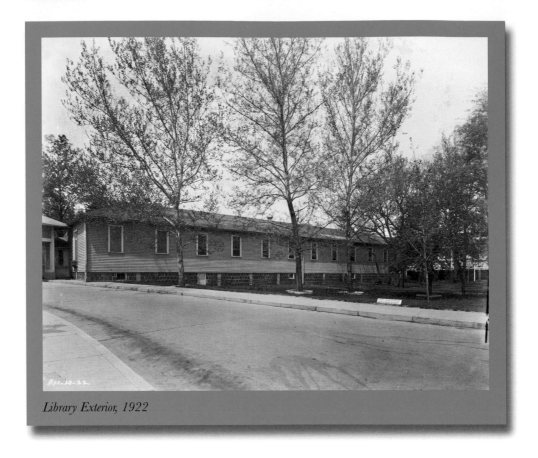

Library Exterior, 1922

idiosyncrasies, he knew definitely what he wanted to do with the now famous hospital entrusted to his management, and he was determined to have only the best available personnel. Miss Lower, like Mrs. Rea, was a volunteer worker during her term as assistant Field Director. From late 1919 until 1922, two male incumbents filled this position, but eventually Miss Lower accepted the responsibility and became a paid representative of the Red Cross.

When it came to selecting a librarian, Colonel Glennan had no more hesitation in pirating the librarian he had known at the Soldiers' Home prior to the war than he had in "recruiting" the head gardener. In March 1920, Mary E. Schick joined the then highly individualistic staff at Walter Reed. Colonel Glennan was extremely interested in the war service library, which was unsuitably housed in the basement of the Red Cross house, and wanted to expand it as a permanent function. Funds were then unavailable for construction of a permanent building, which for convenience should be near the Main Building. Perhaps on an impulse, perhaps because his subtle Irish humor was tantalized by the prospect of having the autocratic chief of the Surgical Service lose a bout with the supposedly weaker sex, the commanding officer offered the new librarian one of Colonel Keller's surgical convalescent wards, appropriately

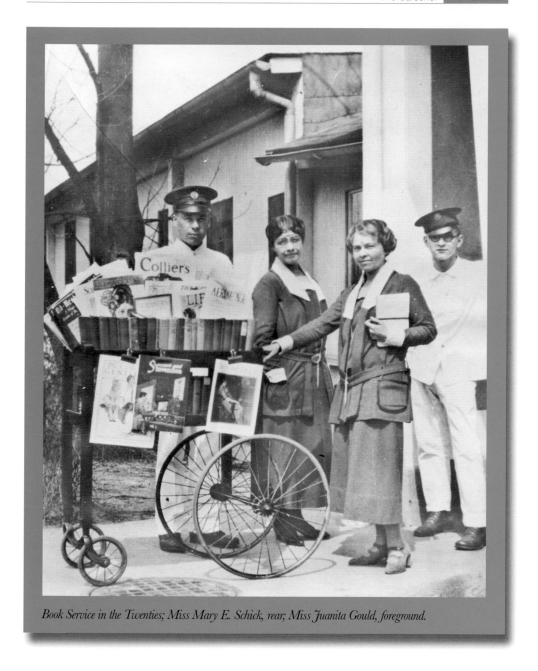

Book Service in the Twenties; Miss Mary E. Schick, rear; Miss Juanita Gould, foreground.

located on "the main drag." On the assumption that possession was "nine points of the law," the move was to be accomplished during the annual Keller vacation. Convalescent patients were pressed into service, and the books were sorted and placed on litters for quick removal from the Red Cross house to the converted ward. The move was not only made with dispatch, but in time the victor and the vanquished became warm friends.[37]

The now legendary stories credit Surgeon General Ireland, a man of warm sparkling personality, with lamenting plaintively that "Noisy Jim" outshone him with the ladies, that he sat back quietly, saying nothing, while the women struggled for his attention;[38] whereas he, Ireland, had to bid for their attention. The tribute to "Noisy Jim's" personality was undoubtedly the only accurate part of the friendly gibe, for old timers well remember the grace, charm and seemingly impartial division of the time he spent making "inspection trips," which conveniently included the afternoon tea hour and the first ladies of the Red Cross and the Library, as these organizations and their directors came to maturity and full bloom under his wise guidance and support.[39]

Catastrophe

The sharpshooter's tree, famous since Jubal Early's raid on Fort Stevens, stood in front of the nurses' residence and across from the Commanding Officers' quarters. Long since recovered from its pruning by Civil War bullets, the old landmark could not withstand the severe ice storm of December 1920, and when it was splintered beyond nature's repair, uprooted and removed, Colonel Glennan grieved as though for a friend. It was, he mused, like an old man that had lived too long.[40]

The year was not to end without further sorrow at the hospital, for on Sunday, December 12, at 11 a.m., a mentally "alienated" patient set fire to a chair cushion in one of the frame barracks assigned to the neuropsychiatric section for the care of shell-shocked and neurotic cases. The patient was removed from the ward promptly, but he eluded his attendants and re-entered the building to lose his life in the flames. Wards forty-three and forty-four, quartering seventy-five patients, were completely destroyed, wards forty-one and forty-two were partially damaged, and several of the patients suffered minor injuries.

The hand apparatus of the Walter Reed fire department proved inadequate for the occasion, and the three-alarm call was answered by neighboring "hook and ladder" companies. Medical Department enlisted men, always drilled for fire action, met the situation bravely, and student and graduate nurses were commended for their heroic action. The potentially hazardous frame buildings had been called to the attention of the Congress, but fiscal appropriations were not forthcoming. It required, therefore, a tragedy to bring the unsafe conditions of the temporary buildings to public attention.[41] In the months immediately following, mental cases from the "forty group" were housed in the "eighty group" of semi-permanent stucco buildings.[42]

It is interesting in this connection, to note that 621 neuropsychiatric cases were

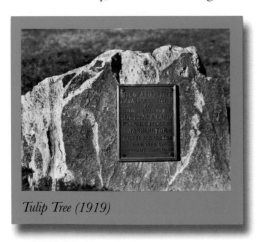

Tulip Tree (1919)

treated during 1920, of which twenty were classed as AWOL cases; twenty-three as cerebro spinal lues; eighty as constitutional psychopathic states; one hundred seventy-five as Dementia Praecox; sixteen as diseases due to alcoholism and drug addiction; twenty-nine for Epilepsy; fifteen for general paralysis of the Insane; twenty-five for Manic Depressive Insanity; five for Mental Deficiency; twenty-seven as "no" nervous or mental disease; twenty for organic diseases of the central nervous system (non-luetic); one hundred eighty-six for psychoneuroses,[43] that wonderfully inclusive term that conceals a multitude of undefined ailments.

The Calendar Changes

Only one hundred twenty more patients were admitted to the hospital in 1921 than in 1920, but two hundred seventy-one more operations were performed, statistical evidence of the industry of the surgical staff and the popularity of the institution.

Although from fifty to seventy-five per cent of all patients were engaged in one or more types of occupational therapy, it was necessary to reduce the departmental staff by September. Some of the aides had been quartered in temporary frame and canvas buildings erected just across Georgia Avenue and above Geranium Street, where a low-cost housing development was built during World War II. After September 1921, such

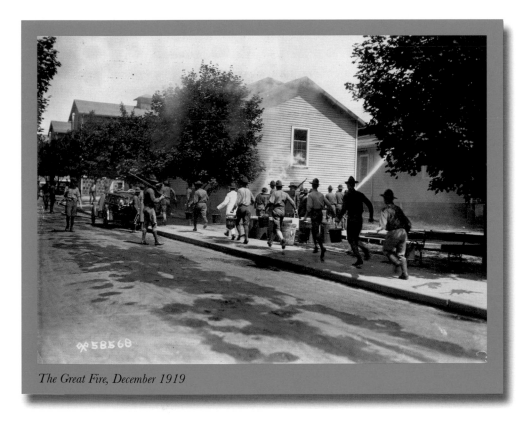

The Great Fire, December 1919

personnel were quartered on the Post in one of the frame barracks formerly assigned to the nurses. In line with the general reduction, such subjects as electricity, and in the fine arts, illustrating, lettering, modeling and painting; sign painting; machine shop practice; mechanical drawing, etc., were dropped from the program. In contrast, the Physiotherapy Department, with only two head aides and twenty-three assistants, gave some 15,400 treatments monthly.

Seventy Regular Army nurses, 60 reserve nurses and 228 students provided nursing services for 5,527 patients at Walter Reed in 1921, where the first class of students was graduated from the Army School of Nursing.

Ten dietitians then were employed in the Mess Department or Food Service, which operated six different messes for a daily average of 1,943 individuals. This department was administered by a Captain in the Medical Administrative Corps and employed forty-three civilians, seven non-commissioned officers and seventy-five enlisted men. The Head Dietician acted as liaison between the department, the medical officers and the ward nurses, instructed student nurses, assigned dietitians and controlled all matters pertaining to the subsistence (feeding) of the sick.[44] Administration of the food service was more complicated than appeared at first glance, for fifty-four per cent of the service was devoted to *regular* or "House Diets"; nineteen per cent to *special diets*; seventeen per cent to *light, soft or liquid diets*; ten per cent to *medical diets*. *Army Regulations* provided that enlisted patients receive the regular garrison ration, usually with a twenty-five per cent surplus to provide for special items required in the care of the sick. In November 1921, this amount was increased to fifty per cent in order to compensate for the seasonal advance in milk, butter, eggs, fresh vegetables, fruits, etc., with the additional expense met by subsidy from the Surgeon General's central hospital fund, composed of accrued savings from unused diets, etc., and from the surplus Post Exchange Fund.[45]

In October 1922, the Army School of Nursing was followed by a school for hospital dietitians, which accepted only two students for the first class, and a school for physio-therapists, with a first class of fourteen young women. Physiotherapists were required to have a pre-requisite of at least a two-year academic course in an approved School of Physical Education. When graduated from the Army Schools, both dietitians and physiotherapists were eligible for Civil Service appointments.

The Laboratory Service was becoming an increasingly busy professional activity, performing, in 1922, some 91,032 examinations; thirty-four per cent of the deaths were autopsied in comparison to only twenty-five per cent of the year before. Basal metabolism readings were used more frequently, with 217 "runs" in comparison to the fifty-two for 1921. The staff was performing experimental work in tuberculosis through animal inoculation. A necessary adjunct to the professional activities, the *Department of Illustration*, staffed by enlisted technicians, was diligently making lantern slides and photographing both operative procedures and patients, especially empyema cases, for use in the clinical training programs.

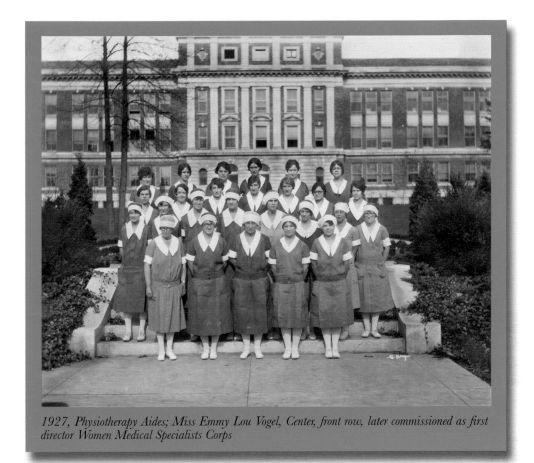

1927, Physiotherapy Aides; Miss Emmy Lou Vogel, Center, front row, later commissioned as first director Women Medical Specialists Corps

The *Office of Supervisor of Clinical Records* was an important and busy function, and although it controlled the entire clinical record system, it was different from similar civilian services in that it was responsible for the discipline, pay, clothing, correspondence, military records, disposition (including the necessary physical examination) and processing of patients leaving the hospital for disability or on expiration of term of leave. As there were many Veterans Bureau patients, a factor that required close coordination with the main Veterans' agency, a separate section secured the appropriate data, prepared reports and carried on correspondence incidental to the hospitalization of the claimants. Approved procedures provided that the Veterans Bureau paid the Army stipulated amounts for the hospitalization of Veteran patients.

The Dental Department treated 5,675 officers and enlisted men in 15,370 sittings; 1,284 "others" in 3,314 sittings and 812 Veterans Bureau patients in 2,064 sittings. A large part of the dental survey work was performed in search for foci of infection; 9,079 roentgenograms were made. Of the 5,286 inpatient admissions in 1922, the majority came from nearby stations, but 217 were transferred from abroad, and 1,069 were admitted from other regions in the United States. Nearly one half were surgical cases, and half again, or 1,223, were EENT cases. Further, an additional 2,319 "minor surgical procedures," such as the injection of salversan, were not added into the total.

The distribution in patient load now showed a marked change from the admissions of 1909–1912, for more civilian dependents were using the hospital facilities:

> *731*   *were officers*
> *1739*   " *enlisted men*
> *146*   " *nurses*
> *1456*   " *Veterans Bureau cases*
> *1214*   " *Civilian dependents.*

This policy not only cultivated good morale, but it was practically essential to the welfare of the low-income enlisted and non-commissioned officer group. Further, it was invaluable to a balanced training program for Army doctors. Like a buxom adolescent, Walter Reed now in the second decade of its growth, was exceeding its original function as "the general hospital for the Eastern United States and as the post hospital for Washington Barracks," as defined in the Surgeon General's earlier reports.

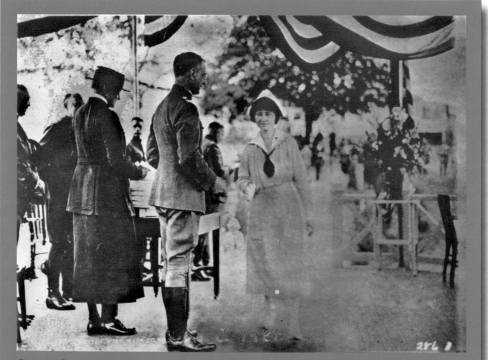

Surgeon General Ireland presenting diplomas, first graduating class, Army School of Nursing; Major Julia C. Stimson, Superintendent of the Army Nurse Corps on the left.

Other Changes

The Come Back, published for twenty-seven months through the courtesy of interested businessmen in the District of Columbia, first planned to release its final issue on March 19. As it had provided practical instruction for a class in journalism, the *Reconstruction Division* effectually urged that this tiny 9x12, four-page publication continue as a Walter Reed newspaper, subsidized from Post Exchange Funds.[46]

The Acts of March 20 and July 1, 1922 provided $94,703.44 and $44,109.22 to pay the adjudicated lands earmarked for the Walter Reed reservation, and the Quartermaster Section of the annual report noted the acquisition of four sets of officers' quarters on Elder and Dogwood Streets and Alaska Avenue. These were, in the strict sense, civilian residences and not regulation government quarters.

A new brick guardhouse was built on the southwest corner of Dahlia Street during the year, and the athletic field bounded by Georgia Avenue, Dogwood and Fern Streets was graded. According to the annual report, Miss Rosalind Wood of Massachusetts donated $25,000 for erection of a range of greenhouses, and on June 28 the contract was let for a Rose House, Carnation House and Palm House adjacent to the formal garden. Although all were completed within six months,[47] there is reason to assume that this amount was insufficient and that the Red Cross allowed a subsidy.[48] Of great significance to the Medical Department as well as to the hospital, a $500.00 contract was let for construction of the long contemplated new Army Medical School building, which, by December 1922, was already thirty-six per cent complete.

"The new year, 1921," said Kean in his diary, "brought a change of administration. The Democratic Administration had apparently outstayed its welcome, and the Army and Navy were joyful over the departure of their former secretaries, Baker and Daniels...

> *The change in administration was not in every way an improvement, however, for the medical profession was amazed at the apparition in public life of a comic little figure, Dr. Charles E. Sawyer, who had been the medical attendant of the President's wife. Although he had never had any military service, he was made Brigadier General in the Reserve and became the medical advisor to the administration on all medical matters, including military and naval medicine, and all questions of medical supply.*[49]

This particular change of administration was of especial interest to the Medical Department, for General Leonard Wood was an unsuccessful contender for the Presidential nomination on the Republican ticket, according to some speculators, because he would make no commitments to the politicians.[50] The new administration was hardly under way when the appearance of the little homeopathic doctor, who frequently accompanied Mrs. Harding on visits to Walter Reed, upset the ranking military medical men in Washington. For reasons best known to the doctors, their tiny five-foot, two-inch contemporary was christened with the Indian-like name of "Pawknee," and almost immediately he and his custom-made boots, custom-made uniform and urgent desire to demonstrate his position in "top-drawer" politics became the subject of many jokes.[51] In fact, it was during his first visit to the hospital that Mrs. Sawyer confided her troubles to interested staff personnel – she had padded her husband's Harrison cap with paper to prevent it from slipping down on his ears.[52]

Distressed because he was only a First Lieutenant, Dr. Sawyer reputedly presented his problem to General Noble, by then back in the United States and serving as librarian of the Army Medical Library, and was informed that the Presidential Executive Order was all inclusive. By a mere stroke of the Executive pen he could be a Brigadier General as easily as a First Lieutenant. Like the acorn and the tree, from little things come big, and some influential medical planners believed that eventual conversion of the 1918 Bureau of War Risk Insurance, with its ultimately controversial Board of Vocational Education,[53] into the Veterans Bureau was facilitated because of "Pawknee's" earnest desire to become a bureaucrat. Further, it was believed that he may have influenced formation of the Federal Board of Hospitalization, responsible for selecting sites and plans for federal hospitals, and his own appointment as Chief Coordinator.[54] The members were representatives from the Army, Navy, Veterans Administration, Department of Indian Affairs, Director of St. Elizabeth's (the Government Hospital for the Insane); and the United States Public Health Service.[55]

Warren G. Harding was the first American president to visit Walter Reed, and the occasion was momentous. Colonel Glennan gave orders that all convalescent patients be stationed around the flag circle. Washed and groomed, dressed in their best, they were to meet the great man. As he stood near his office window watching the gathering crowd, he saw, to his horror, a buxom woman in diaphanous chiffon dress and large picture hat, wandering conspicuously among his interested charges. The Glennan language belied the Glennan reputation, for "Noisy Jim's" monumental calm was shattered when he discovered the "visitor" was the wife of a patient hospitalized for an in-growing toenail.[56]

The School Program

Like all other post-war military medical activities, the Army Medical School program showed some recession, and only thirty-five student officers were graduated at the 24th session, October 1, 1919 to May 28, 1920. Instruction in laboratory procedures was still the main emphasis, but a one-month course in pathology and 14 hours of lecture and 40 hours of laboratory work in food and nutrition were added.[57] The X-ray Section did a rushing business, as patients from the Attending Surgeon's Office, Washington, the Examining Boards, some of the outlying camps and hospitals, and occasionally a selected case from Walter Reed were studied by the Army Medical School experts who performed some 2,190 examinations in 1920.[58] The majority of the trained roentgenologists from civil life had reverted to inactive reserve status, and so the Medical Department

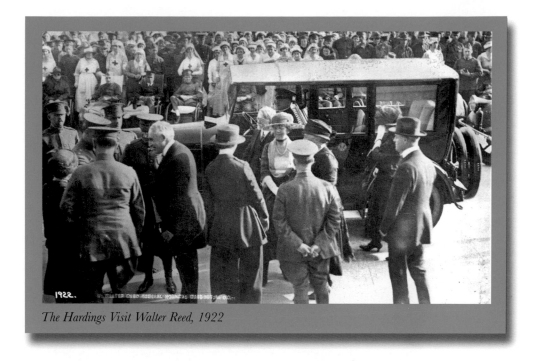

The Hardings Visit Walter Reed, 1922

continued its well established efforts to increase the number of specialists through a twelve-week course in X-ray. The schedule was divided into three four-week periods, with X-ray physics taught in the first period, the students receiving practical work in the roentgenology laboratories of the School and hospital.[59]

The School records for August 1, 1919, show that a sharp division in subject matter was contemplated at such time as a *Field Medical Camp* was selected by the Surgeon General, a change that would permit the relocation of the Army Medical School at the proposed *Walter Reed Medical Center*.[60] Separation of the field and professional activities provided for a redivision of the academic year, with the professional work offered from September 1 until December 31. On April 15, 1920 an Army Veterinary Laboratory was established in conjunction with the Veterinary Department of the University of Pennsylvania. In accordance with the faculty plans for including medical and dental research under one School program, this laboratory was relocated at the Army Medical School on April 15, 1921, and in addition to all phases of veterinary laboratory work, manufactured biological products for therapeutic and diagnostic use. These included such items as bacteriological, serological and histo-pathological diagnostic tests; moreover, the laboratory examination of meats and meat products was taught. As in the case of vaccines for the troops, the Army depended entirely on the Veterinary Laboratory of the Army Medical School for its animal biologics, including intra-dermic and ophthalmic mallein, equine infectious abortion vaccine, shipping fever vaccine and antigens for use in the application of serological tests for glanders.[61] The basic field training for Dental and Veterinary officers was also given at Carlisle Barracks.

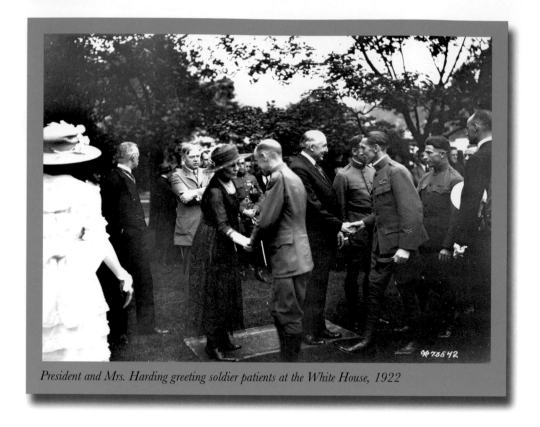

President and Mrs. Harding greeting soldier patients at the White House, 1922

Although not physically relocated, the Historical Division, Office of the Surgeon General, was transferred to the administrative jurisdiction of the Army Medical School on July 21, 1920, where the work of preparing the history of the Medical Department in the World War was continued.[62]

1921

Three classes of enlisted men were taught at the School during the twenty-fifth Session, November 1, 1920 to May 26, 1921. The basic course included such subjects as weights and measures; preparation of stains; preparation of media; care of animals; blood counts; hemoglobin estimation; routine staining methods; recognition of the tubercle bacillus; diphtheria bacillus and gonococcus, etc.; cleaning and sterilizing of laboratory glassware; technique of preparing blood and other smears; technique of collecting blood cultures and the complement fixation tests; methods of securing and preparing pathological material for shipment to the geographical Corps Areas formerly called Departments and to department laboratories. Carefully selected enlisted men were detailed for the advanced course and trained in culture methods and recognition of the more important pathogenic bacteria; recognition of malarial plasmodia, animal parasites, and the ova of intestinal parasites; the technique of serology, including agglutination, precipitin and complement fixation tests; and the technique of immunology,

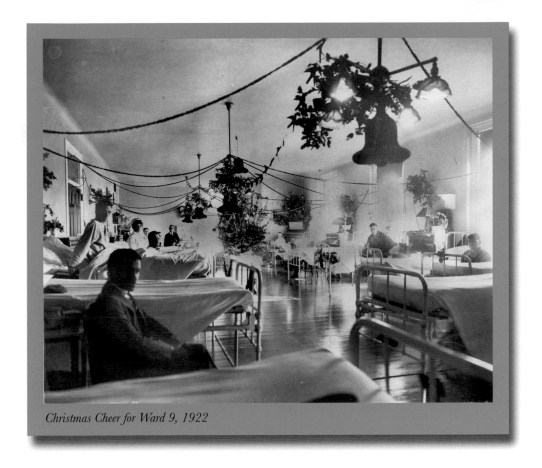

Christmas Cheer for Ward 9, 1922

with applied methods in the treatment of prophylaxis of disease.[63] As the training of enlisted technicians was expanded, thirty men were graduated in the basic course and ten others qualified as expert laboratory technicians. Forty-five X-ray technicians were trained, of whom twenty-two received certificates for special proficiency.[64]

Craig, Siler, Nichols and Callender[65] were the bluebloods among the fourteen medical officers on duty in the laboratory section of the School that year, and all were in some way interested in the continuing intensive research on streptococcus vaccines, protein sensitization, hay fever, food urticaria, skin disease, malnutrition, etc. Supervision of the production of the 1,609,363 cubic centimeters of triple typhoid vaccine and 170,365 cubic centimeters of pneumococcus vaccine occupied much of the staff time.[66] Moreover, some 346 samples of drugs, medicines, laboratory reagents; laboratory, hospital and miscellaneous items were analyzed;[67] and hundreds of physical examinations were per-formed on applicants for Regular Army Commissions, candidates for appointments to the West Point Military Academy, as Warrant Officers, as non-commissioned officers or as citizens military training camp, for promotion, for enlistments and for separations from the service.[68] The *Property Division* controlled the fiscal expenditures, which, in 1921, approximated $125,000.

The Army Medical Department had pioneered in the field of tropical medicine since the Spanish-American War; thus the faculty of the Army Medical School served as a logical spearhead for furthering the study. Colonels Russell, Nichols and Craig, Vedder and Siler were then not only the Army's best informed specialists in tropical disease, but they were probably the outstanding specialists in the United States. Largely as a result of their efforts, the *American Journal of Tropical Medicine* was begun in 1921 and edited by the officers in the Laboratory Division. Similarly, editing the *Abstracts of Bacteriology* became a second literary activity of an Army Medical School faculty member.[69]

1922

There was little change in the overall academic program during this last year of occupancy of the old quarters at 604 Louisiana Avenue. In anticipation of the closer association of the School and the hospital, a more formal organization was under study, with the ranking medical officer of the new center to be called *Commandant*. The responsible heads of the School departments would retain their individuality as Directors, and the faculty nomenclature and positions were to be broadened to include instructors. In consonance with and for supervision of the now five-dimensional training program for doctors, nurses, dentists, veterinarians, and enlisted men, and the special field service training for the male officer categories, the faculty proposed the establishment of a *Training Division* in the surgeon general's office.[70]

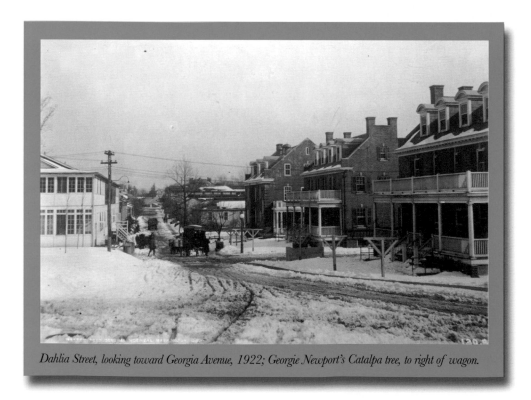

Dahlia Street, looking toward Georgia Avenue, 1922; Georgie Newport's Catalpa tree, to right of wagon.

Research work in the pneumococcus continued during 1922, with extensive studies made on the bacteriology of water; ointments for use in treating syphilis; streptococcus infections, dental caries, etc. As a record high, forty-four individuals were treated for hay fever. The Department of Roentgenology was, as usual, busy, and in addition to the routine work, the X-ray clinic sponsored a repair and maintenance section in order to maintain in good order the apparatus then in use at Walter Reed, Camp Meade, Maryland, and Fort Myer, Virginia.[71]

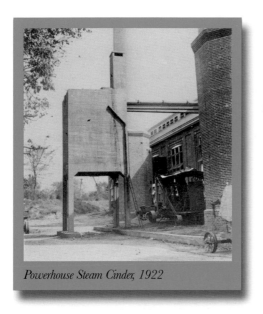

Powerhouse Steam Cinder, 1922

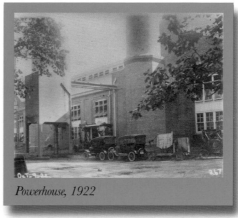

Powerhouse, 1922

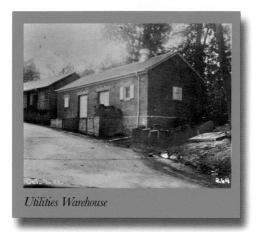

Utilities Warehouse

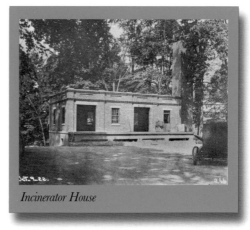

Incinerator House

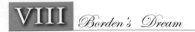
References

1. Hippocrates.

2. Letter from TSG to Hon. Augustine Lonergan, HR, July 8, 1918, SGO 631.-1 (Judge Thompson's files.)

3. See SGO 631.-1, *op cit*.

4. To TAG from TSG, Robert U. Patterson, Sept. 14, 1931. Subj: TSG's Library and the Army Med. Museum. See SGO 631.-1, *op cit*.

5. To TAG from Robert U. Patterson, Sept. 14, 1931. Subj: TSG's Library and the AMM, SGO 631.-1, *op cit*.

6. History of WRGH, prepared in 1921, on file Library, WRAH, pg 25.

7. *The Washington Evening Star*, Feb. 23, 1919.

8. Interview Brig. Gen. A.E. Truby, M.C., Ret., June 27, 28, 1950, and others.

9. Interview Brig. Gen. Albert. G. Love, M.C., Ret., Jan. 24, 1951.

10. *Ibid*, Feb. 13, 1951.

11. SGO 631.-1, *op cit*; *The Washington Evening Star*, 6 Nov. 1920; "U.S. Begins Suit For Reed Grounds."

12. Interview, Col. Herbert N. Dean, MAC, Ret., April 12, 1950; Col. James D. Fife, M.C., Ret., May 26, 1950; Mrs. M.W. Ireland, April 14, 1950; Brig. Gen. A.E. Truby, *op cit*.

13. Personal knowledge of the writer.

14. *The Washington Sunday Star*, June 13, 1926, pt. 5.

15. Dean interview, *op cit*; Annual Rpt, WRGH, 1920.

16. Dean interview, *op cit*.

17. *Ibid*.

18. *Ibid*.

19. Interview with Maj. Gen. Shelly U. Marietta, M.C. Ret., April 25, 1950.

20. Social conversation, Mrs. Anne Duryea Kirk, 1943.

21. *Ibid*.

22. Interview with Miss Margaret Lower, Feb. 14, 1951.

23. Truby, Marietta interview, *op cit*; and others.

24. Interview with Maj. Gen. Robert U. Patterson, M.C., Ret., Aug. 29, 1950.

25. Marietta, *op cit.*

26. Patterson interview, *op cit.*

27. Personal knowledge of the writer.

28. Social conversation with Mrs. Anne Duryea Kirk, 1943.

29. Annual Report WRGH, 1920.

30. *Ibid.*

31. History of WRGH, *op cit*, pg 106.

32. *History of the Medical Department in the World War*, Vol., XV, Pt. II, pg. 591 and 663; 4,212 cases during the war, of that number, 645 were complicated cases of measles, and 2,129 of influenza. Many of these cases became chronic.

33. Social conversation, Colonel James C. Kimbrough, M.C., Ret., Feb. 13, 1951.

34. Marietta interview, *op cit*. Annual Report WRGH, 1920.

35. Fife interview, *op cit.*

36. Fife, Dean, Lower interviews, *op cit.*

37. Conversation, Miss Mary E. Schick, Librarian, Feb. 13, 1951.

38. Interview with Mrs. M.W. Ireland, *op cit.*

39. Interview with Col. Herbert N. Dean, *op cit.*

40. *Ibid.*

41. *The Washington Herald*, Dec. 13 and 14, 1920; *The Washington Post*; Dec. 13, 1920.

42. Annual Report WRGH, 1921.

43. *Ibid*, 1920.

44. *Ibid*, 1921.

45. *Ibid.*

46. *The Washington Star*, March 31, 1921.

47. Annual Rpt, WRGH, 1922.

48. Interview with Miss Marjorie Lower, *op cit*.

49. Biography of General J.R. Kean, MSS on file AML, Washington, D.C. pg 250.

50. Patterson interview, *op cit*.

51. *Ibid.*

52. Lower interview, *op cit*.

53. P.M. Ashburn, *A History of the Med. Dept. of the U.S. Army*, Boston & New York, Houghton-Mifflin, 1929, pg 377.

54. Bureau of Budget Circular 44, 1 Nov. 1921 authorized the Board; Cir. 45, 3 Nov. 1921, named Brig. Gen. Charles E. Sawyer as Chf. Coordinator. Bureau of Budget Cir. 146; JAMA, Jan. 27, 1923; pg 264, 21 Oct. 1924 rescinded Cir. 45 and made Dir. of Vet. Adm. the Chairman.

55. Patterson interview, *op cit*.

56. Lower interview, *op cit*.

57. Annual Rpt, TSG... 1920, pg 482.

58. *Ibid*, pg 485.

59. *Ibid*, pg 483.

60. Proceedings of the Faculty, Nov. 11, 1920.

61. Annual Rpt TSG... 1921, pg 223.

62. *Ibid*, pg 226.

63. *Ibid*, 221.

64. *Ibid*, 222.

65. Minutes, AMS, Nov. 11, 1920.

66. Annual Rpt TSG... 1921, pg 223.

67. *Ibid*, pg 226.

68. *Ibid.*

69. Russell-Welch correspondence, Collection of the Institute of the History of Medicine, Welch Medical Library, Johns Hopkins University, Baltimore, Md. SGO 631.-1 (AMS) GG, War Rec. Div., National Archives.

70. Minutes AMS, Nov. 11, 1920.

71. Annual Rpt TSG... 1922, pg 239.

The Army Medical Center

1923–1925

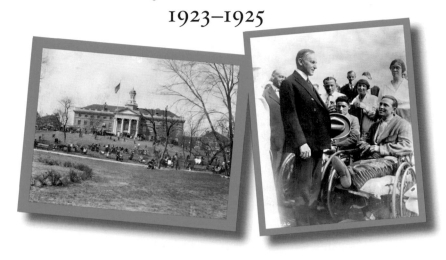

"Man is the only animal that laughs and weeps; for he is the only animal that is struck with the difference between what things are, and what they ought to be."[1]

Some Matters of Opinion

The Red Cross convalescent house was comparatively small, but the furnishings were homelike and the personnel friendly. Thus it was the natural center for organized recreational activities and it played an inestimable part in every phase of institutional life. Its mission was the mission of the national organization whose record of welfare service for the American soldier is unsurpassed by any other volunteer social agency in the world.

Trained Red Cross social workers are essentially liaison agents between the soldier and his community in that they secure for the professional staff, social histories pertinent to the clinical record. The local Red Cross organization, i.e., the Field Director at Walter Reed, may give temporary financial assistance to the destitute; skilled staff workers counsel on housing, legal or personal problems. At the ward level, both trained and volunteer workers supervise recreation programs and act as scribes. The Gray Ladies, so intimately a part of the Red Cross organization at Walter Reed, had, by 1924, a prescribed training course.[2] Applicants were not only carefully selected, but professional staff members provided scheduled instruction in hospital ethics and functions, and the general nomenclature and characteristics of the more common diseases. It was the Gray Ladies who performed the homely unimpressive chores for "the boys" and dispensed many small luxuries and even some necessary items that could not properly be called a Federal responsibility. Their bounty was limitless, but on the whole the men accepted their ministrations as a matter of course. "Griping" is accepted as a basic characteristic of this psychology of soldiers, and the best of them complain happily about the pay, the food, or "the old man." It is not surprising, therefore, that some of the patients accepted the Gray Ladies' attention with affectionate indulgence and others with cynical indifference. For as one wag remarked about the endless supply of razor blades, writing paper, candy and outdated magazines, "Jeez, they're all right, but if they don't give us girls it ain't no use."[3]

There was then a freshness and sincerity influencing the management of welfare activities, and at no other time in the hospital's history was the institutional esprit de corps so great as in the early post-World War I years. Morale was a positive and viable factor rather than an artificial by-product of public relations activities. The patients participated wholeheartedly in the parties, carnivals, corn roasts and entertainments sponsored by the Red Cross and Occupational Therapy workers. They attended social functions at the White House with buoyant enthusiasm. Here at last was evidence of democracy, as commoner and king, soldier and commander-in-chief drank the same kind of brew from the same kind of cup. Rehabilitation of the war-wounded proceeded with genuine rather than professional enthusiasm,

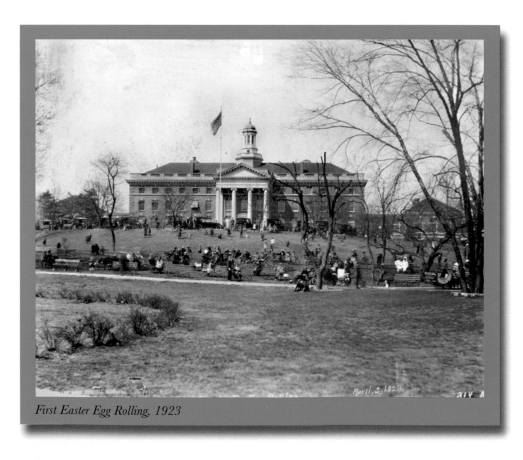

First Easter Egg Rolling, 1923

and whether the project concerned modeling, carpentry, typing or chicken raising near the old Lay Mansion, Walter Reed patients received the warm-hearted manifestations of community interest with enthusiasm, and in their way they returned what they could.

The Red Cross staff sponsored an annual Christmas party for underprivileged city children who were as overwhelmed by the generosity of the Walter Reed patients as the patients were by the generosity of the Washington citizens. The toys and gifts were made at the hospital, under the direction of Miss Bertha York, and more than one young orphan was fondled and loved by "doughboys" homesick for their own "small fry." Hospital workers recall their pathetic yet comical efforts to put some of the more anxious youngsters at ease, especially one legless veteran who fascinated even the most apprehensive young guests by the constant removal and insertion of a well matched glass eye. *The Come Back* was still the medium for inter-ward news, and in that gay December of 1923, it featured a line drawing of a smiling crutch-laden soldier wishing "A Merry Christmas to the Whole World."[4]

The convalescent house was the hub of non-professional activities. There the boys found entertainment and relaxation, card parties and other indoor games,

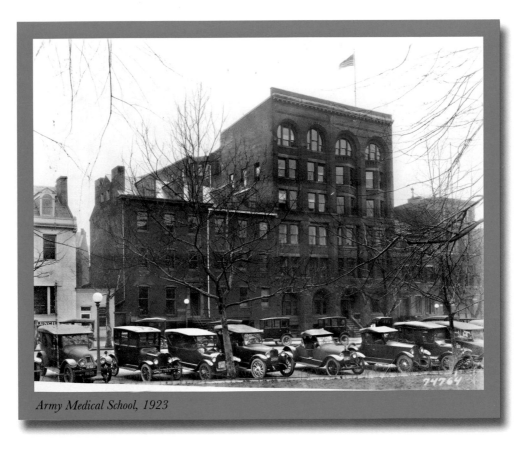

Army Medical School, 1923

a victrola and a player piano. There the Detachment corpsmen had their parties and dances and the officers had their monthly "hops." The main hall was on occasion a chapel, movie house or lyceum, and for several years during the mid-twenties, the annual graduation exercises for the various professional training groups were held in the same hall where Tetrazzine once fainted at the sight of a blind amputee, Schumann-Heink dissolved her audience in tears,[5] and the brasses of the Army Band orchestra shook the very rafters with their rumbling.

The comb-like arrangement of the temporary wards was not attractive, but intra-hospital communication and transportation were comparatively easy. The Post Library was strategically located on the "Main Drag," and its nearest neighbor, arranged T-wise, was Ward 31, where the long-standing chronic cases were treated. The men enjoyed a special sort of community life when on "The Drag," and a group in wheel chairs could always be found out-of-doors when weather permitted. With the characteristic cheerfulness of the amputee, they would sit for hours refighting their old campaigns, swapping risqué stories or commenting on the appearance, especially feminine, of their unsuspecting public. One double amputee, natural leader of the group, invariably managed to get more than a fair share of the attention, for he was the special pet of the Gray Ladies who wandered about dispensing cheer and charity.

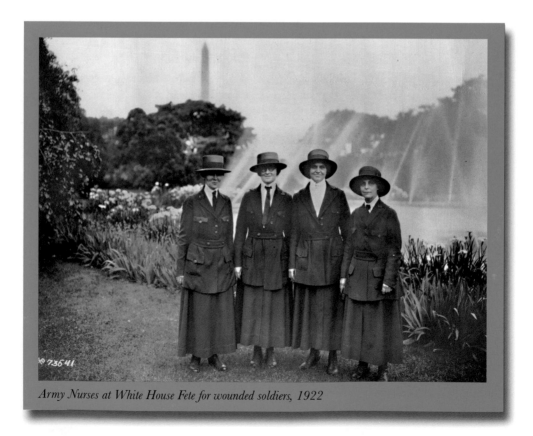

Army Nurses at White House Fete for wounded soldiers, 1922

One fine day as he and his cronies sat sunning, an escort of Gray Ladies conducted several distinguished visitors in his direction. An unpredictable prankish streak prompted him to draw both arms inside his loose robe and leave the sleeves hanging empty. The usual newspaper articles about the "basket cases" at Walter Reed and other hospitals had appeared from time to time, and to the uninformed lady visitor the man appeared as a bona fide case. Thus attention was immediately centered on the apparently helpless victim, as she gave him candy, lit his cigarette and even spoon-fed his ice cream. One of the young women, overwhelmed with pity for the graceless prankster, leaned over to kiss him tenderly on the lips, whereupon nature reasserted itself with surprising speed.

"Oh my God, Oh MY GOD, OH MY GOD," he shouted, throwing both brawny arms around the startled Cleopatra.[6]

All war periods produce countless human interest stories. Some are tales of heroism and daring; some are startling accounts of personal sacrifices. The more spectacular stories make the front pages in newspapers, but the everyday sorrows of the average man are rarely of public interest.

A long-standing and clearly defined rule forbade the association of nurses and enlisted men had, in addition to the social factors involved, a just military basis. Women not only had a difficult time maintaining discipline in the male hierarchy, but nurse leaders then struggling to establish their group on a professional basis[7] were well aware of the social gulf between management and the worker; officer and enlisted status; the doctor and the ward attendant. As nursing was the natural ally of medicine, and as Army nurses had long wanted military status, it was appropriate that rigid standards control their conduct.

Relative rank was granted the Army Nurse Corps in 1920,[8] primarily as a result of the concerted lobbying activities of organized nursing groups,[9] and thereafter the women held a semi-commissioned status, with the grades of second lieutenant through major corresponding in name but not in the identical pay and military privileges accorded male officers. The Army School of Nursing was a favored experimental project of both the organized nursing groups and the Superintendent of the Army Nurse Corps, Major Julia C. Stimson, and so rigid attempts were made not only to train young nursing students to a state of mind and discipline appropriate to military life, but to curb their natural inclination for the ready companionship of attractive males, with or without Sam Brown belts.[10]

As the social value of the military uniform changes in wartime, it was inevitable that some regulations were relaxed. Matrimonial "casualties" as well as student attrition affected the Army Nurse Corps, and Walter Reed had a fair share of war romances of the period. Aides and nurses, volunteers and paid workers alike forsook professional for private life. One of the younger student nurses fancied herself in love with, and married secretly, a handsome, cheery but badly wounded Ward 31 hero. As his prognosis became worse and the first blossom of romance faded, their occasional meetings were insufficient to hold the young girl's interest, and so the soldier's greatest pleasure in life was her daily visit to him on the ward or the "Main Drag". As her interest waned and she came less frequently, he became discouraged and melancholy.

All of the Ward 31 inmates were known to their nearest neighbors, the librarians, and during the last months, when the soldier was slow in dying, depression overcame his reserve and he confided his troubles to the senior librarian, asking her to witness his will. His small estate was bequeathed in escrow to the young girl's uncle, in order to protect her good name and prevent expulsion from the Army School of Nursing. The legal matter was managed with complete secrecy and the man died confidently, sure that his private affairs were unknown.

Surprisingly, at the time of the funeral, Colonel Glennan proposed that the senior librarian accompany a "certain" young nurse to the service. Amazed at his interest as well as his knowledgeable manner, his friend stated that the girl was attending the service with her uncle and aunt and asked why he made the suggestion. The gallant commanding officer not only made no comment, but the young nurse was allowed to finish the course, her supervisor unaware that she had broken one of the most rigid rules of the majority of training schools of the day – the ban on married women. "Noisy Jim," the ironically named, simply didn't talk![11]

In those early and informal days of Post life the majority of the distinguished visitors and sightseers were conducted through the reading room of the hospital library. Others, especially

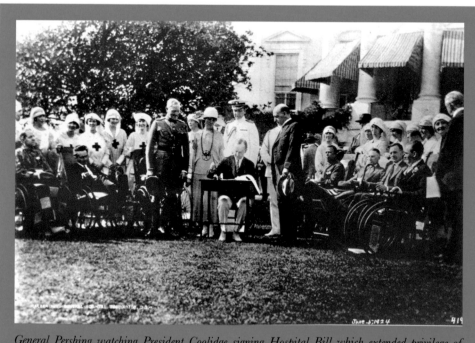

General Pershing watching President Coolidge signing Hospital Bill which extended privilege of Veterans, 1924

those of the military world, passed its portals on their way to and from the clinics. Of all the rather remarkable people who came to Walter Reed during this period, the heroic General John J. Pershing, then Chief of Staff of the Army, created the most excited comment.

The library sorting table faced the door to the main corridor, and although it was not the coolest place to work, it was the most advantageous for viewing the intra-hospital traffic. No one escaped the interested gaze of the volunteer workers, including General Pershing, who almost daily took his careful course to the Dental Clinic. When exactly in front of the door he meticulously doffed his hat, bowed unsmilingly to the ladies, and proceeded somberly on his way. This routine continued for several weeks and then one day he paused momentarily, bowed and smiled dazzlingly at the workers.

After a moment of shocked silence the startled young ladies chirruped as one, "He's got his teeth, he's got his teeth!" and then wondered agonizingly how far the sound had carried.[12]

Professional Pageant

The Surgeon General's Annual Report for 1923 states that

> *No additions or alterations were accomplished at this hospital through the expenditure of "Construction and repair of hospitals" funds, but the Veterans Bureau has expended ... during the present fiscal year the sum of $14,000 for (a) garage, and (b) general repairs to hospital buildings, including electrical equipment, power plant, heating plant, roads, walk, curbs, sewers, drains, etc., $5,000 ... .*

The "Power House Story" is but another illustration of the hospital commander's quiet effectiveness. Early in the Glennan administration a persuasive female engineer, widow of an inventor, convinced the Quartermaster General of the advisability of changing the Walter Reed heating system from coal to oil.[13] General Glennan not only disapproved, but he declined to commit Medical Department funds for what he believed to be an impractical experiment. He agreed, however, to try the new process if the Quartermaster provided the funds and the interested company posted bond for reconversion from oil to coal.[14]

The process in question operated on the principle of flash heat, created by a mixture of oil and water. This was before oil heating was in general use, and as there was no way of serving the plant, an oil line was laid from Takoma Park. Enormous storage tanks were submerged on the ridge above the power house, where Charley Anderson once raised chickens for the hospital mess. The experiment was doomed from the start, for the combustible mixture produced such an intense and uncontrollable heat that it burnt the fire bricks out of the furnaces faster than replacements could be installed. The lady engineer, game to the last, donned overalls and worked at the furnaces with the men. When her funds were exhausted, part of the bond money was used to meet the last payroll.[15] Unfortunately, there is no record of "Noisy Jim's" comments to the Quartermaster General's Office, and on the basis of circumstantial evidence it appears

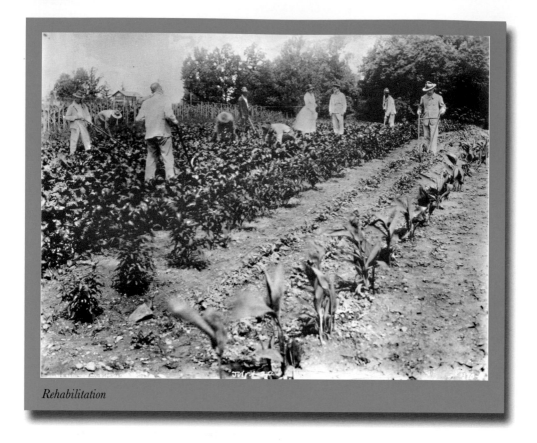

Rehabilitation

that part of the $5,000 provided by the Veterans Administration was used to restore the furnace.

The total bed capacity of all general hospitals was ample at this time, and at Walter Reed, at the end of the fiscal year, June 30, 1923, only 748 of the 1200 authorized beds were occupied, 287 of them by Veterans Bureau patients.[16]

There were, however, 1,568 Veterans Bureau patients admitted to the hospital during the calendar year 1923, and only 1,078 "other" patients from the United States at large. The latter group included both military personnel and their dependents. The organization of the Surgical Service was still substantially the same, and the X-ray Section, Anesthesia and Dental Sections were also under Colonel Keller's general supervision. Numerically, the number of patients admitted on the surgical service had decreased, but the surgeons believed the volume of routine work had not changed appreciably because so many of the chronic cases required extensive surgical dressings and treatment.[17] Colonel Keller continued his occasional demonstration and lecture clinics for Johns Hopkins, George Washington and Georgetown senior medical students, as well as the weekly clinic in military surgery for Army Medical School students, by then reduced from nine to six months.

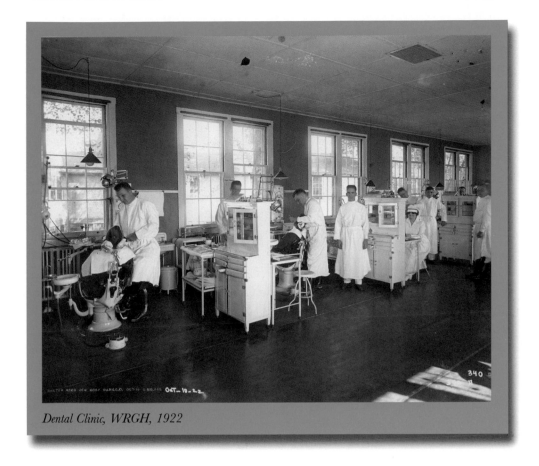

Dental Clinic, WRGH, 1922

Of the 688 orthopedic cases treated in 1923, only fifteen per cent required surgery. On the other hand, some 1,300 cases were seen in consultation from other hospital services or as referrals from the Attending Surgeon's Office, Military District of Washington; and 8,600 plaster of Paris bandages were made in the Orthopedic Appliance Shop, for later use in making body casts. From a strictly statistical evaluation, the EENT section, credited with 1,317 of the total 2,475 operations, Orthopedics, Urology and finally the Obstetrical and Gynecological Sections were the busiest surgical activities.

Citation of statistical facts discloses neither "operating responsibility," i.e., extensiveness or duration of case management, nor experimental therapy. Therefore, to medically interested readers, the evidence of some changes in general therapy is worth noting. The first concerns the sudden rise in the number of laboratory procedures requisitioned by other professional services, and the second concerns the marked increase in the number of post-mortem examinations performed on the military dead. Both changes foreshadow the approach of a new professional era.

In other words, the family doctor, long dependent on the symptomatic diagnosis, was edging over to make way for the laboratory and clinical investigation of disease.

The movement would be slow in coming to a head, but the infiltration of the general practitioner's ranks had begun. The fact that eighty-seven blood transfusions, then mainly prescribed for acute surgical cases, were given at Walter Reed during the year is fully as significant as the 9.4 per cent general increase in laboratory examinations. Hospitalization for extensive dental services was not unusual, and dental activities were increasing in volume as well as in kind, with 16,498 "sittings," 350 restorations, forty-four full dentures, seventy partial dentures and seven dental repairs recorded for 1923. Consequently, if inpatient admissions decreased and the professional services increased, more was being done for the individual.

On March 3, 1919, Government hospital facilities were first authorized for Veterans suffering from service-connected disabilities, many of whom were neuropsychiatric cases. In signing the "Hospital Bill," June 7, 1924, the President endorsed the amendatory legislation called the World War Veterans Act of 1924, which authorized hospitalization for non-service-connected disabilities. In October 1924, the Director of the Veterans Administration became Chairman of the Federal Board of Hospitalization.[18] Walter Reed had not had satisfactory provision for neuropsychiatric cases until this time, and occupancy of the recently constructed new hydrotherapy and occupational therapy sections of the Neuropsychiatric Service early in the year, facilitated the rehabilitation program. Of the physiotherapy students graduated on February 7, ten were appointed as senior aides to fill vacancies in the Physiotherapy Departments in the several other Army general hospitals. Of the eight dietetic student graduates, six received Civil Service appointments. A grand total of 120 graduate nurses then were on duty at Walter Reed; forty-six student nurses were present in the training school and twenty-eight were on indefinite leave of absence for affiliated services in civilian hospitals.[19]

Complaints regarding the average enlisted man's lack of aptitude for military medical duties had prevailed since the Revolutionary War. Technical training was a painstaking business, and hospital commanders often lamented that their institutions received many unsuitable specimens, victims of the recruiting tactics of over-zealous sergeants who assigned recruits unsuitable for field duty to the Medical Department. Coalition of hospital and School had increased the total number of enlisted men in the Detachment to 422, but many of the more expert ones were used to comprise the hundred or so technicians assigned to the detachment for staffing the Army Medical School laboratories. Others performed administrative and clerical duties, had assignments in the Quartermaster and Medical Supply Sections, served as ambulance drivers or worked in the hospital mess. It was not unusual, as Colonel Borden had pointed out, that as a matter of expediency, men were often assigned to the wards who had never before been inside a hospital. In the Walter Reed Detachment one, at least, represented Dr. Borden's contentions.

Lt. Colonel Lloyd Smith was Chief of the Medical Service at the time and thereby nominally in charge of the Laboratory Service. The Army Medical School faculty, with its pursuit of tropical diseases, had stirred considerable interest in the debilitating effects of ascariasis, including a new appreciation of blood dyscrasias. Colonel Smith believed a patient newly arrived from Panama had ascariasis and was treating the man accordingly. Nevertheless, he wanted to verify the diagnosis by examination of the feces and ordered a cathartic in order to collect the specimen during the working hours of the laboratory staff. Unfortunately the patient could not retain the orally administered cathartic and so at great labor, the ward physician administered it intra-venously. For convenience a toilet chair was placed at the bedside, and the corpsman, a reasonably new recruit more aware that "cleanliness is next to Godliness" than of symptomatic diseases, was instructed to deliver the fresh stool to the laboratory as soon after discharge as possible. The laboratory officer and laboratory-trained nurse were directed to stay on duty and await its arrival.

Some several hours later hospital personnel were astounded on seeing the youth march through the halls proudly carrying the toilet chair on his shoulder. Moreover, the laboratory officer was completely overwhelmed when the beaming recruit marched up to him, saluted and deposited a shining toilet chair at his feet. "Here's the stool, Sir," he said with a broad smile, "all fresh and clean."

In contrast to his joy, however, informal "history" credits the discomfited and indignant chief of the Medical Service with literally hopping up and down in a most unmilitary rage![20]

A Milestone of Progress

One of General Ireland's early policy plans for the general hospital program included the assignment of internes, with pay of $60 a month, ration and quarters, and the status of civilian employees.[21] Implementing the program proved to be slower than anticipated and it was not until 1924, when internes were militarized by appointment as First Lieutenants, that a *Director of Training Course For Hospital Internes* was added to the *Training Section*, which had responsibility for such other programs as *Hospital Administration, The Army School of Nursing, The Gray Ladies, Anesthesia for Nurses, Laboratory Technique For Nurses,*[22] etc. Four internes reported for duty on July 15, 1924, and three additional ones before the close of the year for five months of training on each of the Medical and Surgical Services and a two-month period in the hospital laboratory. After June 1924, the course was under the general supervision of Major Ernest R. Gentry, the Medical Department's undulant fever expert and Chief of the Medical Service at Walter Reed. The experiment was not only immediately successful, but Colonel Glennan endorsed the annual training of at least fourteen young doctors who would meet the requirements of the National Board of Medical Examiners.[23]

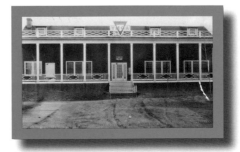

YMCA Hut; site now occupied by permanent barracks.

Of the eight internes completing the course at Walter Reed in 1925

1	*was found qualified and commissioned.*
2	*were found qualified but declined appointment.*
3	*were physically disqualified.*
2	*were professionally disqualified.*
8	

Two others were discharged at their own request before completing the course; one was transferred to Fitzsimmons and twelve were still in training. Thus the percentage of acceptable candidates was extremely low, and the hospital commander noted that not only should a physical examination be made before appointment as internes, but "applicants should only be accepted who desire appointment in the Medical Corps."[24] This indication of general lack of interest in military assignment was similar to the situation immediately prior to passage of the Army Reorganization Act of 1908, and later, after the great war of 1941–1945.

The World War I period was a boon to public health programs. The mass mobilization of men disclosed the unsuspected fact that there were fewer brawny Tarzans in the American population than had been supposed. Concentration of men in training camps encouraged epidemics and increased the venereal disease rate. Mass feeding and quantity cookery required that more sanitary methods of handling food be adopted, the Army leading the way with its more stringent control measures and sanitary inspections. If Walter Reed was an example of the prevailing practices in other hospitals, the food management situation may have been better than that found in the camps, for an ample quota of hospital dieticians and nurses watched eagle-eyed the achievements of the soldier and civilian cooks.

Communication, the key to exchange of information, brought an innovation on January 21, 1924, when regular monthly meetings were instituted for Medical Department officers in and around Washington.[25] Departmental, governmental, civilian doctors and members of the Medical Reserve Corps were invited.[26]

The detailed study of metabolic diseases, just getting under way in 1924, increased by 34.3 per cent the number of basal metabolisms performed. Further, the routine laboratory work increased by 38.8 per cent, with an increasing number of requests for hematological work. Possibly because of the concentrated work in diabetes, the Medical Service reported that "Further experience with insulin confirmed earlier reports, and its use (was) now a well established procedure in the more severe cases of diabetes mellitus. Twenty-eight (28) were admitted during the year with no deaths." As a consequence the laboratory section reported that routine urinalysis increased "out of all commensuration with the increase in number of patients." There had not been a complete recovery from the early post-war slump in surgical admissions, with the result that in 1925 and 1926 there was a noticeable increase in the number of medical cases.[27]

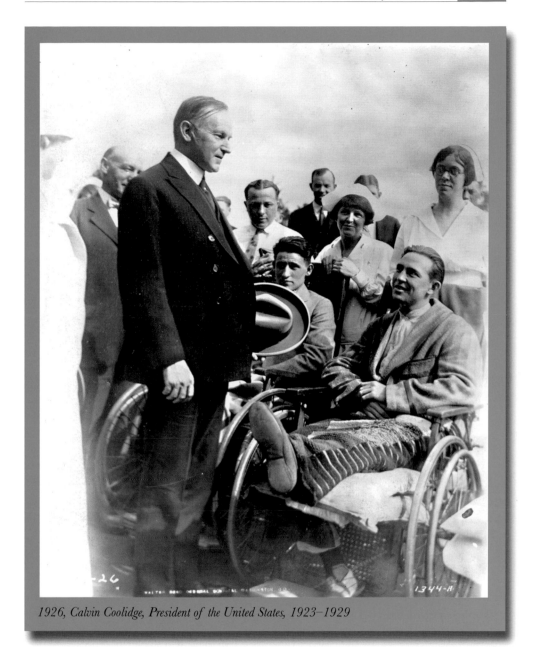

1926, Calvin Coolidge, President of the United States, 1923–1929

The Zihlman Bill, which proposed opening 14th Street through the Walter Reed grounds, was introduced in the House of Representatives during 1924, apparently sponsored by real estate interests and enthusiastic District Commissioners. Representative John J. Rogers of Massachusetts introduced a motion that the extension skirt the hospital grounds, and other Representatives supported him in the struggle to retain the reservation intact, claiming that traffic hazards to convalescent patients would cause removal of the hospital.[28]

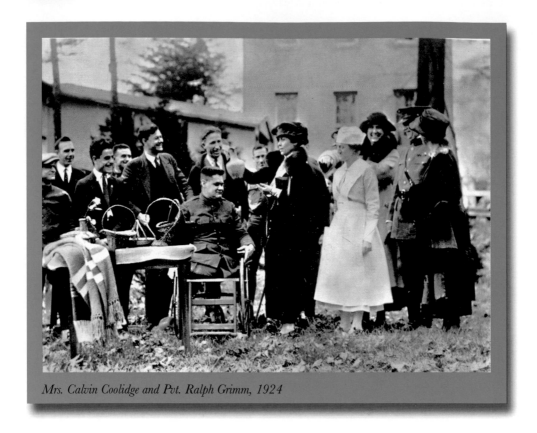

Mrs. Calvin Coolidge and Pvt. Ralph Grimm, 1924

Always an idealist, Colonel Glennan wanted the great tract of land to remain as nature intended, and although the political battle was won at that time, he believed the proposal might be reopened. The most logical way to forestall such vandalism was to erect a building to block this area – but public buildings required time for approval by higher authority as well as money. Thus, as a matter of strategy, he decided to lay a concrete tennis court on the northwest side of the Service Club, an area since covered over by flower gardens. He could then truthfully claim that the land was in use and the project necessary to the welfare of hospital personnel. It was at this time that he unsuccessfully experimented with mixing green coloring in the unpoured concrete. Defeated in his attempt to have the court in aesthetic harmony with nature's own coloring matter, but adamant in his determination to forestall the District Engineers, he directed that the concrete be laid to a depth of twenty inches. He would, according to his principal confidant in this nefarious scheme, have continued the operation indefinitely, but the local Quartermaster's supply of concrete was soon exhausted.[29]

The Hardings had been frequent visitors at Walter Reed, and as the Coolidge administration came into prominence, this custom was continued. Early in his regime General Ireland personally instituted a regular Sunday morning visit to the hospital to see ailing medical officers, old friends and distinguished patients. On the occasion of

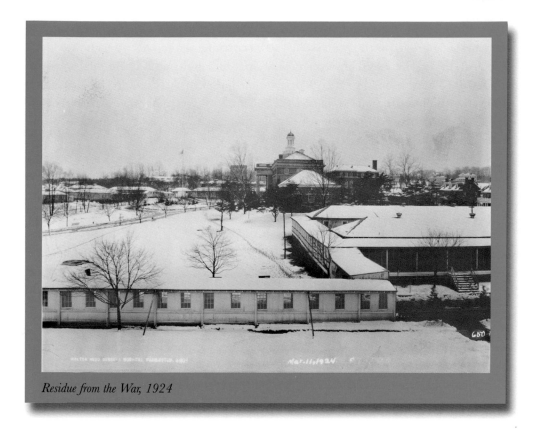

Residue from the War, 1924

the first scheduled Coolidge visit, Colonel Glennan invited the Surgeon General to be present. General Ireland declined, saying it was the commanding officer's "show." The visit passed without any cyclonic ill effects, and General Ireland later asked his friend what he and the President discussed.

> *"Nothing," replied Walter Reed's commanding officer shortly.*
>
> *"What did the President say?" persisted the Surgeon General.*
>
> *"He said, 'Good Morning'," replied "Noisy Jim."*
>
> *"Well, Jim, what did you say?" General Ireland insisted.*
>
> *"I said, good morning, Mr. President," replied the old doctor seriously.*[30]

Exit a Dreamer

More human interest stories were told on the ascetic-looking James D. Glennan than on any of the other nineteen hospital commanders. Perhaps the best but certainly the most noncommittal military hospital administrator of his time, his silence was no handicap when it came to securing improvements for his hospital. A Senator from

West Virginia was a patient at Walter Reed during the Glennan administration, and the Senator so approved of the professional service that he wanted his wife admitted for a medical survey. There was, however, no authority for admitting a senatorial dependent, even with the commanding officer's permission, unless the case was an emergency. Not long after this handicap was explained, the Senator's wife seemingly had an acute seizure while visiting her husband's room. Under the circumstances it was not only humane but necessary that she be admitted as a patient.

When her condition permitted discharge, the Senator voiced effusive thanks and assured Colonel Glennan volubly that he regretted his inability to return the favor. The challenge was tempting, and to everyone's surprise Colonel Glennan announced that the enlisted men needed funds for a new baseball grandstand, as they then sat on a grass bank and watched the game from the rear. In view of the then more reasonable charges for hospital services, the Senator paid handsomely for his family welfare, for the new brick grandstand, equipped with basement showers, dressing rooms and a lounging room, cost him $2200. "Noisy Jim," however, mourned to his Adjutant that the "touch" was so easy he should have asked for more.[31]

Although planned by Colonel Glennan, the gardens and post-war shrubbery planting were for a time the special responsibility of the Occupational Therapy aides, supervised and encouraged by Dr. Lumsden.[32] Prior to erection of the Wood greenhouses, groups of neuropsychiatric patients were daily conducted across Georgia Avenue to the Freeman nursery. There they wandered at will, completing their afternoon outing with a tea party provided by the aides or attendants.[33] After the hospital had its own greenhouses,

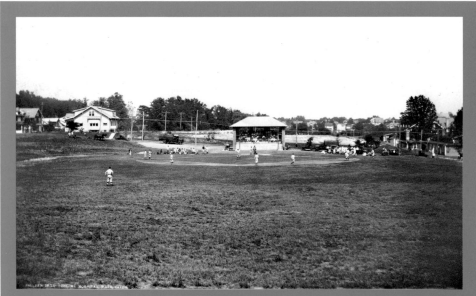

Playing Field; looking toward 14th Street, site now occupied by new Rehabilitation Building, 1924

interested patients were encouraged to raise plants of their own, and many of the wards had competitive flower gardens, for which the Red Cross gave a weekly prize.[34]

Several of the temporary buildings were dismantled during the early twenties in order to provide space for the new School building. By 1925 plans were being developed for razing others in order to attach great new wings to Wards "A" and "B" of the Main Building. It was Colonel Glennan's belief that nature was in itself a therapeutic agent and that ailing soldiers should have easy access to the out-of-doors, especially the beautiful Walter Reed garden. Some of the shrubbery and trees from the Shepherd estate still stood, and he was especially sentimental about a gnarled old apple tree that grew near the "Main Drag," approximately where Ward 9A now stands. As a consequence of this he spent many hours trying to adjust the angulations of the wards in order to save this fruitful relic of the past.[35]

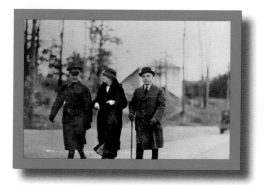 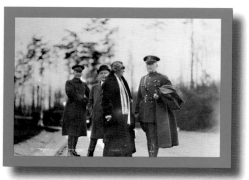

Mrs. Walter Reed and General Glennan, December 2, 1924

In spite of his reputation for almost unbroken silence, the Colonel discussed gardening problems with very little encouragement and during his last year at Walter Reed he spent an increasing amount of time wandering around the hospital grounds. The excavations and blasting for the Cameron's Creek tunnel had uncovered great stones that lay as they fell, and around this natural landscaping he designed the formal gardens. Later, when part of Rock Creek Park was converted into a golf course, many of the displaced evergreens were replanted as a background for this setting, *The Come Back* publishing pictures of the before and after effects of the reclamation. Surplus cherry trees, donated by the Japanese Government for the area around the Tidal Basin, were consigned to Walter Reed and planted on the upper rim of the garden basin, where after 1923, the Post children and their friends came on Easter Monday to roll their colorful Easter Eggs.[36]

The rose garden was the General's especial delight and its luxuriant growth bore radiant testimony to his attentions. Once, while attending a horticultural convention, the old Army doctor chatted happily with an unprepossessing stranger about his plans for a formal garden at Walter Reed. Some months later the Department of Agriculture, whose Bureau of Foreign Plant Industry frequently gave surplus stocks to the hospital, notified the commanding officer that a number of rose bushes from Lyons, France, were in quarantine, gift of wealthy Arthur Decker of Rutherford, New Jersey, who annually imported some for his own estate.[37] The gentle slopes that dropped from the area in front of the flagpole and into the formal gardens formed a natural amphitheater for band concerts, outdoor plays, the graduation exercises of the Army School of Nursing and the Easter Sunrise Services that became traditional occasions at the hospital during these years, and to which the public was invited.

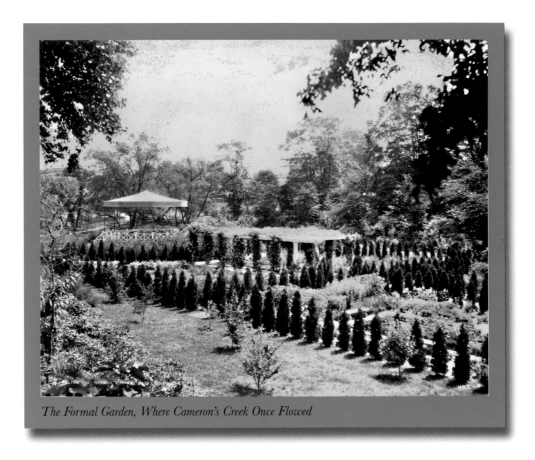

The Formal Garden, Where Cameron's Creek Once Flowed

Samuel "Roxie" Rothafel,[38] popular entertainer of the early twenties, gave a number of benefit performances to secure money for installation of bedside radios at Walter Reed. His campaign was so successful that in July 1925 the first headphone sets were installed connected to a two-way broadcasting circuit located in a basement room of the Main Building. Moreover, the fund was large enough to provide similar sets for some of the other Army hospitals in the East. This represented a progressive step in the occupational therapy of patients and gave the hospital staff just pride in their affiliation with the Army's most modern medical institution.

The Post Commander was promoted to the grade of Brigadier General in February 1925. In March 1926, after a seven-year tenure as hospital planner and architect, dreamer and benevolent friend, James D. Glennan retired for age. In relinquishing the most influential factor in his daily life, command of the Walter Reed General Hospital, he likewise relinquished his will to live. Two years later he succumbed to pernicious anemia, the invading blood disease which had gradually changed his formal military appearance to a look of almost ethereal asceticism. Man, the mortal, was no more, but for as long as the hospital should stand the spiritual influence of "The Gardener" would be evident as a loving reminder of his presence.

The Little Red School House

The Army Dental School, established in Washington, January 6, 1922,[39] began its first session within the week, and the first graduation class, June 22, 1922, held joint exercises with the Army Medical School at the New National Museum. The new army Medical School building, still incomplete at this time, was not officially transferred from the custody of the constructing Quartermaster of the Military District of Washington to the installation Quartermaster of Walter Reed until June 15, 1923. The Army Medical Center was formally recognized September 1.[40] The tract then comprised almost 110 acres, and

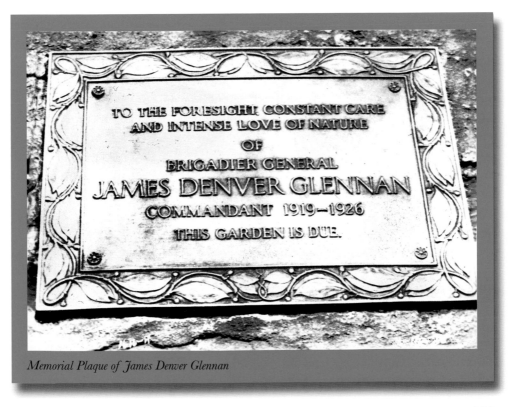

Memorial Plaque of James Denver Glennan

*All public lands included within the boundaries of the military reserva-
tion located in the Takoma Park section of the District of Columbia and
occupied principally by the Walter Reed General Hospital (were) known
as the Army Medical Center, Washington, D.C.*[41]

Beginning in August 1917, the Veterinary Corps had given a series of short courses in Chicago; authority for the Army Veterinary School was provided by WD Circular No. 271, 16 July 1920, and established at the General Supply Depot, Chicago, Illinois, but given the name of the Veterinary School of Meat and Dairy Hygiene, changed to Army Veterinary School of Meat and Dairy Hygiene, changed to Army Veterinary School by AR 350-105, February 11, 1922. Relocated in Washington on July 7, 1923, like the other Medical Department professional training programs, it was grouped under the one administrative canopy of the Army Medical Center. Each sub-school managed its own internal administrative affairs.

The first section of the School building, an approximate one-third its ultimate size, was hardly more than four walls at the time of occupancy, as there were no cupboards or work tables and few items that could be called permanent fixtures. Some of the old laboratory equipment used at 604 Louisiana Avenue was installed intact, and even a number of the so-called "Walter Reed" and "Russell" tables, dating from the early days at the Army Medical Museum, were repaired and kept in use for historical reasons. Still, the students attending the 28th Session, January to June 1924, had less scientific equip-ment than they needed, and this first year of occupancy was not without problems. One, at least, was obviated as a result of the farsighted planning of the vaccine laboratory staff, which had anticipated both housing and administrative problems and prepared surplus quantities of vaccine to have on hand for emergency use.

In spite of the complications that usually attend the moving day of any household, Stephen Foster himself could not have been prouder of the new location, for after thirty years of wandering, the Army Medical School faculty at last had a home of its own. Located on the little knoll occupied by the tent-sheltered Hospital Company "C" in April 1909, the new School building was monarch of all the other structures. If patients from Washington bemoaned the long ride "out" to the hinterland occupied by Walter Reed, to Post duty personnel the walk "up" to the School or "down" to the headquarters was proportionately as bad.

Regardless of the fact that the Army Medical School was the older professional activity, the hospital was the better known, both because of its professional reputation and its heroic name. Thus Walter Reed was literally the Center, and the center was Walter Reed. From the public information viewpoint, the earlier concept of the new professional coalition as *The Walter Reed Medical Center* was probably a more appropriate and certainly a less confusing title than the chosen name, and its selection might have discouraged some over-zealous recruiting sergeants from persuading academic-minded but insolvent recruits to enlist in the Army on the promise of a federally subsidized

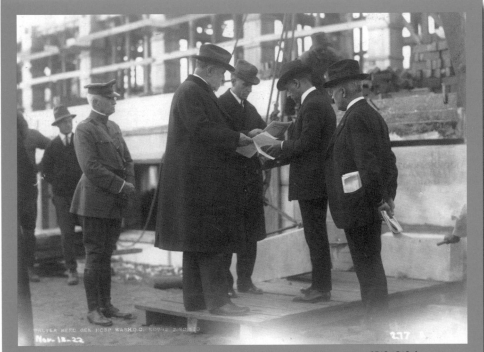

Laying Cornerstone, Army Medical School, General Glennan and Secretary of War Weeks

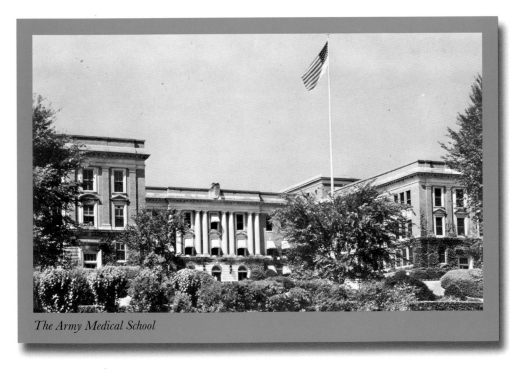

The Army Medical School

education at the Army Medical School. Such promises were a favorite recruiting hoax[42] during the Center's first ten years, and a number of superior young men arrived at the Post only to be assigned as bottle washers, laboratory technicians or as members of a "ground force" clean-up squad, for practically all of the installation support activities were maintained by military personnel. Patients were counted as members of the organization, for once transferred to the hospital, and for the duration of their stay, they were a direct responsibility of the hospital commander. Thus, maintaining a Post with a personnel complement of some 2,000 [43] individuals, at least half of whom were bed cases and convalescents, kept the recruiting sergeants as well as the Staff "on their toes."

The closer physical association of the School and hospital was particularly advantageous to the clinical program, for the hospital staff delegated some of the X-ray and much of the laboratory work to the faculty, which found the case histories valuable teaching assets. In return, the faculty directors of the departments of laboratory and roentgenology served as consultants to the hospital staff, as well as members of a Center consulting board.[44] Thus they formed the professional teams proposed by earlier medical planners.

Civilian medical education had improved markedly since 1893, and newly commissioned officers were better prepared for general practitioner duties. Public health and epidemiological studies were necessary to the successful maintenance

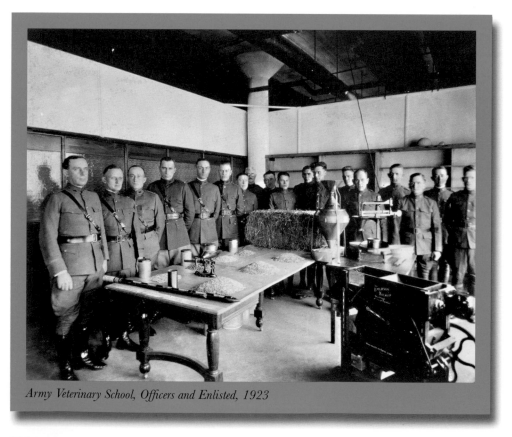

Army Veterinary School, Officers and Enlisted, 1923

of a worldwide military force, and the Army Medical School courses in these subjects then were irreplaceable by any standard. An entirely new concept of domestic public health measures was taking shape, which ten years later, under the "New Deal" influence and the rapidly growing United States Public Health Service, would change the medical history of the nation.

Responsibility for military public health rested with the Medical Department, with its allied functions of dentistry, veterinary medicine and nursing. The male officers in the first two groups attended the same basic course in preventive medicine and clinical pathology as given the doctors. Colonel Siler had long advocated strengthening the advanced medical course, usually given only to a selected group of older officers, for he believed more emphasis should be placed on medicine and surgery, with the latter course including intensive work in gross pathology and more practical work in urology.[45] Insofar as the Army was concerned, past experience seemed to prove that specialists in roentgenology required a broader foundation in clinical medicine and pathology than usually given, but that few of the Army doctors with aptitude for X-ray work selected it as a specialty, and few who selected it as a specialty had the aptitude.[46] Thus the faculty had come to believe that the advanced training should cover a six-month period in the general hospitals, with exemption from all administrative duties.[47]

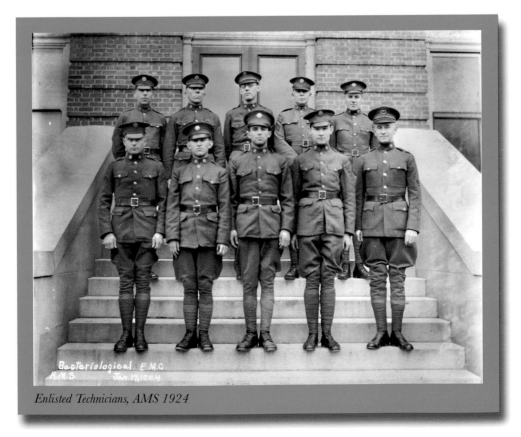

Enlisted Technicians, AMS 1924

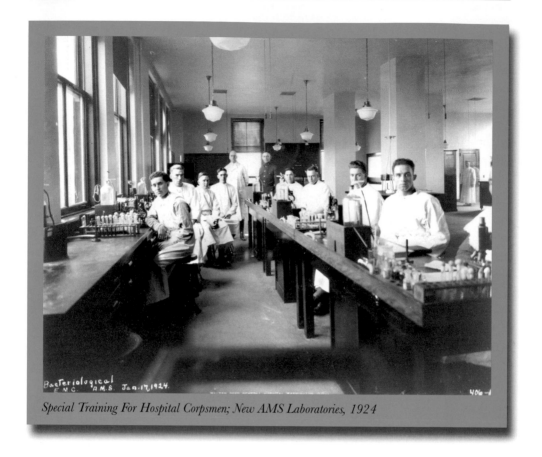

Special Training For Hospital Corpsmen; New AMS Laboratories, 1924

In 1922 Major Henry J. Nichols published *Carriers in Infectious Diseases* and Major Harry L. Gilchrist, lecturer at the Army Medical School and already recognized as a specialist in the medical aspects of chemical warfare, published *Reports on the After Effects of Warfare Gases*. Hospital clinical programs and School investigative programs were partially cause and effect. It is interesting, therefore, that in 1925 the hospital laboratory service reported an increasing number of sputum examinations for tubercle bacillus, and at the same time Lieutenant Colonel Edward Bright Vedder published *The Epidemiology of Sputum Borne Diseases and Its Relation to the Health of the National Forces*. Colonel Siler and other Army epidemiologists influential in establishing and staffing the Tropical Disease Board in Manila, confirmed earlier research findings that dengue or break bone fever was transmitted by the *Aëdes aegypti*, the same insect that carried yellow fever, and they were writing prolifically on this topic. In 1924, Major Kirk, Chief of the Orthopedic Section at Walter Reed, published his first edition of *Amputations*.

The *Army Medical Bulletin*, a Surgeon General's Office publication published at Carlisle Barracks after 1922, was busily indoctrinating its readers on subjects of general military medical interest. Medical Supply, for instance, which received its first real impetus from Darnall's standardizing and testing experiments,[48] first conducted when the School was housed with the Museum, received a surprising amount of printed space. Even discussions of the medical regiment, medical tactics and medical sanitation were still of interest to the Corps of 1925.

The clinical investigative program was at best a slow process, and some medical officers believed the compulsory reassignment of all personnel, required under the "Manchu Act" of 1912, should not apply to the scientists. Major Nichols, whose service was invaluable to the School faculty, and others were perforce required to take their two-year-in-six duty with troops regardless of the challenge of undiscovered viruses, the work begun by Colonel Hans Zinsser of the Medical Reserve Corps with preliminary skin tests,[49] and idiosyncrasies of the Aëdes Egypti. Many of them were never able to understand why this mandate should apply to personnel at the Army Medical School but not to all personnel at the hospital.

Regrouping of the hospital and school as the Army Medical Center resulted in the adoption of a shield, used for a number of years without a motto. Of the heraldic symbols on this shield, the cadeuceus represents the Medical Department; the year book and flaming torch represent knowledge. The crest is the helmet of Minerva, the patroness of medicine. The Medical Department colors, maroon and white, form the relief.

The motto, as finally chosen, was selected from popular suggestions offered by officers, nurses, aides, dieticians and enlisted men from the Troop Command, Army Medical Center. Three mottos were screened for special consideration, of which the one proposed by the late Lieutenant Colonel Henry J. Nichols, once of the Army Medical School Faculty, was selected – "To the spirit of science and the instinct of service."

The wise and beloved Jefferson Randolph Kean, Medical Department sage for over half a century, was asked to interpret the motto and disclaimed the phrase "instinct of service." At his suggestion the line was revised to read *Scientiae Inter Arma Spiritus*, the spirit of science and of arms,[50] a dedication for a great military hospital responsible for the care of as well as the prevention of casualties of war.

References

1. William Hazlett.

2. Interview with Miss Margaret Lower, February. 14, 1951.

3. As told to the writer.

4. *The Come Back*, Nov. 9, Dec. 21, 1923; Conversation with Miss Mary E. Schick, 1941.

5. Lower interview, *op cit*.

6. Conversation with Miss Mary E. Schick, 1941.

7. Florence A. Blanchfield, *Organized Nursing and the Army in Three Wars*, MSS on file HD SGO.

8. Act 4 June 1920 (41 Stat. 767).

9. Blanchfield, *loc. cit.*

10. Worn by officers only.

11. Conversation with Miss Mary E. Schick, 1941.

12. *Ibid*; General Pershing was a frequent "official" visitor during this period; *The Come Back* for March 19, 1926, notes that he is a patient.

13. Annual Rpt WRGH, 1922.

14. Interview with Col. Herbert N. Dean, MAC, Ret., Apr. 12, 1950; Power House employees, April 1950.

15. *Ibid.*

16. Annual Rpt TSG... 1923, pg 107, 108.

17. Annual Rpt WRGH, 1923.

18. Annual Rpt, 1933, U.S. Veterans' Administration, pg 11; BOB Cir. 46, October 21, 1924.

19. Annual Rpt WRGH, 1923.

20. Interview with Jessie M. Braden, June 26, 1950.

21. Memo for C/S from TSG, 20 February 1920, File 210.1-1 (M.C.) C.C. and WD Cir. 177, 13 May 1920. (quoted)

22. Annual Rpt WRGH, 1924.

23. *Ibid.*

24. *Ibid*, 1925.

25. Medical Dept. Officers Meet, Jan. 21, 1924, *The Come Back*, Jan. 25, 1924.

26. SGO Circular Ltr., 28 Dec. 1923.

27. Annual Rpt WRGH, 1925, 1926.

28. *The Washington Evening Star*, May 13, 1924.

29. Dean interview, *op cit.*

30. Interview with Mrs. M.W. Ireland, April 14, 1950.

31. Dean interview, *op cit.*

32. *Ibid*; See *The Come Back*, on file Library, WRAH.

33. Lower interview, *op cit*.

34. *The Washington Sunday Star*, July 5, 1925, Pt. I; See *The Come Back*, 1922–1925.

35. Dean interview, *op cit*.

36. *The Come Back*, April 2, 6, 1923.

37. *The Washington Sunday Star*, June 13, 1926.

38. *The Come Back*, March 26,1924; April 11,1924; April 18, 25,1924; August 1,1924.

39. 1st Ind. AGO, 6 January 1922, File 352.-1 (ADS) GG; War Department General Order No. 15, 8 April 1922, Sec. VI; AR 350-105, 11 February 1922. (quoted)

40. WD GO #33, August 31, 1923.

41. Annual Rpt TSG... 1923, pg 246.

42. Personal knowledge of the writer.

43. Annual Rpt WRGH, 1924.

44. Annual Rpt TSG... 1925, pg 309.

45. Minutes AMS (On file Office of Commandant), Sept. 11, 1923.

46. Annual Rpt TSG... 1922, pg 257.

47. Minutes, *loc cit*.

48. Interview with Brig. Gen. Albert G. Love, MC, Ret., Feb. 13, 1951.

49. Annual Rpt TSG... 1924, pg 251.

50. *Service Stripe*, July 27, 1946.

The Pride of
the Medical Department

1926–1929

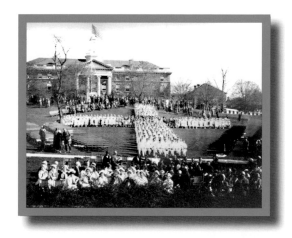

"I did not know how to value (the life)
of a sick or wounded soldier by any pecuniary standard."[1]

The Congress apparently failed to visualize permanent extension of the Veterans Administration into a gigantic adventure in socialized medicine. As the Army Medical Department was anxious to replace the temporary war service buildings at Walter Reed with permanent structures, an arrangement was worked out whereby the Veterans Administration supported the construction program, on the understanding that Veterans beneficiaries would be hospitalized on pro rata costs, changed, in 1926, to a flat rate of $4.15 per inpatient day.[2]

The rather generalized hospital cost accounting system used by the Medical Department included charges for the pay and allowances of officers; pay, allowance, and subsistence of nurses; pay, subsistence and clothing of enlisted men; pay of civilian employees, and rations when provided; subsistence (for sick in hospital only); medical supplies; and miscellaneous items such as laundry, utilities, light, water, heat, telephone services, maintenance and repair of buildings and grounds. The total of all accountable items enumerated, divided by the number of inpatients, established the cost per inpatient day. This was, in 1926, $4.83.[3]

Thus the Medical Department apparently lost on the cash emoluments incident to hospitalizing Veterans cases, but from the long-range viewpoint the ledger remained "in the black," for during the 1925–26 session of Congress, $1,050,000 of a total $2,000,000 was appropriated for permanent construction at Walter Reed

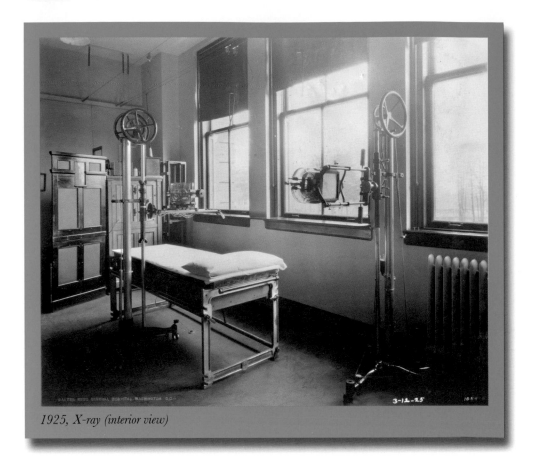

1925, X-ray (interior view)

alone,[4] and other Army general hospitals profited similarly. The temporary wards immediately behind the Main Building were removed during the year, in order to make space for the laboratory requirement of a regular ward for basal metabolism work, where patients could spend the night, and a mortuary chapel and receiving room, out of sight of the hospital wards.[5] The old stone gatehouse, landmark of the Shepherd dynasty, was razed, and some of the stones were used for walks in various parts of the grounds.[6] On July 2, 1926, the last issue of *The Come Back* appeared; old times and old landmarks had changed.

The bed capacity of the five general hospitals then operated by the Medical Department remained relatively constant during this period. Of the 1200 permanent or, in Army parlance, "fixed" beds allotted to Walter Reed, with a stand-by or expansion quota of 360,[7] the fiscal accounting of June 30, 1926, showed that 758 were occupied.[8] War Department General Staff planning figures for bed authorizations usually provided a fifteen per cent dispersion factor for emergency overflow, and so during the tranquil late twenties the hospital was able to admit all eligible applicants. By and large, however, the number of Veterans' beneficiaries equaled the combined military admission of both officer and enlisted men.

Some of the medical officers on duty at Walter Reed during this period believed this group of patients more of an administrative liability than a professional asset. It was customary

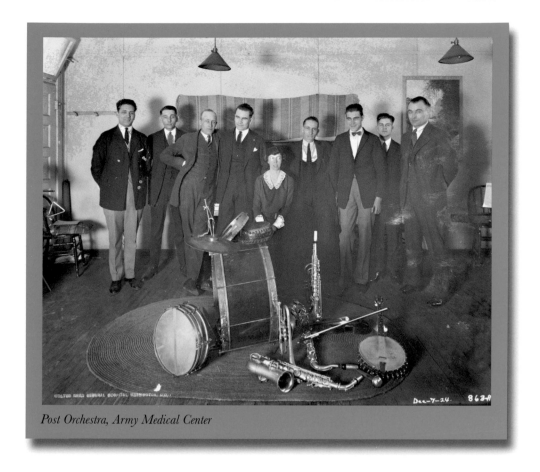

Post Orchestra, Army Medical Center

practice to use ambulatory enlisted patients for light ward duties, such as carrying specimens to the laboratory, pushing wheel chairs or acting as messengers, and such tasks were usually discharged with good will and a spirit of helpfulness. The situation was occasionally different with Veterans, however, for military disciplinary channels were no longer operative. Some, as was to be expected in any large group, were malingerers, and they cared little for routine ward work; others were notably anxious to prolong their period of hospitalization, for Walter Reed was known for its excellent food service and pleasant surroundings. A few were always sensitive to fancied wrongs, which were referred to sympathetic Congressional supporters.

Unlike civilian hospitals, with their appreciably shorter periods of hospitalization, the intimate personal relations between doctor and patient, and the divergent classes of patients admitted, military patients were predominantly a homogeneous group as to sex, occupation, salary and social security. Thus the mores and behavior pattern of the well soldier to a large extent were unchanged by transfer to the medical Post. Harmless-appearing card games became high-stake blackjack games when the ward officers or nurse disappeared in their private offices, and on occasion "Hiram and Johnny Walker" snuggled under more than one pillow or carelessly draped lounge suit in bed-cupboard.

Regardless of stringent *Post Regulations*, there was usually a willing visitor or nimble cab driver who could be persuaded to carry contraband, including narcotics, and so the twelve-hour duty for the medical officer-of-the-day was far from tranquil, and many became as adept with the stomach pump as General Arthur had been in his early days at Vancouver Barracks. It was not unusual to have benevolent metropolitan police-men deliver to Walter Reed's "noble façade," patients who were not only inebriated but indigent—for want of a better place to send them. Fearful and quavering was the young doctor who inadvertently admitted such cases, especially repeaters, and then had to justify his lack of judgment to his praeceptor, the canny Ernest R. Gentry, for once admitted the men were difficult to discharge. Only a few of the cases were misances, but many were chronic, requiring domiciliary care. After their value as teaching mate-rial, the staff preferred new clinical problems.

During 1926, there were 751 patients on the Neuropsychiatric Section.[9] Diagnostically, the cases were preponderantly dementia praecox, psychoneurosis and constitutional psychopath. The malarial treatment for paresis and cerebro-spinal syphilis was used in nineteen cases, therapy that held "out more hope for good than any other form of treatment heretofore used."[10]

The total number of medical admissions decreased during this period; nevertheless the clinical investigative program reflected the progressional advances in therapy used in civilian hospitals. Recognition of Diabetes Mellitus, once a hopelessly debilitating

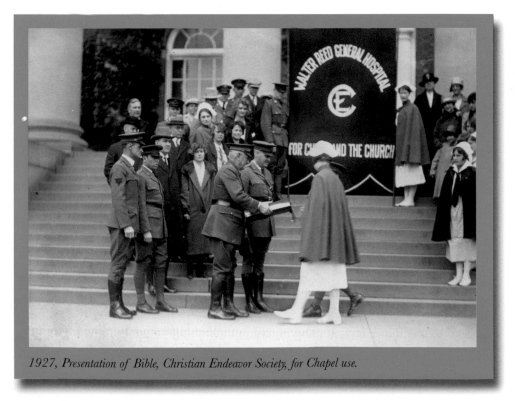

1927, Presentation of Bible, Christian Endeavor Society, for Chapel use.

disease, was increasingly easy and forty-eight cases were reported as improved under treatment and dietary care. Further, the cardiovascular section performed 210 electrocardiograms, and the laboratory completed 132,495 procedures.

Of the 3,343 surgical operations, 2,080 were EENT; 108 were genito-urinary; and 157 of the 270 gynecological patients had some form of surgery. The Dental Service, still under administrative supervision of general surgery, had departments of clinic dentistry, prosthesis, oral surgery and dental roentgenology, and during 1926 treated a total number of 2,376 military patients in 12,646 sittings, and 3,093 "others" in 10,826 sittings.[11] In harmony with the general trend toward more complete clinical investigations, the Department of Roentgenology, renamed from X-ray, made 10,387 examinations and gave 623 Roentgen ray treatments.

The Personnel Quotient

Medical Department Tables of Organization and Equipment,[12] provide specific allowances of personnel for installations of stated bed size. Thus the assignment of doctors, nurses, enlisted technicians, orderlies, etc., is not a haphazard affair but is controlled at the source of manpower intake – the Surgeon General's Office. The current T/O provided 516 enlisted men for duty at the Army Medical Center, with the detachment strength averaging only 510 for the year. The enlisted men not only performed technical and nursing

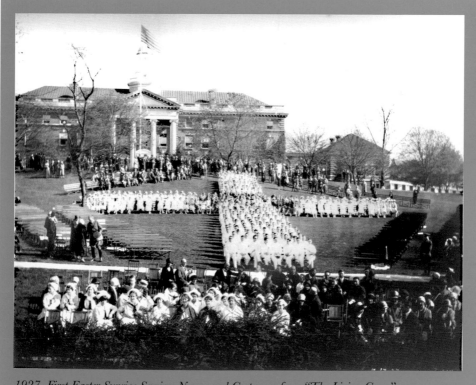

1927, First Easter Sunrise Service, Nurses and Corpsmen form "The Living Cross"

duties, but they also maintained much of the equipment and serviced various Center activities. Manpower was not in short supply, and approximately forty per cent of the corpsmen completing their enlistment re-enlisted at their home station.

The Hospital Corps barracks at Walter Reed, Building No. 7, was superior to many such accommodations on other military posts. The building was attractively furnished, the food service good, and if the Regular Army monthly "take home" pay seemed meager in comparison to the cash salaries of civilians, the money was clear, for clothing, food, medical service and other amenities were provided by the government. Civilian clothes could be worn in off-duty hours, and while amusements were available on the reservation, the Georgia Avenue street car line provided easy access to the city. Duty at the Center was unusually pleasant, and if some of the young ladies of Washington learned to their surprise that their handsome dates from the hospital were not doctors, as they may have been led to believe, few seemed to have cared. To some of the short-haired, long-waisted "flappers" of the day, the ability to do the Charleston was of more consequence than the prestige of a learned profession.

The Rea swimming pool was usable only during the summer months. First provided as part of the rehabilitation program for World War I patients, the schedule was by then so arranged that all classes of Post personnel used it freely. Movies were shown at the Red Cross House and the YMCA, but the Knights of Columbus Hut was used only for religious services, by the resident priest, and on Sundays. The Post Exchange, in the basement of the Red Cross, was renovated and a lunch counter and soda fountain were added. A restaurant was operated as part of the Service Club or Guest House management, maintained for the families of sick patients. Of the two barber shops on the Post, one was in the Red Cross House and the other was in the main barracks, for the easy accommodation of the men.[13]

Recruit training was based on Section III, General Order No. 4, 1921, and Medical Department Bulletin No. 18. The 120 hours of instruction covered a six-month period and included orientation in such subjects as military courtesy, the Articles of War, Army Regulations, personal hygiene, physical training, first aid, anatomy, physiology, nursing, school of platoon, shelter tent pitching, personal equipment, functions and relations of the Medical Department to the line, litter drill (loaded and unloaded) general orders of a sentry, guard duty and guard mount. Special instruction was given for promotion as junior non-commissioned officers and to candidates for sergeancy. On-the-job training for assignments as technicians for the X-ray, laboratory and dental (including property) sections was conducted by the various hospital departments in question, with the successful competitors given appropriate technical ratings or promotions on recommendation from the departments. "The general health of the command (was) good," stated the Post Commander in the Annual Report. "The number of sick days lost in hospital (was) due to the time cases (were) detained rather than to the number of new cases admitted."[14]

The Happy Hours

For years there had been innumerable complaints from the Dietetic Department over the lack of food storage space, which necessitated day to day buying, as well as the penetrating odors that seemed to steep certain portions of the Main Building with a permanent aroma of cookery. On December 28, 1927, the north annex to the Main Building was opened and provided not only ample space for storage, but a commodious kitchen and dining hall, Mess II, wards for the Ear, Nose and Throat department, and space for a permanent hospital library.

Securing adequate space for the library had become a pressing question, for the old Ward 32 was foredoomed to make way for the new east wing of the Main Building. Further, the collection of books in the officers' waiting room, adjoining the Commanding Officer's Office and known as the Medical Library, had long since outgrown its space.[15] Opened on April 1, 1928[16] and occupying a 50 x 100 foot section below the new Eye, Ear, Nose and Throat wards, the new Library was a gem of architectural planning. The open book shelves were so arranged that one-fourth of the room was partitioned off to form a professional library, which while not sound proof, was at least an off-bounds area for all but professional personnel.

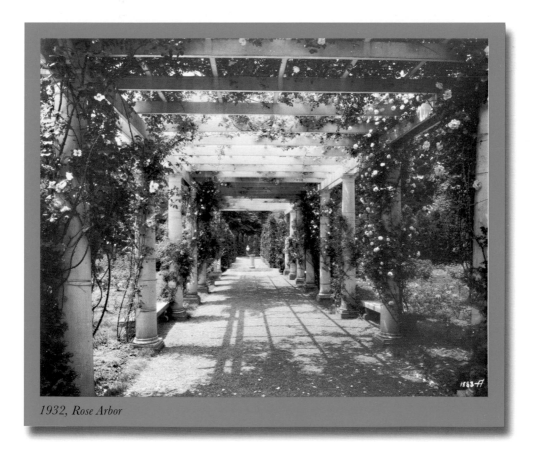

1932, Rose Arbor

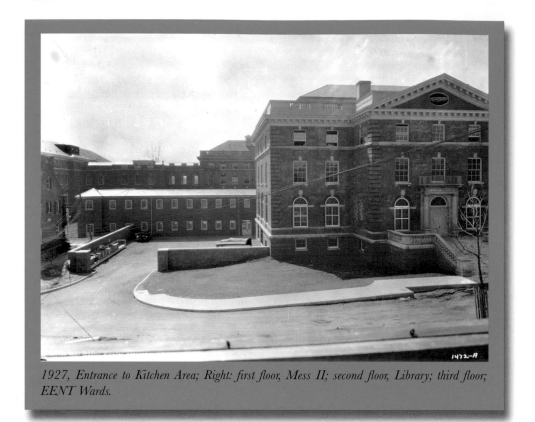

1927, Entrance to Kitchen Area; Right: first floor, Mess II; second floor, Library; third floor; EENT Wards.

The Library and librarians, Misses Schick and Gould,[17] occupied a special place in the hospital activities, for more often than not some of the doctors and favored patients stopped by for afternoon tea, a delightfully informal little back-room ceremony that marked the close of a long day on the wards. The longer stay of military hospital cases encourages a comradeship and familiarity with the staff less easily secured in the hurried and impersonal atmosphere of the great civilian hospitals. And regardless of the large number of technical library procedures carried on behind the scenes or in the early morning hours, the librarians always managed to appear unhurried and gracious. The dilettante scholars and musicians among the patients and staff came to feel that The Library was their own serene sanctuary, and there was always a select group of congenial spirits to discuss literature and the arts. Some discussed the Wall Street news and soul-shaking world events, and some discussed their own soul-shaking problems. If they leaned too long on the lectern, they were gently and graciously dismissed without quite knowing how or when the turn in small talk reminded them of other obligations.

There were few medical librarians as such at this time, for Library Schools offered no special courses in this field. And in spite of Miss Edith Kathleen Jones' book on *Hospital Libraries*, there was not such a marked pseudo-scientific trend toward bibliotherapy as that which began to develop in the late thirties. The average librarian's medical knowledge was like the gaps in a crossword puzzle, for medical nomenclature and a somewhat haphazard knowledge of clinical symptoms was self-acquired through handling of medical journals issued to the staff or cataloging medical texts. The Walter Reed Library was one of the largest and best organized in the reconstruction program, and Miss Schick was well known to her contemporaries in the hospital library work.[18]

One unusually shy but attentive bachelor officer member of the Library group visited regularly for some weeks while undergoing a physical survey, then suddenly his daily trips ceased. If the librarians noted his absence, they assumed that he had been reassigned to duty on his former post. When he reappeared some three weeks later, pale, wan and walking with a one-sided gait, it was an occasion for rejoicing, and he endured a jovial scolding over his long neglect. Embarrassed over the friendly attention and hedging his answers, the young man finally confided that he had been one of Colonel Keller's surgical patients. "Oh-oh, an operation!" exclaimed the self-educated library student of the medical arts, "Well, it's better to have it behind you than in front of you," she said, and wondered at his shocked expression and at his hasty departure.[19] This occasion marked the shy young officer's last visit to the Post Library, and it was several weeks before his one-time confidante learned that he had undergone a hemorrhoidectomy, the then popular high compound enemas and all.

Installation Support

A new Red Cross building was also completed, but not released to the government until 1928. The East and West wings to Building No. I were still incomplete, but the Quartermaster was alert to his responsibility for such a large and increasingly complicated construction program. Cost data, reports and blueprints were brought up-to-date, and all building systems over and under ground were appropriately identified as governmental or commercial. Reservation maps and a block plan were made for separating steam, water, gas, electric, sewage and drainage systems.[20] Sewage was removed by the District of Columbia system and the garbage by city trucks. All water used at the Center came from the Potomac, through the Washington aqueduct of the U.S. Engineer Department, and it was both potable and adequate.[21] All trash and refuse was burned in the Post incinerator, and, since some horses were still stabled on the Post, the manure was stored in concrete pots, sealed for fermentation and later used as fertilizer.[22]

Post Headquarters administration apparently presented few problems at this time, and the principal grievance of the Post Commander concerned the old and inadequate laundry equipment. Standard medical supplies were requisitioned from the Medical Supply Section of the New York General Depot, and the allowance was adequate. Moreover, the monetary allowance provided by the Surgeon General's Office, under the two-year Replacing Medical Supplies fund established in 1906, was adequate for all needs.[23] It was used mainly for the purchase of nonstandard items such as drugs and new equipment which the testing laboratories had not had time to approve and add to the

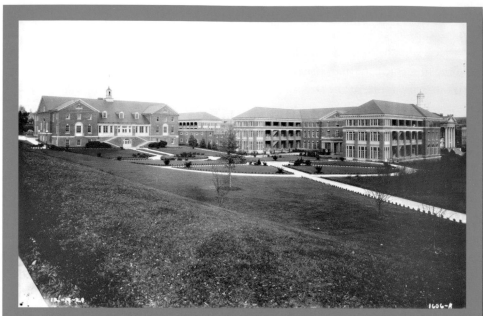

1929, New Red Cross Building and West Wing, Main Building

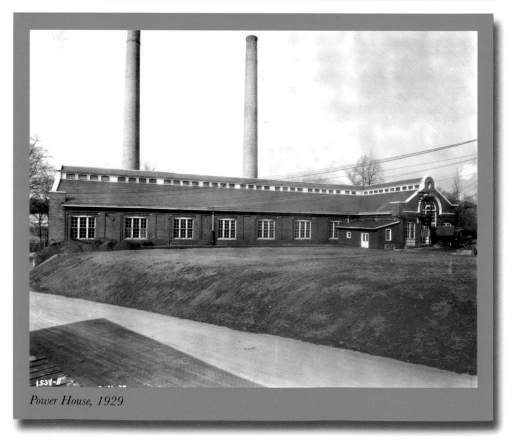

Power House, 1929

Surgeon General's catalogue of standard supplies. War surplus supplies were gradually being exhausted, including the much-deplored paper bandages,[24] and the new supplies were considered vastly superior. In 1928, when furnishings and equipment were purchased for the new wards, the bedrooms were equipped with Simons metal furniture. The solariums received the then popular wicker furniture, which soon proved a burden to the exterminator experts. Even the old wooden refrigerators were being replaced by electrical equipment that was "a big improvement over the old unsanitary ice box."[25]

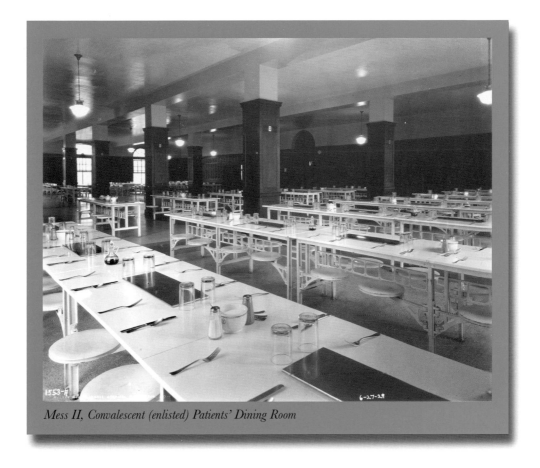

Mess II, Convalescent (enlisted) Patients' Dining Room

Six separate messes (food services) were in operation; the Post had four miles of roads of which more than fifty per cent were concrete, and a concrete-curbed parking lot adjacent to the formal gardens. Of the male personnel assigned to the Army Medical Center in 1927, 322 officers and 535 enlisted men were assigned to Walter Reed; eleven officers and forty-nine enlisted men were assigned to the Army Medical Center Headquarters; and fifteen officers, sixty-eight enlisted men and thirty students were assigned to the Army Medical School.[26]

The Quartermaster's work orders, that is current maintenance, showed that 5,325 shop activities were completed during the calendar year 1927. The Fire Department, usually considered an inactive group, extinguished fifty-six minor fires, most of which resulted from careless disposal of cigarette butts and matches. This section was staffed by civilians, but the principal labor force was drawn from the Walter Reed detachment, whose versatile qualities were eulogized by the Quartermaster officer:

> *The enlisted medical personnel have proved themselves good apprentices, willing and ready at all times to carry on their work. The enlisted men on the paint detail have done exceptionally good work. In many cases they have applied as much paint and covered as much surface in as neat a manner as the painters working for a commercial firm.*[27]

Officer Pavilion No. I, a medical ward during World War I, was converted into a general Post Exchange. Conveniently located across from the one-time "Pest House," so-called in Colonel Birmingham's day, but by 1927 a separate and well-equipped obstetrical ward, it was near to both the permanent and the frame barracks, and in time it became the off-duty social center for the Detachment. Extensions were added to the Medical Supply Warehouse and to the Guard House. The deep scar of Cameron's Creek had long since been covered[28] over by the formal garden, but a further "face-lifting" occurred in 1928, when a gleaming white pergola was added.[29] By 1929, Building No. 34, the old mortuary, was demolished, and some of the early permanent quarters were razed to provide space for a new Isolation Ward or Infectious Disease Section.

The East Wing of Delano Hall, the nurses' residence destined to be the envy of all the Army hospitals, was completed in November 1929. As it was designed for gracious living, it provided single rooms, with a connecting bath for each two rooms assigned to the general staff nurses, and a suite of living room, bedroom and bath for the Chief Nurses. Final completion of the structure in 1934 included well furnished sitting rooms, lounges, recreation rooms, kitchenettes, pressing rooms, and a grand ballroom of unusually magnificent proportions.

Mrs. Julia O. Flikke was Chief Nurse at Walter Reed during the late twenties and early thirties, and her staff, on December 31, 1928, included 104 Regular Army Nurses. As the principal Chief Nurse, Mrs. Flikke held the relative rank of Captain, Army Nurse Corps, and the eight Chief Nurse assistants held the relative grade of First Lieutenant. Eighty Regular Army Nurses in the grade of Second Lieutenant and fifteen reserve nurses performed the principal bedside nursing duties for 7,448 patients.[30] They were, however, generously assisted by the hospital corpsmen and to some extent by the one hundred eighteen student nurses then on duty at the hospital.[31] Of the 1200 beds, the maximum occupancy occurred in the "pneumonia months" of January, February and March:[32]

Month	Officers	Nurses	EM	VB	Civ.	Total
January	67	4	313	436	112	932
February	80	8	297	440	114	939
March	91	8	318	412	113	942

Re-evaluating Subsidized Education

In spite of the bedside nursing service rendered by the students, the Army School of Nursing had become something of a morale and administrative burden to the Medical Department.[33] Nearly one-fourth of each class remained away from the parent institution in order to complete affiliated training in subjects not adequately provided at Walter Reed but required for examination and licensing by the various State Boards of Nurse Examiners. This was not only a costly procedure for the Medical Department, but of the 755 students who graduated from 1921–1929, only 182 accepted appointments in the Army Nurse Corps, and twenty-three of this number were appointed in 1927–28. Of the 182, only fifty-four were still in the Corps,[34] slightly more than nine per cent of the total number of 509 Regular Army Nurses (supported by an additional 190 reserve nurses[35]). Thus the Army School of Nursing was not contributing markedly as a replacement factor for nursing personnel but was benefiting the civilian communities.

The academic program provided for the students had, moreover, affected the morale of the regular nursing staff at Walter Reed to some extent, for the School had a separate educational director, rules, regulations and working hours which some of the Regular Army Nurses considered unnecessarily favorable. The Superintendent of the Army Nurse Corps, Major Julia C. Stimson, was a well-known figure in the nursing education circles of the national nursing organizations, and many of the older Army Nurses, graduates of the regular three-year training programs, believed that the Army School of Nursing was of greater interest to her than other Corps problems.[36]

Mrs. Flikke apparently had only an administrative association with the Army School of Nursing, in spite of being the senior nurse on the staff. A precise, soft-spoken woman, she was in no sense an agitator for educational reforms, and many of her contemporaries believed she accepted the nurse's role as functional rather than military and that she did not believe women should be an integral part of the Army. Reserved, trim and immaculately groomed, she was particular about minute details and ably managed her staff with a detachment that some nurses found exasperating.[37]

Prior to World War I, nurses had not mixed socially with the medical staff to any great extent.[38] Social trends had changed for the better, however, and the relative rank status of the Army Nurse Corps, secured by the national nursing organizations, gave the women a more definite military standing. These factors, plus Surgeon General Ireland's warm championship of Major Stimson, affected the prestige of the Army Nurse Corps as a whole. Mrs. Flikke was both personable and tactful, and so she undertook what was essentially the role of official hostess for Major Stimson. Thus under her expert management Sunday dinner at the nurses' residence at Walter Reed was a pleasantly anticipated ritual for the families of older medical officers in and around Washington.[39]

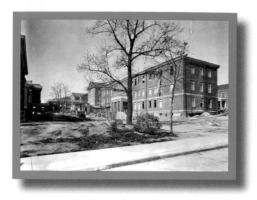

1929, Construction of new Isolation Ward; tree in left rear, behind truck, is Georgie Newport's Catalpa tree

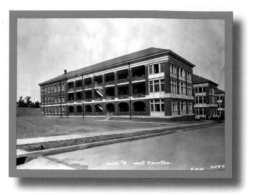

1930, Medical Wards (enlisted); lower floor, third building, extreme right later used as Out-Patient Clinic

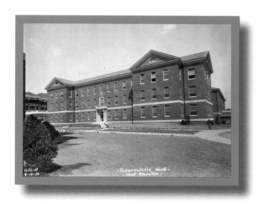

1930, Tuberculosis and Venereal Disease Ward, one floor later converted for use as an Obstetrical Ward

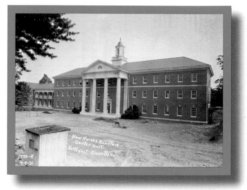

1931, First Construction at Delano Hall

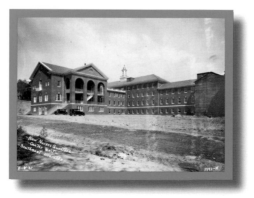

Delano Hall, center unit, rear

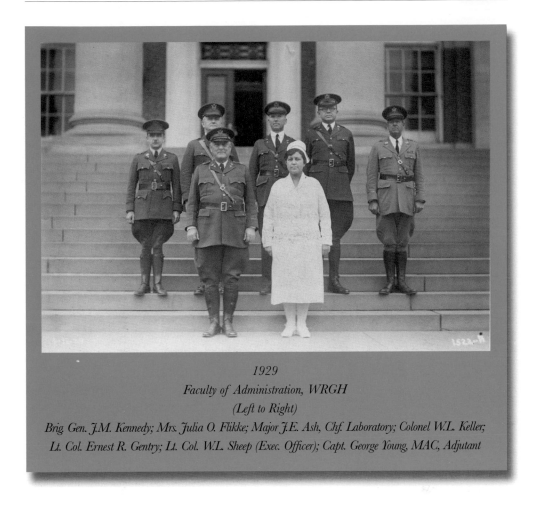

1929
Faculty of Administration, WRGH
(Left to Right)
Brig. Gen. J.M. Kennedy; Mrs. Julia O. Flikke; Major J.E. Ash, Chf. Laboratory; Colonel W.L. Keller;
Lt. Col. Ernest R. Gentry; Lt. Col. W.L. Sheep (Exec. Officer); Capt. George Young, MAC, Adjutant

Post Commander Number 12

Brigadier General James M. Kennedy, Post Commander from March 1926 until December 1929, was a bluff, hearty man.[40] Long an intimate friend of General Ireland, he was one of the elite members of the "official family."[41] Although Kennedy had some success as a surgeon he was undoubtedly better known as a hospital administrator.[42] Kindly, jovial and deeply interested in patient care, he took infinite trouble to provide the small niceties that added so much to the comfort of the sick.[43]

General Kennedy had been Chief Surgeon of the New York Port of Embarkation during the war, and it was generally conceded that he was both a capable administrator and a good sanitary engineer.[44] Shortly after the war he became the Chief Surgeon of the Philippine Division, and it was to his office that the overworked and mentally exhausted editor of the Index-Catalogue, Fielding N. Garrison, by then a commissioned officer and Lieutenant Colonel in the Medical Corps, was assigned. It was therefore Garrison, the indefatigable letter writer, who in the early twenties provided a word-picture of the man later to command the Army Medical Center. "Colonel Kennedy, our Chief is a man of broad mind and generous disposition, with the sweetness of temper that big broad-gauge men of large physique usually have, and he has given me some extraordinary work to do."[45] The extraordinary work, for Garrison had never practiced medicine, was cooperative work with the Army's third Tropical Disease Board, whose members arrived in Manila in September 1922; and to another friend he wrote, "I have the good fortune to have a military chief who is an aristocrat and a gentleman, a man who is used to having vassals. Working for such a man, certainly the nicest man I have ever worked for, I find my duties intriguing and engaging."[46]

Convivial and cheerful, General Kennedy tried with almost child-like anxiety to be a model of all the virtues which "Noisy Jim" had represented, and so he asked his executive officer to remind him quietly when he showed signs of straying from the path of dignity, which tried his inclination for bluff, warm-hearted comradeship.[47] He may have lacked his predecessor's fine sensitiveness to nature, but he carried out, to a large extent, the carefully laid plans for beautifying the grounds.[48] The hospital was famed for its beautiful gardens and well stocked greenhouses, and General Kennedy instituted the practice of sending flowers to all women and children on the second day after admission to the hospital, and of having flowers placed on the caskets of all destitute and friendless soldiers who died at Walter Reed.[49] He was not well during his last year as Post Commander, but as General Ireland was approaching the retirement age, "Big Jim" remained on duty regardless of his own infirmities. In December 1929, he requested transfer to Letterman General Hospital, which he had once commanded, and he died there in October 1930.

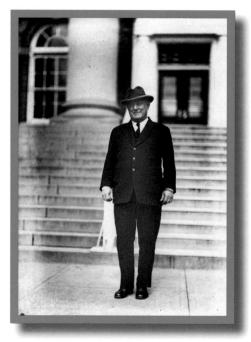

Brigadier General James M. Kennedy, 1926

In the Course of Progress

Special Orders No. 47, Army Medical Center, April 7, 1926, authorized a *Professional Board* for coordinating the scientific investigations of the School faculty and student instruction with prevailing clinical practices at the hospital. General Kennedy was nominally President of the Board; actually, Colonel Henry C. Fisher, then Commandant of the School, served as chairman of the group, called the Faculty Board. The members included, from the School, the Director of Laboratories and X-ray, with the Librarian, a medical officer, serving as recorder, and the Chiefs of Medicine and Surgery from the hospital.[50]

Doctor R.L. Kahn, Sanitary Corps Reserve, was assigned to the School for a two-week period of active duty in 1925, to begin his now famous work with the Kahn precipitation tests for detection of syphilis. In June 1926, the Serology Section of the School laboratories again began performing all of the Wasserman work for the hospital.[51] On August 27, AMC General Order No. 8 placed both laboratories under the direction of the School. The Kahn-Wasserman comparative evaluation series continued of paramount interest until 1928. By that time the 13,000 cases studied supported the recommendation that both tests be used by the Army Medical Department.

Twelve full-time instructors, including one dental and one veterinary officer, and twenty part-time instructors were assigned to the School in 1926. In addition to the preparation and issue of the stock vaccines, which had justly earned distinction for the Medical Department, the laboratories were now preparing scarlet fever streptococcus toxin for the Dick Test for immunization against scarlet fever. Major Nichols was that year completing his last assignment as Director of Laboratories and had begun a study of chemotherapy in bacterial infections, which was later prepared for publication by Major James S. Simmons, a still little-known Army epidemiologist who was then writing energetically on a number of special problems. Nichols was not only concerned with the malarial treatment of paresis, but he was still deeply involved in studies of yaws, begun some sixteen years before. Lt. Colonel Craig, Director of the Department of Laboratories, published *A Manual of the Parasitic Protozoa*, followed, in 1927, with seven independent articles.

Laboratory work of such an exacting nature required well-trained technical assistants. This was an old and annoying problem to the faculty, for the training and retraining of personnel absorbed an undue amount of time. Colonel Fisher proposed, therefore, that fixed allotments of specialist ratings for enlisted men would encourage a more permanent interest in the work.[52] Although not especially interested in the details of the professional programs, he was a canny administrator, and during 1926 he inaugurated a program of "constructive economy" that saved some $10,000.[53]

Many of the Army Medical School students were in the younger age brackets, men having recently completed Medical School and internships, and it was becoming increasingly difficult to interest them in the basic professional courses, which included medicine, surgery and other subjects covered in the undergraduate schools. Their critical attitude was shared by some of the older students and a "goodly proportion of the staff, including Generals Kennedy and Fisher, and others to such an extent that abandonment of the school or at least the part other than post-graduate work was recommended to the Surgeon General." The primary value of the course evolved from the instruction in public health and tropical medicine, which were essentially military problems, but such courses were either condensed or omitted from the usual Medical School curriculum. In 1927 a meeting was held in the Surgeon General's office to consider closing the basic school course. The viewpoints of the Medical School and Medical Field Service School faculties and students were weighed carefully, Surgeon General Ireland finally decreeing a rearrangement of the work so that the two branches would supplement each other. Public health and preventive medicine theories

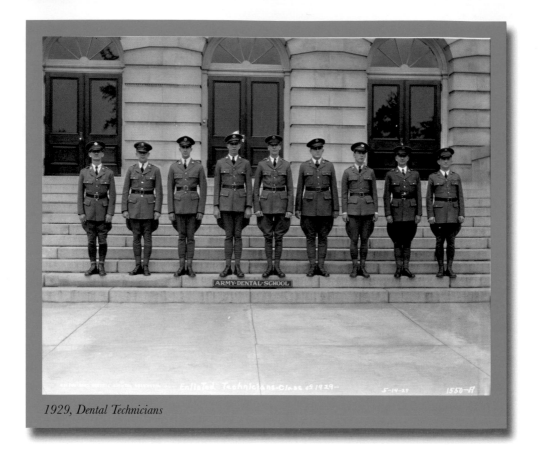

ARMY-DENTAL-SCHOOL

Enlisted Technicians-Class of 1929-   5-14-29   1550-A

1929, Dental Technicians

would be emphasized at the Army Medical School, with the practical application featured at Carlisle. By 1929 the instruction in clinical medicine and contagious diseases was omitted, and emphasis was placed on clinical psychiatry and electrocardiography. In the former, special consideration was given to the preliminary examination and rejection of mentally unstable military applicants.

Aviation medicine was arousing considerable interest by this time, although it was not then a regular part of the Army Medical School curriculum. A year later, however, lectures on aviation medicine and gas warfare were introduced.[54] By 1929 the lectures were supplemented by a tour of Bolling Field Air Base, including a brief flight over the city,[55] and a special demonstration at the Chemical Warfare School at Edgewood Arsenal, Maryland. Colonel Harry L. Gilchrist, a one-time medical officer, had achieved distinction in this branch, ultimately becoming a Major General and Chief of the Chemical Corps.

The Army Medical School research program was already well known, but the Army Veterinary School was just beginning to pioneer in its own field. Major Raymond A. Kelser, V.C., not only demonstrated the principle but published, in 1926, a thesis showing that surra, an equine disease prevalent in the Philippines, was transmitted under natural conditions by the Tabanus Stratus fly.[56] In 1927 he published the first manual

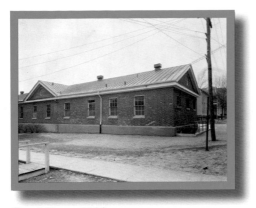

Guard House, 1929

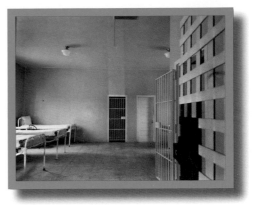

Guard House, Interior View

of Veterinary bacteriology, and in cooperation with the Philippine Insular Bureau of Agriculture, he produced a vaccine for rinderpest. At about the same time, Captain Francois H.K. Reynolds, V.C., began working with Major Simmons and Captain Joe H. St. John, M.C., to demonstrate that the aëdes aebopictus was a second dengue vector and that the egg of an infected mosquito could not transmit the virus to the next generation.

Studies on dental caries had for some years been of interest to dental officers assigned to the various Army hospitals, and at Walter Reed the Medical Service was always alert for related foci of infections. From 1926 to 1929, Major Fernando E. Rodriquez of the Army Dental Corps performed investigations on the bacillus acidophilus theory of dental caries, and he was one of the first dental investigators to isolate the lacto bacilli from carious teeth.[57] The relationship between the hospital and School investigation is well illustrated by the seven per cent increase in dental work at Walter Reed during 1929.[58]

The *Army Medical Bulletin*, published at the Medical Field Service School after 1922, served as a literary vehicle for medical officers. It was by no means ample enough to include all of the military-medical scientific articles and manuals produced, and by 1929 the *Army Dental Bulletin* appeared as a supplement.

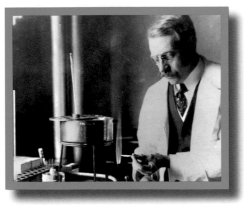

Colonel Russell in Laboratory, AMS.

Within the thirty-six year period from 1914–1950, only the ten years of the Glennan-Kennedy administration was one of serene and untroubled progress. There was no American war, and the great economic recession of the thirties had not set in. The joint Army-Veterans Administration hospitalization program made

Congressional funds easier to secure, and the Medical Department experienced its first great peacetime building boom. Army doctors were writing on widely different subjects, producing articles, manual and texts, and the volume of their literary output compared favorably with the work published by civilian scientific foundations having similar research objectives.

In addition to the individual assets of some of the outstanding men such as Siler, Vedder, Dunham, Craig, Nichols, Russell, Gentry and Keller, there were certain departmental assets that lent prestige to the Corps: five well equipped general hospitals and a great many excellent post or station hospitals; a post-graduate medical school and six allied health schools, and the Field Service School at Carlisle. The Post Surgeon and dispensary doctor were comfortingly familiar figures, men interested in the organization to which assigned whether it was Infantry, Cavalry or Artillery. Corps morale was good, pay was adequate if not ample. Seniority and experience mainly influenced assignments, and for the most part specialization and seniority were inseparable. The select few who showed a decided scientific bent were, as scholars ever are, held in awesome respect by their juniors. Regardless of the attractive nature of some administrative assignments, the distinction of being a hospital commander or the chief of a division in the Surgeon General's Office, the admiration and respect accorded the outstanding scientists of the School lingered in memories longer than the exploits of their more active but less erudite brother officers. Every effort was made to insure their success, for others shared Surgeon General Sternberg's belief that "Every man in the Corps that had ambition and ability should have his chance."[59]

References

1. Statement of the Causes which Led to the Dismissal of Surgeon General Hammond, pp, New York, 1864, p 6.

2. Annual Rpt TSG... 1926, pg. 292.

3. *Ibid*, page 296.

4. *Ibid*, page 295.

5. Annual Rpt WRGH, 1926.

6. Interview with Col. Herbert N. Dean, MAC, Ret., April 12, 1950.

7. Annual Rpt WRGH, 1926.

8. Annual Rpt TSG... 1926, pg 294.

9. *Ibid*, pg 354.

10. Annual Rpt WRGH, 1926.

11. *Ibid*.

12. Called T/O & E.

13. Annual Rpt WRGH, 1927.

14. *Ibid.*

15. "Medical Library in Main Bldg., To Be Moved to Post Library," *The Come-Back*, April 9, 1926.

16. Annual Rpt WRGH, 1928

17. Mary E. Schick; Juanita Gould.

18. "Post Librarian Speaks at 20th Century Club Luncheon," *The Come-Back*, April 19, 1926.

19. Conversation with Miss Mary E. Schick, 1941.

20. Annual Rpt, WRGH, 1928.

21. *Ibid*, 1926.

22.. *Ibid.*

23. *Ibid*, 1927.

24. Interview with Miss Margaret Lower, February 14, 1951.

25. Annual Rpt, WRGH, 1928.

26. *Ibid*, 1927.

27. *Ibid.*

28. See photograph in *The Come-Back*, June 1, 1923.

29. Annual Rpt WRGH, 1928.

30. Annual Rpt TSG... 1928, pg 328.

31. Annual Rpt WRGH, 1928.

32. Annual Rpt TSG... 1928, pg 328.

33. Florence A. Blanchfield, *Organized Nursing and the Army in Three Wars*, MSS on file HD SGO; Interview with Maj. Gen. Robert U. Patterson, MC, Ret., Aug. 29, 1950; Interview with Brig. Gen. A.E. Truby, MC Ret., June 27, 28, 1950.

34. Annual Rpt TSG... 1928, pg 326.

35. *Ibid*, pg 264.

36. Blanchfield, *op cit.*

37. Patterson interview, *op cit*; Interview with Jessie M. Braden, June 26, 1950; Miss Dora Thompson former Supt., ANC; Lt. Col. Nellie V. Close, ANC Ret; Misses Frances Poole and Mildred Johnson, ANC, Ret., June 26, 1950; and others.

38. Interview with Lt. Col. Elida J. Raffensperger, ANC, Ret., June 26, 1950.

39. Personal knowledge of the writer.

40. Interview with Col. James F. Hall, MC., Ret., April 17, 1950.

41. Conversation with Brig. Gen. J.E. Bastion, MC, Ret., Sept. 14, 1950; Hall interview, *op cit*.

42. Hall, Dean interviews, *op cit*.

43. Conversation with Brig. Gen. William L. Sheep, MC, Ret., April 26, 1951.

44. Dean interview, *op cit*.

45. Garrison to Welch, Oct. 27, 1922, Collection of the Institute of History of Medicine, Welch Medical Library, Johns Hopkins University, Baltimore, Md.

46. S.O. No. 38-0, W.D. 19 Feb. 1922, and S.O. 85-0, W.D. 12 April 1922, See *Army Med. Bull.* 1929, pg 135, et seq; quote from Ltr Garrison to H.L. Mencken, Collection, *op cit*.

47. Conversation with Brig. Gen. Charles Walson, M.C., Ret., June 25, 1951.

48. Interview with Mrs. Merritte W. Ireland, April 14, 1950.

49. *Washington Post*, Aug. 18, 1929.

50. Annual Rpt TSG ... 1926, pg 317; SGO 631.-1 (AMS) GG, War Rec. Div. Nat'l Archives.

51. Annual Rpt TSG... 1926, pg 320.

52. Annual Rpt WRGH, 1926; SGO 631.-1 (AMS) GG, War Rec. Div. Nat'l Archives.

53. SGO 631.-1 (AMS) GG, War Rec. Div. Nat'l Archives.

54. Annual Rpt TSG... 1928, pg 315.

55. *Ibid*, 1929, pg 309.

56. Synopsis of the work of the Army Medical Research Board in the Philippines, AMB, 1929, pg 171-173 (quoted).

57. F.E. Rodriquez, *Studies in the Specific Bacteriology of Dental Caries*, Military Dental Journal, Dec. 1922, Vol. V, No. 4 (quoted).

58. Annual Rpt WRGH, 1929.

59. Ltr from Mrs. George M. Sternberg (the Grafton Hotel) to Col. Borden, April 1, 1920, handwritten, filed in Borden scrapbook.

Time Marches On

1930–1931

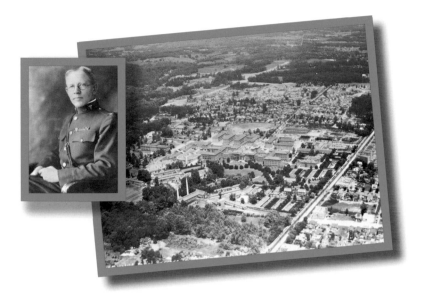

"History never repeats itself exactly, because the world moves." [1]

Carl Rogers Darnall

He was the sort of quiet unspectacular looking man who so frequently influences the course of history but leaves little tangible evidence of his passing. He was deeply devoted to his family and his snub-nosed old Franklin car. And his knowledgeable enthusiasm for old glass, his gentle manners, droll humor [2] and his unfailing kindness assured him an affectionate respect and consideration [3] not always accorded some of his more politically agile contemporaries. He served as chemistry instructor and secretary of the Army Medical School from 1903–1913, and until the "Manchu Law" finally compelled a change of station. He had, during his long stay at the School, developed the Darnall Field Filter, later replaced by the Lyster bag, as well as a process of water chlorination that proved of inestimable value to national as well as military public health. Some considered that the treatise on "The Purification of Drinking Water for Troops in the Field" by Captain Carl Rogers Darnall, Assistant Surgeon, U.S. Army, was the most significant paper published in *The Military Surgeon* during 1908. [4] This, however, was but the prelude to his really monumental discovery of a method for purifying water by utilizing compressed anhydrous chlorine, which could be released from cylinders in controlled amounts. To prove this "liquid chlorination method" practical he invented the chlorinator, a complex mechanical apparatus for delivering "liquid" chlorine into city water supplies, swimming pools and sewage treatment systems.

Darnall's method and apparatus was patented in the United States and in thirteen other countries and is now used throughout the world, but he gained little financially from his invention. When faced with the alternative of resigning to become a manufacturer of chlorinators or continuing his Army medical career he chose the latter course and sold his patents outright to the Wallace-Tiernan Company. His article "The Purification of Water by Anhydrous Chlorine," which appeared in the *Journal of the American Public Health Association* in November 1911 was undoubtedly the most important of his several published works. Some years later legal priority for this invention was established when the company won a civil suit against the city of Philadelphia for infringing on the Darnall patents.

He began the practice of testing medical supplies and equipment for the Surgeon General's Office during his first assignment at the Army Medical School, while it was still located in the old Museum-Library building. Therefore it was principally due to the efforts of this phlegmatic, methodical physician-chemist, fondly called "Old Wooden Face" by his contemporaries, that the Medical Department was saved thousands of dollars and the humiliation of being the victim of well-meaning but impractical inventors and over-zealous salesmen.[5] Finally, as a result of the chemical and structural analysis of drugs and equipment, the Medical Department established a separate testing laboratory.[6] When he was promoted and reassigned in Washington during World War I, Colonel Darnall devoted full time to medical supplies, and as Kean, the recorder, noted, under his "efficient management everything was ready for shipment at a moment's notice."[7]

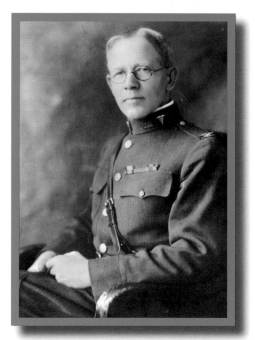

Carl Rogers Darnall, Post Commander Dec. 12, 1929–Dec. 31, 1931

Like many scientifically inclined men, Colonel Darnall cared little for social life, and although a close friend[8] and associate of General Ireland, he apparently paid little attention to Corps politics. He served for a time as executive officer in the Surgeon General's Office, taking, in his quiet and efficient way, a load off the Surgeon General's shoulders, thus freeing the gregarious, politically astute General Ireland of many routine duties. It was a comfortable and pleasant association, for the Surgeon General felt that he could "safely leave the office and that affairs would go on as usual, or at least not be tangled."[9] His two-year command at the Army Medical Center, as a Brigadier General, came at an inconspicuous time for any extraordinary achievements. As the depression had set in he had no opportunity to alter the status quo.

Progress Versus Recession

The building program, long planned as a Medical Department activity, was then nearing completion, and on December 30, 1930, the last temporary wooden buildings were abandoned for ward use.[10] The 1919 fire had not been forgotten; thus the newly opened neuropsychiatric building[11] attracted attention from the press.[12] Only fifty-four of the 104 beds were occupied at the time of the official opening[13] and structurally it was not without drawbacks, although such matters were not published. For instance, the building had four floors and an elevator, but the elevator was not long enough to accommodate a wheeled litter, and patients had to be carried from one floor to another by hand-litters. An underground passage connected this section with the main part of the hospital, but the Section Chief, whose patients were troublesome, to say the least, believed that chaperoning the patients to the laboratory and the various clinics was an administrative hardship[14] in that such a practice necessitated the assignment of extra attendants.

Regardless of some drawbacks, the modern building was a vast improvement over former facilities. By August 1931 it not only shared in the hospital's public address system, but the strictly closed wards housing the disturbed patients had their own arrangements for movies, shown by Red Cross personnel. The inexorable advance of the depression was noticeable in the 148 more neuropsychiatric cases admitted in 1931 than in 1930.

The hospital registrar's office maintained careful statistics on admission and discharges. Thus the number of admissions by nomenclature of disease, the number who died, who were returned to duty, who were retired or separated from the service on the Certificate of Discharge for Disability, familiarly known as the CDD to enlisted men, is an accurate means of gauging the general physical condition of the military population of the Regular Army. Laboratory diagnostic methods were becoming increasingly accurate, and in 1931, encephalograms were used as a diagnostic aid in fifteen cases, with the clinical recordings of the staff physicians at Walter Reed indicating a growing awareness of the so-called psychoneurotic disabilities of young American males. For instance, as some

> *228 military patients (were) discharged on certificates of disability from the section (NP) during the year. The fact that a very large proportion of these discharges were for functional disturbances that existed prior to enlistment, provides a strikingly unfavorable commentary on our recruiting system. One is impressed with the enormous amount of time and money that was fruitlessly expended in recruiting, clothing, subsisting, attempting to train, and finally in hospitalizing and affecting the discharge of these individuals.*[15]

The Medical Service staff was concerned with the average number of days that patients spent in the hospital prior to discharge or transfer to another institution. For instance, definitive care was not provided for tuberculous patients, for the Army maintained Fitzsimons General Hospital for this purpose and the Veterans Bureau had its own facilities. Nevertheless, the average tuberculous patient waited twenty-seven

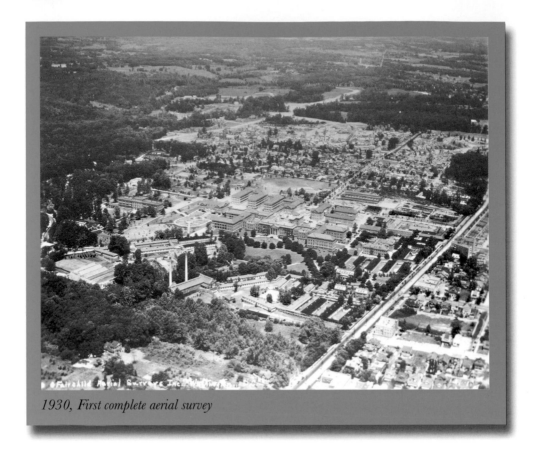

1930, First complete aerial survey

days between the day of request for transfer to another hospital and the day of departure. The average neuropsychiatric patient waited thirty-two days; and soldiers under permanent separation orders waited as much as forty-two days.[16]

Operational Affairs

The new Clinic Building, which housed dentistry, X-ray and the physical therapy rooms, represented the most modern hospital planning. Roentgenology occupied the second floor but had an additional completely shock-proof X-ray unit in the main building, near the operating room, and a special unit in the Genito-Urinary Clinic. During 1931 and in these three clinics, some 17,350 cases were examined by X-ray, 1,572 received treatment.[17]

Of the 7,200 total new admissions to the hospital in 1931, 2,774 were Veterans Bureau cases and 1,747 were patients from the United States at large.[18] The distribution in class of case was much as usual since the acceptance of Veterans' beneficiaries; roughly, the number of officers, nurses and others (civilians) equaled the total number of enlisted men admitted, but the number of Veterans' cases was always in excess of the number of enlisted men.[19] The normal bed capacity had dropped from 1,200 to 1,000 fixed

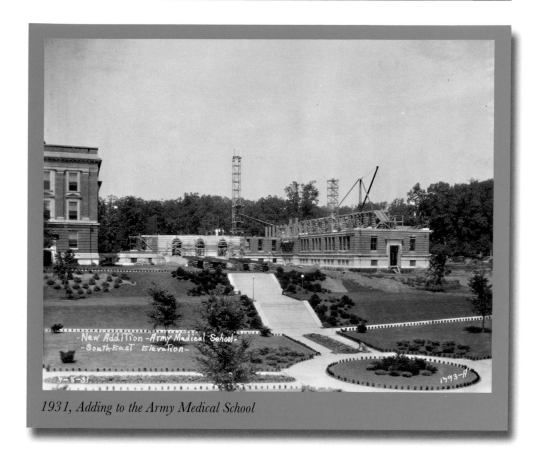

1931, Adding to the Army Medical School

beds,[20] but the Dietetic Department reported that 1,772 individuals were fed daily, this number including the nurses, dieticians, aides and the personnel fed in the detachment cafeteria. It was cause for concern in the Dietetic Department that the ration had a fluctuating but consistently low value, as, for instance, 0.33 in October 1931, and that approximately sixty per cent of the bulk was represented by meat, a high cost item. The dietetic service therefore suffered a hardship in proportion to the change in commodity prices, and it was forced to exercise the strictest economy in order to stay within the budget. Post Exchange dividends were low or nonexistent by this time and could provide little in the way of subsidy. Thus staffing and serving Mess I, for patient-officers, with tray and table service; Mess III, the detachment's own cafeteria; and Mess IV, the Nurses' Mess, which provided table service, was a dietary and administrative undertaking deserving the highest praise.

The new professional concept of transfusing patients with bloodstream infections was reflected in the 117 blood transfusions given in 1931. The 1,422 local anesthetics, 1,769 general anesthetics, and 467 spinal anesthetics, in the latter case an increase of 250 per cent over the 162 spinal, illustrated the changing trends in operating room techniques.[21] The Walter Reed hospital then was using a Sanborn portable bedside electrocardiographic machine and one stationary Hindle #3. In January 1931, a pulse wave recorder and a Tycos Dermatherm machine were added.

In 1930, the Chief of the Laboratory Service, which was working in conjunction with the Army Medical School laboratories, complained more loudly than usual over the paucity of replacements for laboratory personnel. Only three enlisted men on duty January 1, 1929 completed the year. Four laboratory-trained men accepted civilian positions, a matter easily understood as only three of them received a cash salary of as much as $50.00. So, said the laboratory chief, "the constant training of green men is a continuous grind" and in order "to offset the rapidly changing enlisted force more nurses were secured."[22] It was even proposed that a small group of nurse technicians be trained for reassignment in the various general hospitals. This would doubtless have been acceptable had War Department funds been available for increasing the strength of the Corps, for so many civilian nurses were out of work a year later that the Army School, then on the verge of closing, adopted the slogan of the national nursing groups "Fewer and Better Nurses."[23]

Army Medical Center

The average monthly strength of the Troop Command in 1930 and 1931 was approximately 530, with the majority of the men assigned to ward duties in the hospital. Manpower was readily available, as a result of the dearth of civilian jobs, and

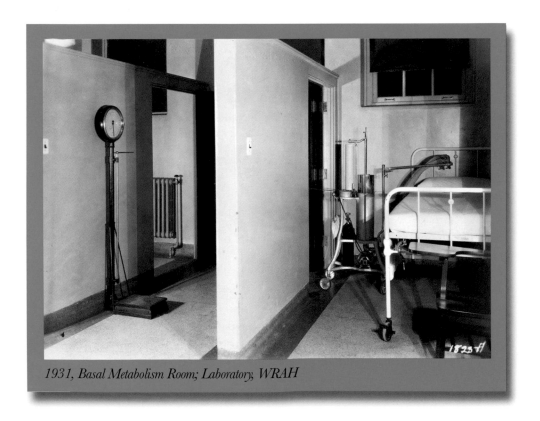

1931, Basal Metabolism Room; Laboratory, WRAH

after November 1, 1931, War Department policy restricted enlistments to men reenlisting within three months after discharge. At the Army Medical Center company commanders were showing a decided agreement with the newer concepts of personnel administration, such as shorter working hours, which, of course, required more personnel to perform the usual duties. This was an administrative disadvantage, for it represented a vital decrease in the detachment strength and thus affected the ready discharge of hospital duties. In addition to shorter working hours, more frequent furloughs were thought to encourage reenlistments and strengthen morale.

The general unemployment situation apparently curtailed desertions, which dropped from forty-nine to forty-one, and AWOL's, which dropped from 163 to 117. However, not even economic distress affected the venereal disease register, for there was only one less case reported than in the previous year.

Station reenlistments at the Army Medical Center increased from sixty to eighty-seven, and the men appeared to be well satisfied both with living conditions and the kind of work performed. Church-going was not an all-absorbing pastime, but the welfare and recreation officer stressed athletics, and judging from the increase in book circulation at the Post Library, it was cheaper to improve the mind than to wander far afield in search of amusement.

Reorganization

Army Medical Center administrative functions were reorganized in 1931. The staff then consisted of the Commanding General, an Executive Officer, an Adjutant, a personnel adjutant and the chiefs of all installation support activities such as Quartermaster, Finance, Signal, the Surgeon (hospital commander), Chaplains, Medical Supply, and the Recreation Officer. The assistant commandant was responsible for all matters of instruction, but he was not concerned with the administration or discipline of the School personnel.[24] Surprisingly, there were three Commanding Officers of the School in a one-year period: Colonel Henry C. Fisher, July 1, 1929 to October 6, 1929, Colonel Charles F. Craig, October 7, 1929 to May 18, 1930 and Colonel Edward B. Vedder, May 19, 1930 to June 30, 1930.[25]

The various School functions were now so well organized that the professional work was almost routine, even stereotyped. Lack of laboratory space was again a major problem, but the proposed expansion of the School building was expected to remedy the situation. Relocation of the School on the Army Medical Center grounds had, however, increased the number of administrative duties required of the staff members, and details as Officer-of-the-Day, to Courts Martial and Boards absorbed a great deal of time heretofore devoted to scientific work. Colonel Russell, who had retired in 1919 and affiliated with the Rockefeller Foundation, was still interested in Army Medical School activities. As an internationally known expert he was familiar with world health problems and research projects, and regretfully, it seems, he called attention to the fact that the School was not maintaining its past record for research. In

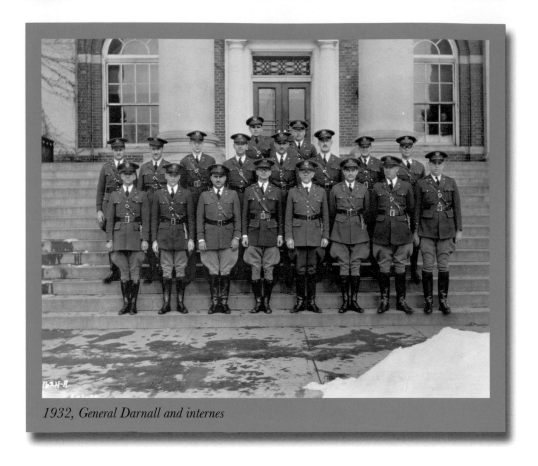

1932, General Darnall and internes

addition to an apparent lack of interest, however, he also named such restrictions as the "onerous" property responsibilities and the increase in the teaching load that may have modified or curtailed the faculty output.[26] Certainly there was less original research work and writing undertaken at the Army Medical School during this lean two-year period.

The uncertain economic condition of the country as a whole, the general movement toward a reduction in the total supply of nurses, and the cost of operating the Army School of Nursing, finally brought orders for its closure. The Superintendent of the Corps had successfully resisted earlier moves to close the School, and General Ireland, soon to be out of office, delayed rather than create undue friction in his staff. Some of the General Staff officers, friends and military classmates of the incoming Surgeon General Patterson, warned him informally that the Army School of Nursing would be closed by higher directive if he didn't undertake a "housecleaning" of his own accord.[27] Therefore, as one of his first official acts, General Patterson suspended the training school on August 12, 1931, with orders for closure on January 31, 1933, with graduation of the last class.[28] Thus there ended, insofar as the Medical Department was concerned, a costly private lesson in subsidized education. In the development of the nursing education program, however, it would long stand as a monument to progress.

The thirty-fifth session of the basic course for Medical Department officers began at the Army Medical School on September 2, 1930 and ended January 30, 1931, with graduation of forty-eight officers who then proceeded to Carlisle, Pennsylvania, for the course in field medicine. The work in Sanitary Chemistry had gradually become less important in thirty years, for the majority of the civilian undergraduate medical schools were by then teaching this subject. Thus during the last year of his administration, the course that Carl Rogers Darnall had taught at the Army Medical School in 1903 was replaced by toxicology. The course in pathology was lengthened, and brief instruction was offered in the medico-legal aspects of post-mortems. Among other changes, the course in surgery was itemized for each day and was "made more practical by eliminating very largely the lecture system."[29]

The tenth advanced course, beginning on February 2, 1931 and ending on May 28, was drastically modified. Whereas the School had previously offered (a) Preventive Medicine, (b) Clinical Medicine and Surgery, and (c) Roentgenology, the Training Division of the Surgeon General's Office proposed that student officers elect a preferred subject. Of the six officers in attendance, one elected a special course in internal medicine and clinical medicine, two elected clinical medicine, and three elected clinical surgery.[30] Specialization was more marked in the elective graduate training of civilian doctors, and the Army was showing definite signs of following the trend. Therefore, considerable effort was made adequately to prepare the students as functionaries in a post medical service, where it was obligatory that the Army doctor have knowledge of more than a single field.

Colonel Keller not only occupied a nearly duplicate set of quarters to that occupied by the Post Commander, but his evaluation of the professional abilities of young medical officers influenced their careers. The professionally able Chief of the Medical Service, the intransigent, energetic red-haired Lt. Colonel Ernest R. Gentry, was allegedly the only man in the hospital who could hold his own ground with the militant surgeon. When a member of the Training Division, office of the

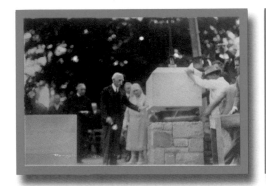 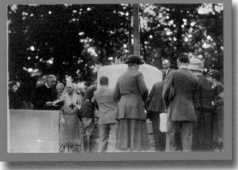

Left Picture: Andrew Mellon, Secretary of the Treasury. Right Picture: Mrs. Walter Reed at right with officer. Laying Cornerstone, Memorial Chapel, May 28, 1930.

Surgeon General, persistently advocated a rotating service for doctors in the general hospitals, better to prepare them for Post life, Colonel Keller "bucked" the program at Walter Reed and refused to have internists rotated to his service. If the training officer persisted in furthering this heretical plan, declared the Chief of the Surgical Service whimsically, it would serve him right to sometime have an internist operate on him.[31]

The Tabernacle

A mortuary chapel had long been a necessity for the Post, a quiet dignified place out of sight of the morgue refrigerators and other grim evidence of death. Dr. Borden had planned for such a building, but in the years when the hospital was small and public funds were scarce, all improvements were directed at housing the sick.

One of the more obvious needs for a sanctuary was evident during the influenza epidemic of 1918, when the mounds of caskets were piled under a tent fly placed behind the morgue. After the YMCA and Knights of Columbus erected temporary structures during the World War I building boom, there were places, even if inappropriate, for funerals, an occasional wedding, and for church services. When these buildings were razed to make space for the new Clinic Building and the "Section," the adaptable Red Cross Recreation house accommodated such services as a matter of course. With chameleon-like rapidity it could be changed from a public auditorium suitable for the graduation exercises of the Army Medical School, into a moving picture theater or a Sunday School room for the Post children. In 1922, spurred by Miss Lower and supported by General Glennan, the Gray Ladies began to plan for construction of a Memorial Chapel.[32]

The northeast corner of Dahlia and Fourteenth Street was the first choice of locations, but this area included some of the condemned civilian houses then being used as officers' quarters, and so the opposite corner was selected in 1924. According to the records, a cash donation of five dollars, given by an ex-soldier-vaudeville entertainer, formed the nest egg for the Chapel fund. Other gifts varying from twenty-five cents to $32,000.00 were obtained by the energetic Gray Ladies,[33] but it always seemed to be Mrs. Rea, their fairy godmother, who provided a much-needed donation at the opportune time. The nurses, hospital corpsmen and Red Cross workers contributed the proceeds from an amateur performance of *Believe me, Xanthippi*; Poli's Theater used D.W. Griffith's famous picture *America* for a benefit performance. The nurses at Walter Reed raised money by cake sales and off-duty chores, and various wealthy benefactors chipped in. After formation of the Altar Guild in 1932, the wives of the military personnel shared in the responsibility for all future activities.

Fifty thousand dollars was first thought to be sufficient for the building fund,[34] and so the Gray Ladies sought the official blessing of such military dignitaries as the Surgeon General, the Chief of Staff of the Army, and on the Chief of Staff's requirement, Congressional authority, in order to build on Government property. The new project was widely advertised, and Mrs. Walter Reed was among the distinguished visitors invited for the ground-breaking ceremonies on November 11, 1929, "on the eleventh hour of the eleventh day of the eleventh

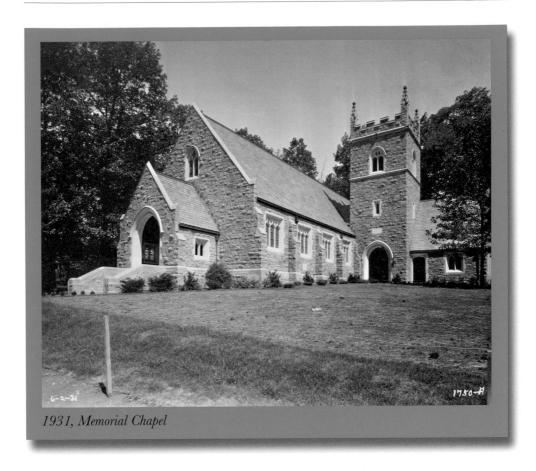

1931, Memorial Chapel

month of the eleventh year after the Armistice."[35] She was under the impression that, like the hospital, the Chapel was a specific memorial to her distinguished husband, and she came to the ceremony prepared to consecrate the ground in his memory.[36]

In the ensuing months the excavations uncovered military relics of the Battle of Fort Stevens, such as minnie balls and lead bullets left by McCook's and Early's men.[37] As in the case of the hospital, it was therefore singularly appropriate that the Chapel, "a memorial to the men who gave their lives to service,"[38] was erected on ground once defiled by war. The corner stone was laid on May 28, 1930, and it enclosed an appropriate record of the vari-ous Post activities. On May 16, 1931, five days before the Chapel was formally dedicated, a wedding ceremony was performed. On May 21, 1931, the day of dedication, the infant son of a medi-cal officer was baptized. Three services were held on June 7: the first, a 7:30 AM Protestant communion service for the Gray Ladies; the second, an 8:30 AM Roman Catholic High Mass and the third, at 10:30, was a general consecration of the building as a non-sectarian chapel. The organist, Major Cyrus B. Wood, Medical Corps, Instructor in Chemistry and Toxicology at the Army Medical School,[39] was assisted by a choir composed largely of Post personnel. The first funeral conducted in the Chapel was that of an Army Nurse, one who had long been a hospital patient, victim of a malignant disease.

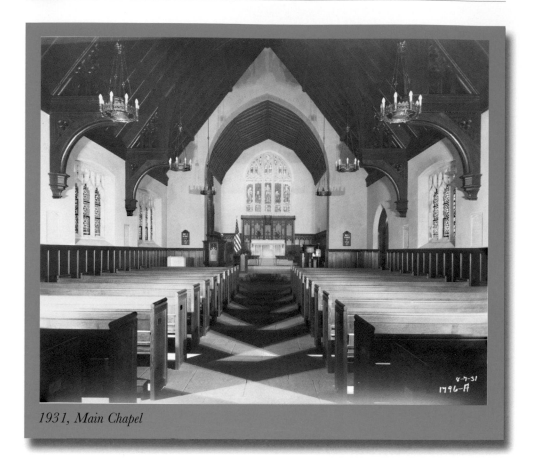

1931, Main Chapel

When the construction bids were examined in October 1929, the $50,000 estimate had increased to $84,900 without the windows, the organ, the altar, the handsome flagstone floor and foundation, or the Glennan memorial tower. When finally completed, the building cost $161,000.[40] The original five-dollar bequest was supplemented by an impressive list of memorial gifts, one of the most beautiful being the "Little Chapel," or mortuary chapel, designed for small religious gatherings, weddings and funerals. It was equipped by the McCook family, in memory of the fighting McCooks "who served their country in the war for the preservation of the Union,"[41] a gift singularly appropriate because of Alexander McCook's participation in the battle of Fort Stevens. The small sanctuary as a result of the more frequent use, in time became primarily a Roman Catholic sanctuary. The Gray Ladies collected old silver for the solid silver communion service, made by Private Ralph Grim, a double amputee patient who became an expert silversmith in the rehabilitation shops at Walter Reed.

An article by Jean Eliot from *The Washington Herald* of November 25, 1936, lists some of the more interesting facts regarding gifts and donations to the little building.

This is a personal little church. Everything in it is memorial to someone much loved. The altar was given by Mrs. Blair Spencer for her Mother, Mrs. John A. Johnson. Princess Boncompaigni gave the organ in memory of her father, Gen. Wm. F. Draper. The exquisite rose window was brought from England by Mrs. John W. Davidge to honor her father and mother, John W. Weeks, once Secretary of War, and Mrs. Weeks. Another window was given by the late Representative John Jacob Rogers, whose widow Edith Nourse Rogers, is an enthusiastic Gray Lady. Still another was presented by the nurses at Walter Reed and has a sentimental history, since they earned the money off duty, with laundry work, polishing shoes, baking cakes, even by hauling trunks and furniture in a push cart. The Gray Ladies themselves gave the church bell. The tower, reminiscent of the one on the church at the entrance to Plymouth Harbor, England, is a memorial to Gen. James D. Glennan, who was in command at Walter Reed for eight years. Every stone (actually given by the Misses Elizabeth and Harriet Riley from their farm), every lovely bit of glass, every inch of carved wood is a contribution of affection or representative of individual sacrifice.

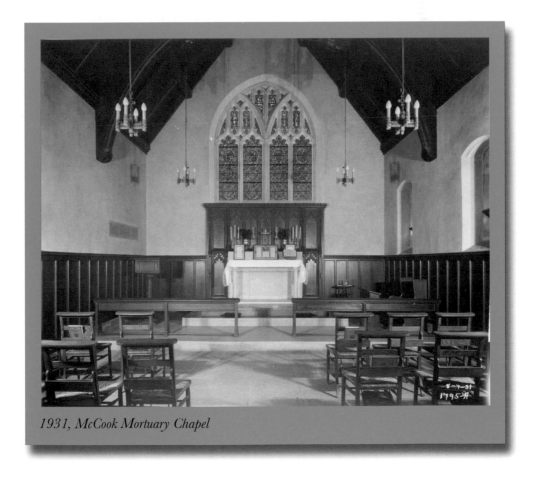

1931, McCook Mortuary Chapel

Although a gem of Gothic loveliness, the Memorial Chapel is the only building on the reservation that fails to harmonize the colonial architecture of the Borden plans. Aloof and secluded, it was often deserted in fact, a lonely sentinel to the wishful thinking of past generations of Gray Ladies and Army Chaplains, who visualized it as a busy tabernacle for the ill and the oppressed. On occasions such as Christmas and Easter it is filled to overflowing, and the congregation is reminiscent of a prearranged DeMille setting. Soldiers in Class A uniform, patients in maroon or blue lounge suits, afoot and on crutches, patients in wheel chairs and now and then one on a litter, nurses in white, nurses in khaki, a few officers but more frequently, their wives, and an occasional squirming and inattentive child form the picture. During the first ten years of its life pews were practically empty, for the exacting demands of a twenty-four hour professional service to patients leaves the duty personnel little free time for church going, and so more than one discouraged Post Chaplain came to believe that the "road to Jerusalem" was unduly rough if it detoured through the Army Medical Center.[42]

When a military transfer to a Southwestern station interrupted Major Wood's duties as organist, Miss Mary E. Schick, the Post Librarian, agreed to fill the place temporarily, but she remained until the pressure of World War II activities interfered. Securing a choir that would be sure to appear on Sundays was a masterly accomplishment. Some of the enlisted choir members would come to rehearsals, but, tempted, by a weekend pass or some off-the-Post amusement, they blithely remained away on Sunday.

There was then neither adequate stipend nor prestige attached to being a chorister, nor was there much joy in singing to row on row of empty pews. In fact it was remarkable that the organist and the chaplain maintained their own morale, for at the time there was little evidence that their services were valued. At one time the choir stalls were entirely empty, and the Chaplain had no assistant to ring the tower bell, that final warning to wandering sheep that the service would start with or without them. Anxiously he came to the organist to explain his dilemma, urging her not to start the processional hymn without him.

Then, with vestments flapping wildly, he rushed out to pull the bell rope and warn the errant of the passing time. Spiritually undaunted, with clothing properly rearranged, he presently marched solemnly into church singing lustily, sans choir support of any kind.[43] Such was the interest in church attendance in the Memorial Chapel during the late thirties. It was, for a time, practically a two-man affair with the Chaplain and the organist as the sole interventionists between the wanderers and the Lord.

References

1. P.M. Ashburn, *A History of the Medical Department of the U.S. Army*, Boston & N.Y., Houghton-Mifflin, 1929, pg 128.

2. Interview with Brig. Gen. Wm. L. Sheep, M.C., Ret., April 26, 1951.

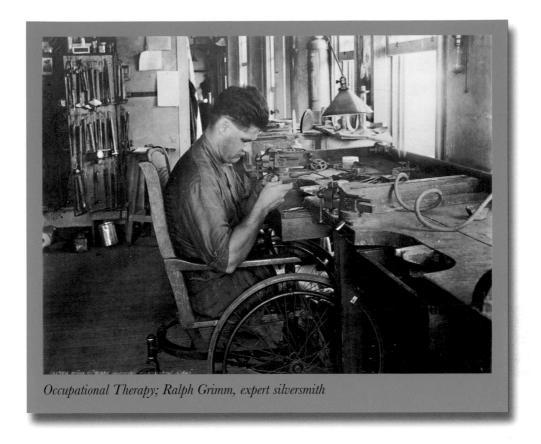

Occupational Therapy; Ralph Grimm, expert silversmith

3. Interviews: Maj. Gen. Robert U. Patterson, M.C., Ret., Aug. 24, 29, 1950; Col. John Huggins, M.C., Ret., April 20, 1950; Maj. Gen. Morrison C. Stayer, M.C., Ret., June 10, 1950; Mrs. Margaret Gardner, March 16, 1951.

4. Edgar Erskine Hume, *History of Association of Military Surgeon of the U.S., 1891–1941*, pg 47.

5. Interview with Brig. Gen. Albert G. Love, M.C., Ret., Feb. 13, 1951.

6. *Ibid.*

7. Biography of Gen. J.R. Kean, MSS on file AML, Wash., D.C. pg 99.

8. Interview with Mrs. Mathew Reasoner, April 17, 1950.

9. Interview with Mrs. M.W. Ireland, April 14, 1950.

10. Annual Rpt WRGH, 1931.

11. Hereafter called The Section.

12. "Last Fire Trap at Hospital Barracks," *The Washington Evening Star*, Dec. 31, 1930.

13. *Ibid.*

14. Annual Rpt WRGH, 1931.

15. *Ibid*, pg 67.

16. *Ibid*, 1931.

17. *Ibid.*

18. *Ibid.*

19. Annual Rpt TSG... 1931, pg 362.

20. *Ibid*, pg 361.

21. Annual Rpt WRGH, 1931.

22. Annual Rpt TSG... 1930, pg 339.

23. *Ibid.*, 1931, pg 359.

24. Annual Rpt WRGH, 1931.

25. Annual Rpt TSG... 1930, pg 317.

26. SGO 631.-1 (AMS) GG – War Rec. Div., Nat'l Archives.

27. Patterson interview, *op cit.*

28. Army Medical Bulletin, No. 52, April 1940, pg 104.

29. Annual Rpt.... TSG, 1931, pg 350.

30. *Ibid*, pg 350.

31. Interview with General J.E. Bastion, Sept. 14, 1950, (to perform, he said, specifically, a hemorrhoidectomy).

32. Feltman S. James (comp) *The Story of the Memorial Chapel...* published by the Chapel Guild, nd., on file Library, WRAH.

33. *Ibid*, pg 11.

34. *Ibid.*

35. *Ibid*, pg 13.

36. Interview with Miss Margaret Lower, Feb. 14, 1951; Mrs. Rea, founder of the Gray Ladies, was accorded this honor.

37. Mrs. William J. Graham presented The Library with a large collection of such relics, collected at the time the Chapel was built.

38. James, *op cit*, pg 15.

39. Minutes of AMS, on file office of the Commandant.

40. *Ibid*, pg 17.

41. James, *op cit,* pg 38.

42. Conversation with Miss Mary E. Schick, 1941.

43. *Ibid*.

Replacing the Old with the New

1932–1935

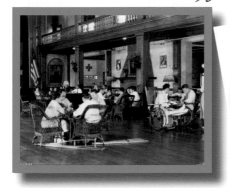
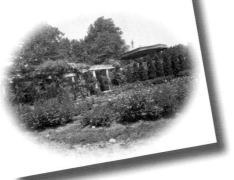

*"An obstacle that would
halt a cab-horse is a jump to a thoroughbred!"[1]*

A Hard Assignment

Robert Urie Patterson, a warm friend of Patrick J. Hurley, the Secretary of War, had upset the forecasts as well as the wagers of Medical Department officers by receiving the appointment as General Ireland's successor when he retired for age on June 1, 1931.[2] A "dark horse" of unknown potentialities, General Patterson began a four-year tenure with the usual administrative house-cleaning.

General Darnall had not been well during his last year at the Army Medical Center, where the administrative burden became increasingly heavy, and so the Surgeon General persuaded Colonel Albert E. Truby, then executive officer in the SGO, to prepare for the line of succession at the Center by serving as Darnall's under-study.[3] This rearrangement of personnel required considerable administrative finesse, for the Secretary of War wanted Colonel Keller, then senior officer at the hospital, to have the forthcoming vacancy of Brigadier General when "Old Wooden Face" retired. In fact, until personally reassured by Colonel Keller, who believed rank and command were inseparable, Mr. Hurley refused to accept General Patterson's statement that the Chief of the Surgical Service preferred continuing in professional work.[4]

Colonel Truby was not released from the Surgeon General's Office until three months after his appointment as commandant of the Army Medical Center, but as one of his first official acts he issued an order designating Colonel Keller as the commander of Walter Reed General Hospital. In the meantime, the Surgeon General

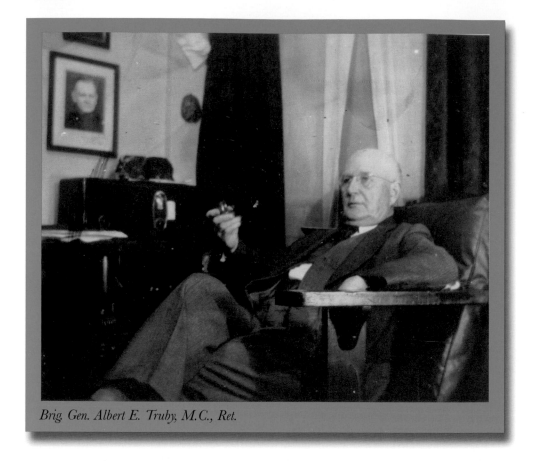

Brig. Gen. Albert E. Truby, M.C., Ret.

> *Requested orders for Colonel (William H.) Moncrief, who was an experienced hospital commander, to report for duty at Walter Reed Hospital. When he came, however, he was not allowed to command the hospital because he was junior to Colonel Keller, and so he was assigned as executive officer and performed the mass of administrative work. In practice this plan worked, but (it) was not altogether satisfactory. It was not possible to assign a senior medical officer as commanding officer of the hospital and consequently this system was not perfect.*[5]

By contrast, Colonel Keller was not especially enthusiastic about devoting his professional time to administrative duties. In fact, he disregarded some of the routine but important details and the Adjutant General finally sent word to him informally that literally he must sign the officers' efficiency reports regardless of whatever else he did or did not do.[6] As commanding officer of the hospital he was responsible to the Post Commander for the functions of the Executive Office, including the Adjutant, Inspector and Registrar, and the professional services of surgery, medicine, laboratory, nursing, dietetics, and the Red Cross. Supervision of these activities consumed time that he believed better spent in surgery.

Albert Truby had wider interests than the exclusive practice of medicine.[7] A brilliant undergraduate student in Medical School, his Army career had been both successful and dramatic. He had been in Cuba during the Kean-Gorgas mosquito eradication campaign; he had known and served with Major Walter Reed;[8] and he had served the usual tours of duty on Army posts, which were the lot of the average Medical Officer prior to World War I. Moreover, following the Spanish-American War, he had commanded the old "Company B" of the Hospital Corps.

Among his other duties he had commanded an evacuation hospital; he had, like Colonel Philipps, been superintendent of the famous Ancon (Gorgas) Hospital in Panama; he was once Chief Health officer in Panama; he had duty as the Chief of the Medical Division of the Air Service. Like General Kennedy he had been commander at Letterman General Hospital on two different assignments. Like others in the long line of his professional forebears, he had been a Department Surgeon (Chief of the Division) in the Philippines.[9] Small and rotund but with a brisk walk reminiscent of the proverbial rolling gait of the sailor, during his early years in the Army he was nicknamed "Cupid." This appellation was earned during a tour of duty at Alcatraz Island, with an Infantry Division recently returned from the Philippines, where he frequently served as best man at weddings. The name was well chosen, for cheerful-looking and with an enviably ruddy complexion he invariably bore a more marked resemblance to his decorative progenitor on the Valentine than to a seaman or a soldier. A careful administrator, scholarly and humane, his administration was one of credit to the Medical Department.

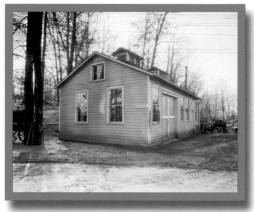
Blacksmith Shop

There was some administrative friction between the hospital and the School activities at the time of the Truby appointment, with the hospital personnel concerned with many unrelated administrative functions.[10] And so he was off to a troubled start – personnel problems and a lean exchequer for operating expenses. The test of an able administrator is not what can be accomplished with a great deal of money but how the financial ends can be made to meet when they seem hopelessly far apart. If Albert E. Truby was affectionately called "Cupid" because of a benign engaging manner it was a case of mistaken identity, for his pleasant, affable ways concealed a shrewd judgment that stood the Army Medical Center in good stead during the lean years of the depression.

As one of his first administrative responsibilities, he persuaded Surgeon General Patterson that the Center should be established on a sound military basis; this could be accomplished by removing from the hospital administration such functions as utilities, transportation, the Post Exchange, landscaping, etc.

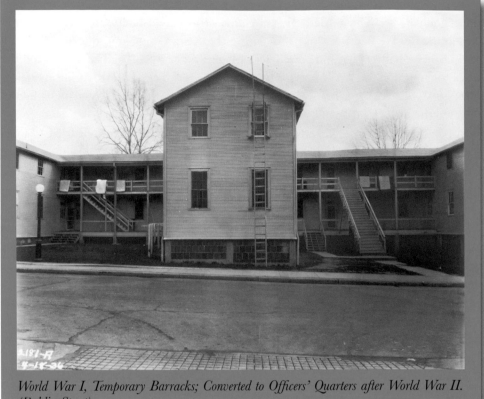

World War I, Temporary Barracks; Converted to Officers' Quarters after World War II. (Dahlia Street)

There had always been complaints and friction, especially during and after World War I, and the work of the commanding officer became most exacting and difficult. Much of this trouble was caused by the improper alignment of functions. Therefore, it was (his) idea that the hospital should be commanded by the senior medical officer on duty at the hospital and that he would command the Center. This arrangement proved to be most satisfactory, as previously the commanding officer of the hospital had been greatly overworked. With the support of the Surgeon General, therefore, all of the proper functions of the Center and necessary personnel were gradually withdrawn from the hospital. This improved the morale of the Schools, which had never been satisfied with their status at the Center.

(He) felt that the Center commander would have plenty of work, and that the hospital commander could better meet the many complaints and demands on his time by War Department officials, members of Congress, and other people who practically required his personal attention to matters pertaining to the sick… under (this) arrangement, hospital authorities immediately investigated the complaints; corrections were made, and if action was required by the Center commander, he was notified and made his own investigation.[11]

Daily informal inspections were made to some unit, with a formal or military inspection made on Saturday. Thus every unit of the command was covered completely at least once a month. It was during this period that the extensive excavation and regrading of the area in front of Delano Hall was accomplished, with the road cut through to 16th Street. Much of the small shrubbery was saved, transplanted to new locations and thus contributed to the ultimate beauty of the Post. Like General Glennan, he was an enthusiastic nature-lover and purchased boxwood and other decorative shrubbery. A central steam connection was made from the Post Power plant to family housing units by using soldier labor and local Post funds. The two principal sets of quarters, on the Main Drive, were remodeled and improved, and built-in garages were constructed. As he was an excellent amateur carpenter,[12] his natural interest in the detail work served him in good stead in planning hospital construction.

Mrs. Truby, gentle, energetic and business-like, devoted a great deal of her time to Post welfare activities. She assisted in organizing the Chapel Guild in 1932, and she showed an unusual degree of consideration and interest in the families of the junior officers.[13] The Post-World War I expansion of the Army was an episode of the past, but military personnel was loosely identified as Old Army and New Army. As the general had been commissioned during the Spanish-American War, the Trubys were Old Army, almost the last of a generation that valued the traditional customs of the Service. And so it was they who had prepared for issue to the Army Medical Center personnel, a booklet called *Social Customs*, whose cover bore an appropriate quotation from Burke:

> *Manners are more important than laws. The law teaches us but here and there – now and then. Manners are what vex and soothe, corrupt or purify, exalt or debase, barbarize or refine us by a constant, steady, uniform, insensible operation like the air we breathe.*

Like the leavening of the Old Army with the new, social concepts were undergoing changes during this period, and the records of the Truby administration clarify the changing concept of the military general hospital as an overflow for battle casualties into an institution for the everyday use of military personnel. Thus the mounting emphasis on professional specialization and the concept of medical care as a right rather than a privilege for Army personnel are both noticeable.

The singularities as well as isolation of frontier life had required that the dependents of military personnel receive medical care, but this was a friendly understanding between the Surgeon General and the line commanders and in no way required by law. After 1901 those hospitals having female nurses, sufficient medical service personnel and adequate bed space admitted dependents, at the discretion of the commanding officer. Such patients were assessed a nominal sum for maintenance, usually the amount of the ration plus a small overhead charge applied to the payment of female custodial employees required in servicing the wards. Thus custom assured provision for bed space for dependents and if some nurses objected to the arrangement, the doctors considered the variety of cases a professional asset.

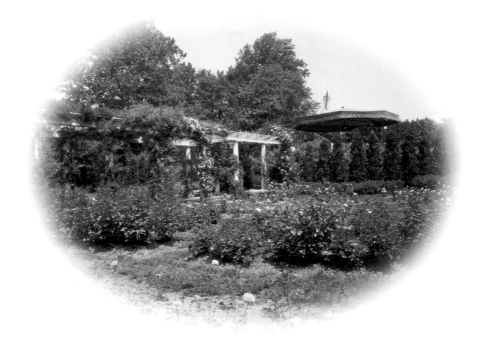

1932, The Rose Garden

As a consequence, the proportion of civilian dependents admitted to Walter Reed increased steadily through the years and, with the Veterans Bureau patients, composed approximately one-third of the total admissions. For instance, of the new admissions during 1932, almost one-fourth were civilians:

New Admissions[14]

	ACTIVE DUTY	RETIRED	TOTAL
Officers	451	74	525
Warrant Officers	25	6	31
Enlisted Men	<u>1989</u>	<u>62</u>	<u>2051</u>
	2465	142	2607
Nurses	61		61
Student Nurses	<u>86</u>		<u>86</u>
	147		147
Veterans Adm.	2774		2774
Civilians (All classes)	<u>1672</u>		<u>1672</u>
	4446		4446

Grand total: 7200

A Change in Specialists

On May 26, 1932, Lt. Col. Shelley U. Marietta replaced Lt. Colonel Ernest R. Gentry as Chief of the Medical Service.[15] One of the few Army doctors who was both a doctor of medicine and doctor of dentistry, Lt. Col. Marietta was an indefatigable worker. He was not only an excellent clinician, but he was one of the earlier Army doctors to become intensely interested in endocrinology. Quiet and reserved, he had the reputation for keeping abreast of current medical literature with the devotion of a high priest.

Organizationally the professional services were substantially the same. The Medical Service supervised the admission and classification of patients, and it was divided into a general section including Officers and Women, Cardiovascular-Renal, Gastro-Intestinal, Tuberculosis, Skin and Infectious, and Neuropsychiatric.[16] Interestingly, for administrative economy, the prison ward operated as a part of the general medical service, although there is no record that a woman was admitted, even on legitimate business. In many hospitals the type of cases represented by the Officers' and Women's section would not have been separated from the general medical service, but the difference in social status of military patients, involving the officer-enlisted man, and the long periods of hospitalization, made this arrangement practicable.[17]

The general clinical program was obviously becoming more detailed. For instance, some 2,005 electrocardiograms were made at Walter Reed that year;[18] eighty to ninety per cent of all the inpatients received some attention at the Dental Clinic; twenty-four per cent of all the patients received some form of physiotherapy. Although the Laboratory Service was still pleading for a civilian technical staff in order to obviate the turn-over in personnel, it nevertheless performed 170,172 procedures and autopsied more than seventy-five per cent of all the deaths.[19]

Administration of so busy an institution was complicated, for unlike civilian hospitals, where the average patient enters at will and leaves anxiously because of the high cost of medical care, the Post Commander had many rarely seen personnel problems. This was particularly true in regard to enlisted patients and Veterans, whose

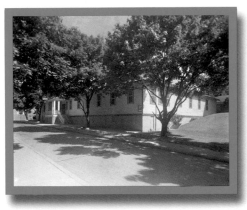

Post Exchange, WRGH, formerly Officers' Pavilion No. 1 in World War I

physical presence on the medical post established them as numerical members of the command. In the case of military personnel this included discipline, travel orders, furloughs or leave, as in the case of the Troop Command assigned for maintenance of the organization.

Receptacles for clothing and personal articles were provided for the ward patients, but this practice encouraged uncontrolled freedom and absence without leave, as well as encouraging the easy storage of liquor and other contraband.[20]

There were fewer nurses per patient on convalescent wards than found in the average civilian hospital, for the corpsmen were able to discharge the non-professional nursing duties. Still, lack of constant oversight by a nurse-officer or non-commissioned officer permitted a certain laxity in discipline. In contrast, the wide dispersal of wards necessitated a higher ratio of custodial personnel to patient than might otherwise have been expected, and unavoidably some attendants could always be coaxed to serve as intermediaries between the patients and the pleasures of the outside world.

The wards in the Main Building were designed with large private rooms, but each ward had an open cubicle, with beds for about six convalescent patients, and they were troublesome to service. Cleaning was not the only problem, however, for the assignment of beds in cubicles was a sensitive point Colonel Marietta finding that where officers or women were involved there was "much difficulty experienced in caring for the seriously ill and aside from the question of the seriously ill, officers and women usually accept(ed) open ward accommodations reluctantly. Although theoretically the matter of rank and prestige should not enter into the assignment of beds," said the Chief of the Medical Service, "it is in reality a practical and troublesome problem that has to be met daily."[21]

General Truby apparently disapproved of using an Army hospital as an experimental station for new pharmaceuticals, even if the required quantities were issued gratis by the civilian drug houses, for he realized that proper listing of experimental data would be laborious, time-consuming and require auxiliary personnel already in short supply. Trained in an era where the art and practice of medicine was a rite, he disapproved of the growing tendency among Army doctors to use proprietary drugs rather than write their own prescriptions.[22]

In-Service Problems

The Veterans Administration was expanding its own hospitalization programs, and whereas in 1931 the Army Medical Department provided 2,265 of the total number of 9,732 beds available to veterans in other governmental facilities,[23] a gradual reduction in the use of Army facilities had set in. Legislation passed on March 20, 1933 denied admission to many Veterans formerly eligible under the largesse authorized in June 1924, for sixty-two per cent of the cases treated in the intervening years were for non-service connected disabilities. The total admissions for 1933 were only eight per cent less than in 1932, but the cut was spread to the non-Veterans' hospitals and Walter Reed felt the pinch when the auxiliary funds were withdrawn.[24]

The Veterans Administration was prepared to hospitalize practically all of its own cases by 1933, a change in policy that would have created a large deficit in unoccupied military hospital beds had the Army not been authorized by Executive Order No. 6101, April 5, 1933, and Circular No. 3, Civilian Conservation Corps, May 12, to treat non-elective cases.[25] The admission of a generally younger age group of men changed the type of case treated, the Annual Report for 1933 recording that:

There was a definite loss in stomach and gall bladder surgery, in cases presenting kidney and bladder pathology, in the surgical derelicts which are passed from hospital to hospital, in old fractures with mal- and non-union, in acquired deformities, in the crippling arthritis, and in chronic chest infections. There was a marked increase in acute fractures, traumatism to soft parts of the extremities, infected wounds, acute abdominal conditions, inguinal hernia, traumatic eye conditions and acute empyema.

Staff physicians at Walter Reed were observing an increase in the number of cancer cases, and as the bed situation in Army hospitals then encouraged the ready admission of dependents, in 1931 the Surgeon General's Office issued Circular No. 25, proposing an annual voluntary examination of adult women residing at or near Army stations, for the early detection of cancer. Many other remediable physical conditions were observed, and by 1933, although the admission of surgical cases from the United States at large remained practically the same, there was a marked increase in the amount of female surgery performed at Walter Reed.

Further, in spite of the changing character of the clinical material provided by CCC cases, the inpatient admission of 7,122 in 1930 dropped to 6,431 in 1934. Notwithstanding the numerical decrease in patients, the number of laboratory procedures performed increased from 99,833 to 199,158 in 1934. Routine requests for blood counts were beginning to constitute a bottleneck in the discharge of laboratory work, for often as many as 150 day were requested.[26]

As the four-year fellowship program was in effect Colonel Marietta believed that the

Rotation of officers for training purposes (was) an important function of the Medical Service, officers without previous experience in a general Hospital being so rotated as to afford them two or three months experience in each of the various departments; senior officers of the rank of Major are taken into the office of the Chief of Medical Service for one month of administrative training.

If the Commandant of the Army Medical School, by then Colonel P.W. Huntington, believed he had a legitimate complaint over the amount of time the faculty members spent on routine administrative duties, Colonel Marietta likewise believed the ward doctors on his service were penalized, for they spent considerably more time at meetings of the CDD Boards, Disposition Boards, Section VIII Boards, Court Martial, physical examination of applicants for the U.S. Military Academy and instruction of officers at the Army Medical School than appeared advisable to the best interest of the professional services. During 1934, thirty-four ward doctors at Walter Reed gave 146 hours of the scheduled course at the School, primarily at the clinic and ward level.[27]

Colonel Marietta was considered to be one of the best internists in the military medical service, and like Colonel Keller he gave unstintingly of his time to both patients and staff. As the administrative requirements were creating a critical situation, and, in his opinion, jeopardizing patient care, a year later he reported that

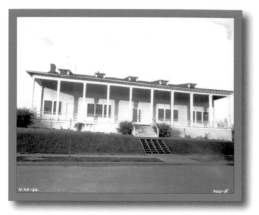

Post Gymnasium, 1933; site later occupied by permanent barracks

Clinical instruction makes a major demand on the time of the officers of the Medical Service. It is believed it could be better carried out by trained teachers in the subjects listed who could devote their full time to clinical teaching and the necessary preparation that is demanded for good teaching. Such activity could be combined with clinical research in contradiction to laboratory research.[28]

Allergy studies were increasingly a part of the general diagnostic survey of patients, and one medical officer was trained in this specialty at the New York Post Graduate School.[29] In June 1932, an Allergy Clinic was not only opened on the first floor of the Main Building, but an additional specialist was being trained for relief work. By 1934 an air filter had been installed in one of the private rooms on the Officers' Section as a diagnostic measure in the treatment of pollen asthma and hay fever. The care of diabetic patients, fifty per cent of whom were chronic and for a time had their own dining room, were assigned to this section and instructed in routine urinalysis and insulin dosage.[30]

In 1932, 2005 electrocardiograms were made at Walter Reed General Hospital, the tracings showing a wide variety of clinical conditions. During the first part of the year, when the majority of patients were veterans, there was a preponderance of degenerative heart conditions with a "generous sprinkling of purely leuitic cases." With the advent of the Civilian Conservation Corps and a younger group of men, a larger number of rheumatic heart lesions were found in the 1303 tracings of a year later.

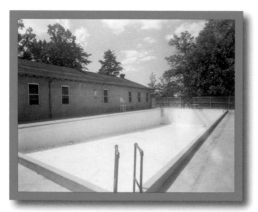

Rea Swimming Pool later assigned to Officers Club use.

Only 1303 CCC cases were admitted to Walter Reed during 1933, but by the end of 1934, a total of some 3,000 case histories had been handled by the Registrar's Office. This was not only a tremendous volume of work, but seventy-five per cent of the records were defective in some way, thereby requiring a careful check of interviews, additional telephone calls, or the return of the records to other stations in order to secure accurate information.

For the Sick

Appropriations for the new laundry, bakery and Quartermaster warehouse were secured in 1931, with the buildings completed during 1932.[31] In 1933, the old open cage elevators, installed in the Main Building at the time of construction, were replaced with modern cabs in enclosed shafts. The temporary wooden structures were demolished during the year, and two auto parking spaces were constructed for staff use, one between the Laboratory and Isolation Ward and one in the northeast court of the Main Building. A much-needed apartment for eighteen families of non-commissioned officers was built on the Fern Street side of the reservation and occupied in December 1933. As replacement for the rapidly deteriorating temporary structure surrounding the Rea swimming pool, General Truby proposed a new pool, one connected with the gymnasium.

The Post Exchange surplus fund, used to subsidize various welfare and recreational activities on the Post, provided no dividends in 1932,[32] a factor which sharply curtailed book purchases for The Library. The Army-Veterans Administration contract system permitted assignment of some of the funds for welfare and recreation activities, including the purchase of library books and the payment of a certain number of civilian employees. In accord with the general reduction in Veterans Administration activities at Walter Reed, some civilian aides were necessarily suspended from duty for want of Medical Department Hospital Funds to pay them. In April 1933 The Library book fund was eliminated,[33] and with the reduction of patients during the summer months, one civilian librarian was suspended for a five-month period. Similarly, the senior bracemaker from the Orthopedic Brace Shop was discharged in 1933 but rehired in 1934.

Social effects of the depression were felt in various ways. For instance, admission requirements for appointment in the Army Nurse Corps were strengthened in 1934, no doubt as part of the general curtailment of the over-production of nurses during the late twenties. Possibly because as the Army School of Nursing had adopted the national slogan of "Fewer and Better Nurses," and there was some feeling among Regular Army Nurses that the School graduates received preferential treatment, a number of the Regular Army Nurses, although holding three-year appointments, began attending night school in order to comply with the requirements of high school graduation or its equivalent, imposed on new members of the Corps. A similar enthusiasm for education was manifest among the enlisted men, and a specific appropriation was finally made from Post Exchange funds in order to provide for the purchase of appropriate texts for the student groups.[34] Other signs of retrenchment were significant; for example, in 1931 the Chief Physiotherapy

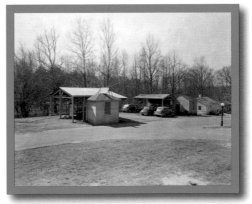

First Gasoline Station, AMC

Aide was paid $2500 annually but by 1934 this sum was reduced to $2100. The head aides by then received only $1620 and the aides only $1440 per annum, with deductions made for quarters and rations as the young women resided on the Post.[35]

General Truby was, of course, distressed that circumstances compelled curtailment of many activities that were amenities to the sick. He was well aware that sudden withdrawal of the CCC funds would create a situation similar to that resulting from withdrawal of the Veterans Administration during the year before, and he protested vigorously that the proportion of Regular Army patients and their dependents treated at Walter Reed justified a more stable payroll situation. The professional staff was not only engaged in research and teaching, a never-ending responsibility in the training of doctors, but he believed that "an institution of (its) size and standing should not be dependent on incidental funds for the payment of vitally important work in the treatment of the sick."[36]

As Affecting Morale

General Orders #26, Headquarters, Army Medical Center, July 22, 1933 placed all of the Post enlisted complement in one Detachment, under the jurisdiction of one Detachment Commander. For administrative purposes the Detachment was divided into A Company for headquarters administration; B Company, auxiliary manpower for the professional services; and C Company for assignment to the Army Medical School. The authorized enlisted strength at this time was 576, with an average strength of 581.[37] The unstable civilian work situation favored the Army in one respect, for a higher type recruit was obtainable in 1932, some with college education and many with two or more years of high school.[38] The situation appears to have changed in 1933, for the Troop Commander noted that "the physical condition and development of the enlisted personnel (was) below the standard of the line organizations due to the long hours of duty, the confining work and the shortage of personnel necessary to carry on activities."

No internes were trained at Walter Reed in 1933, and the Army School of Nursing was closed officially on January 31. The 137 Regular Army and Reserve nurses present on December 31, 1932 dropped to 106 by December 31, 1933. This decrease was more theoretical than actual, for on August 2, twenty-five civilian nurses were employed with CCC funds.

General Orders No. 15, Headquarters, Army Medical Center, June 5, 1934, effective June 30, reorganized the Detachment into two distinct organizations rather than three companies. The Walter Reed Detachment provided enlisted men for the hospital, including attendants for ambulance call and the enlisted mess. The Headquarters Service Detachment provided personnel for all non-nursing and administrative functions using enlisted personnel.

Meeting the requirements for the sick is necessarily a never-ending responsibility for hospital personnel. Although the enlisted men worked a twelve-hour day, a requirement deplored by the hospital commander, the Detachment strength was usually considered

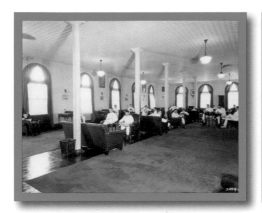 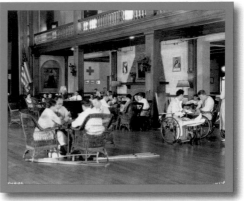

Hospital Corps, Lounge, Main Barracks, *Recreation at the Red Cross "Hut"*
1933

inadequate for current needs. Civilian hospitals were using an increasing number of WPA (civilian) workers for auxiliary services during this period, and the Army, long dependent on the services of soldier-labor, was unknowingly in the process of following suit. At various times during 1934, some forty-seven enlisted men were replaced by civilian operators, janitors and food service employees, through use of CCC and VB funds.

The corpsmen were encouraged to participate in athletic activities, and in spite of the long hours of work, the Detachment morale continued to be "fairly high." According to the command, more liberal furloughs, better housing conditions and shorter hours further would improve it.[39] As in all strata of American life, a social change was setting in, but it was not apparently recognized as such.

Of Interest to the Medical Department

As one of his first official acts as Commandant of the Army Medical Center, General Truby presided at the last graduation exercises of the Army Medical School to be held in the Red Cross house, January 29, 1932. With the exception of a short but intensive course offered two flight surgeons in roentgenology, ophthalmology and otorhinolaryngology, orthopedic and general surgery,[40] few radical changes had been made in the curriculum since the war. The Army Dental School, then housed in one the semi-permanent buildings erected during World War I, continued certain collaborative research work with the United States Bureau of Standards. The most spectacular medical research work of the depression years occurred a year later when an immunizing substance was isolated from pneumocci, using the Felton Method. Pneumonia prophylaxis, tried in all the CCC camps, was evaluated to determine its usefulness in protection against types I and II pneumonia.[41]

CCC fatalities from pneumonia in the winter months of 1933 equaled 12.5 out of every hundred cases but were reduced almost fifty per cent after pneumonia vaccine and oxygen therapy were used with the serum.[42] Work in the Army Medical School

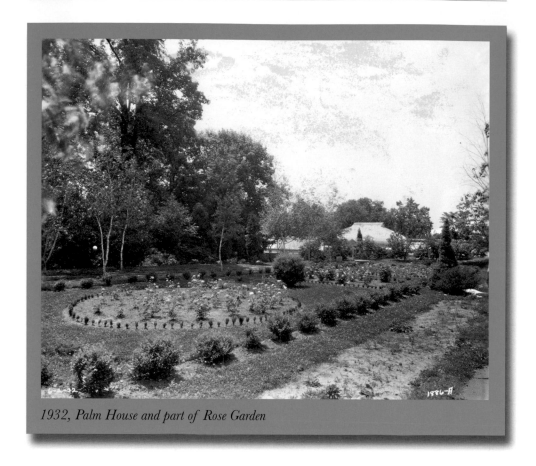

1932, Palm House and part of Rose Garden

vaccine laboratory was interrupted during the year when some of the old sterilizers and equipment, relocated from Louisiana Avenue in 1923, were replaced.[43] Further, the center and North Wings of the School building were completed and occupied during the year,[44] thus providing, along with additional office and laboratory space, a handsome auditorium named for the one-time Surgeon General Sternberg. In spite of the lean state of the Army Medical Center budget, General Truby was successful in securing handsome red velvet drapes for the windows, an accomplishment not to be overlooked in view of the general curtailment of spending.

Major Raymond A. Kelser, V.C., who first demonstrated that the bite of the Aëdes Aegypti mosquito transmitted equine encephalitis, was still at work on this problem. By 1933 he had not only identified seven additional species as capable of transmitting the disease, but he had demonstrated that the human race was likewise susceptible to encephalitis, with mosquitoes as the transmitting agent.[45]

The suspended research activities at the Army Medical School during these years was not unlike the national income, and there is no better index to the state of affairs than the Surgeon General's usually ample report, which in 1935 reduced the space allotted to the Army Medical School to slightly less than three pages.

The Thoroughbred

Hospitals, like people, show definite characteristics, especially those institutions where the personnel is permanent or semi-permanent. And so it was at Walter Reed, where some staff members, like Colonel Keller, remained on duty continuously for a number of years. Others were repeaters, for many of the specialists served their four-year tour, then transferred to other general hospitals to wait out the restrictions imposed by the Manchu Law. Washington was a pleasant place to live, and there was always enough "hot" news of impending international calamities and Capitol intrigue to keep even the poorest listener busy sorting fact from fancy. Young doctors new to the Army coveted the Walter Reed assignment; doctors who had grown old in the Army were reluctant to leave.

In 1930 Norman T. Kirk returned from a two-year tour in the Philippines to resume his place as Chief of the Orthopedic Section at Walter Reed and his pleasant association with his praeceptor, Colonel Keller. He attacked professional problems with his usual zeal and proceeded to treat cases transferred from other institutions with a sure, deft touch, noting in the Annual Report that the profession as a whole was inadequately trained in treating fractures and first aid splinting for transportation.[46]

Colonel Keller was known as a martinet and hard taskmaster, and his young satellite as a temperamental instrument-thrower. As if two individualist surgeons were not enough for the nursing staff and corpsmen to cope with, the third, James C. Kimbrough, Major, Medical Corps, was assigned Chief of the Urology section in 1930. After arrival of the tall Lincolnesque Tennessean, the Urology Section pre-empted first place in the Walter Reed "Hall of Fame" reserved for surgical prima donnas. For in him there were combined all the most marked characteristics of the other two "K's," plus some additional ones that were pure Kimbrough.

It was a poor day when he failed to toss at least two sounds back into the instrument tray or rumble and grumble in well-feigned rage that he could never get his personnel trained to suit him. Amazingly, he could enter the cystoscopy room like March's proverbial roaring lion and leave it as meek as a ewe lamb. Now and then someone crossed him, and a few had the courage of nurse Clytie Reynolds, who indulged his mercurial moods and endured the long hours of work for some four years, and then quietly requested transfer to another hospital "where she could rest."[47] Sergeant Ralph Green, "Doc" Green to old timers, was hardier and stayed on duty in the Genito-Urinary Clinic for thirty years. He quietly patched up the pieces when the current explosion was over; for him the "Kernel" could do no wrong.

Although long a bachelor, when Jimmy Kimbrough finally married, he was one of the most domesticated of husbands and indulgent of fathers. There was seldom a conversation that failed to include Pauline and Jane, or Jane and Pauline, depending on whether the wife or young daughter was uppermost in his thoughts at the moment. A diligent and prolific writer on professional subjects, he was also an avid history scholar and general reader. A favorite of the senior librarian; who invariably saved the most recent accessions for his perusal, he was sure to make at least one daily visit, especially after the relocation of the Urology Clinic from the second floor center of the Old Main to the section adjoining the Library. This routine became firmly established, and when he returned to Walter Reed in the late thirties as a repeater, he once remarked in stentorian tones for all to hear that "By God" he sometimes had difficulty telling which he loved more, Pauline and Jane or Miss Schick and The Library – but he couldn't do without any of them![48]

It was not unusual for him to amble into the Library for a last-minute review of some new urological technique, prior to going to surgery, and then regale the librarian with his latest story, shaggy dog or otherwise, to the intense interest of all readers within hearing, for there was no auditory privacy in the Medical Library, merely a convenient regrouping of book shelves. There was a period, during his first tour at Walter Reed, when doctors were discussing privately and the press was hinting publicly, that monkey gland treatments were amorously more effective than a drink from the Conquistadores' "Fountain of Youth."

As the popular discussion of this operation became more open, "Big Jim" had many pleading requests that he become a dispenser of lost virility. As he was a conservative surgeon, one who took no unnecessary risks, the suggestions made him irritable![49] He came stomping into the medical section of The Library one morning, requesting a full bibliography on the subject. While thumbing through the current periodical literature, he described the operation in detail, to the delight of the over-the-bookstack-listeners. It was, the librarian meditated later, a little like a story she once heard on Mr. Coolidge. On his return from church the laconic President faced his inquisitive wife, who asked him the topic of the minister's sermon.

"Sin," answered her taciturn husband briefly.

"What did he say?" persisted Mrs. Coolidge.

"He was agin it," said the President.

And that expressed the current opinion of the Chief of the Urology Section exactly, at least on the subject of vasectomies.[50]

A tall man, with a jointed-doll gait, "Big Jim" had a habit of rocking back and forth on the balls of his feet as he talked. He often peered at his listeners over the top of his bifocal glasses or, head back and chest out, squinted at them owlishly through the lower half. Noted for his good stories and a bookshelf collection of trinkets erotica, contributed by amused patients, his habit of unhesitatingly voicing his opinion earned for him the reputation for being severe. Slow-footed internes faced their three-month rotating service in the Genito-Urinary Clinic with apprehension, for even the most agile had difficulty in meeting the pace set by "the old man."

More often than not patients were well indoctrinated with Kimbrough-lore before arriving at the Genito-Urinary Clinic. As they were unaware of his gentle and skillful

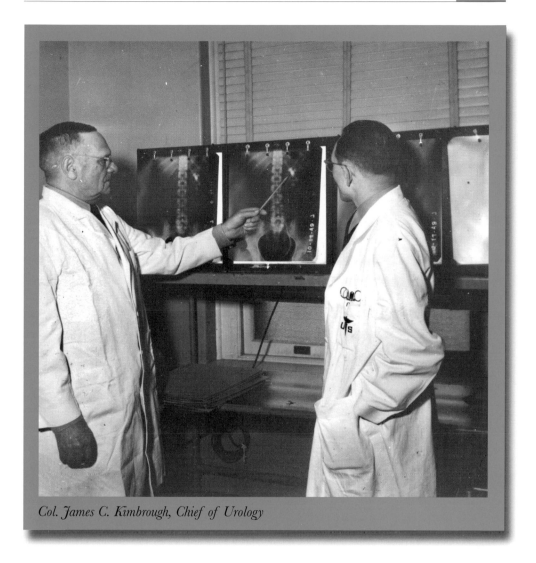

Col. James C. Kimbrough, Chief of Urology

technique, some faced the urological examination with fear and trembling, only to learn that his gruffness was a shield for hiding his immense sympathy for human suffering. Perhaps the only time in his life that he was ever completely nonplussed was when a frail and trembling little old lady of seventy, scheduled for a cystoscopy, faced him like an infuriated bantam hen, and before he could say a word, announced in quavering voice, "I'm not scared of you, I'm not scared of you a bit!"

Born on a farm near Madisonville, Tennessee, a small town later made famous by his cousin, Senator Estes Kefauver, Jimmy Kimbrough early began to make his own way in life. As one of several children he learned the give and take of daily adjustments along with the rugged philosophy of his native region, where a little money and a little moonshine whisky each went a long way. Honest and unpretentious, he was never known to take part in Service intrigue or in any way to put his own welfare ahead of that of his Corps. His dry salty humor and well calculated posturing as a "toughie" formed a natural smoke screen that concealed his warm-hearted affection for his fellow man, and a thinly overlaid crust of hard-shell Baptist doctrine.[51]

But recently graduated from medical school at the onset of World War I, he was, like thousands of other patriotic young Americans, impatient to be off to war. While he was in Chattanooga on a weekend trip, one of his classmates persuaded him to take the examination for the Regular Army, and he complied in jest. He had not heard the results of the examination when the 17th Engineer Unit began assembling at Fort McPherson, Georgia, but he packed most of his personal possessions in a new cowhide bag, treasured graduation present, bought himself a uniform, and went along.

His knowledge of American history and especially the Civil War, when the command had loose control of men and the muster rolls, had shaped his ideas of Army life. When the regiment was ordered from Fort McPherson to New York for embarkation to France, young Dr. Kimbrough, still with no commission, climbed on the troop train, new bag and all. As the troops embarked on the transport, the men were deprived of their personal luggage, which was tossed on a rapidly mounting pile, and issued duffle bags. Parting with his most valued possession was painful, for it seemed doubtful that a poor boy from his section of Tennessee would soon have another so handsome. As he wandered around the port deck for a last minute glimpse of New York, he saw his shining new suitcase roll to the base of the luggage pile. The temptation was too much. He made a quick trip down the gangplank, recovered his property and smugly departed for France, the only man aboard with a cowhide bag.

His anxiety to get "over there" in a hurry brought other complications, for it had not occurred to him that regimental officers were issued personal orders. He was not accustomed to having much money so the absence of funds during his first three months in Europe didn't bother him much. There was always a good poker game under way and he held his own with contemporaries in the National Army. This idyllic situation didn't last, however, for as a good many Regular Army sergeants and enlisted men received temporary promotions as officers, they invaded the poker games – and invariably won. When reduced to his last dollar, he presented himself to the Paymaster, learning to his amazement, that insofar as the Army was concerned, James C. Kimbrough of Madisonville, Tennessee, was not commissioned nor was he in France! When the matter was finally cleared-up, Lt. Kimbrough learned that he had passed the examination creditably, but his official papers had not been forwarded after his unceremonious departure.[52] According to other Kimbrough legends, he was just as eager to be off to war in 1942 and though older, he was not a more cautious man. As Chief of Professional Services for the European Theater of Operation, comparable to Colonel Keller's World War I position with the AEF, the indomitable Jimmy rushed ashore from a heaving landing barge while more timorous associates awaited "time and tide." He wanted to be the first medic ashore in France and airily disregarded the barge commander's threat of court martial!

Known for many years within and without the Medical Department as an outstanding urologist, he was, like Ernest R. Gentry, well able to retain control of professional affairs in his own section. Whereas some other Army surgeons branched out into general surgery in order to become eligible for the position of chief of a general hospital surgical service, Jimmy Kimbrough remained with his specialty. He seemed unconcerned that some men he had trained as lieutenants inherited the higher administrative positions, and when the Medical Department "promotion-pattern" changed noticeably after World War II, and some less well known specialists were rewarded with general officer grades, he shruggingly chalked the circumstance up to the fortunes of war. And so he began his third tour of duty at Walter Reed in 1946, saying if the Army would only leave him alone he could be happy until he died. Retired by statutory regulations in 1948, he continued on active duty through a yearly contract arrangement with the Surgeon General's Office.

Many distinguished men were his patients, and regardless of the difference in accommodations provided by bed assignments for general officer or soldiers, each case received the same degree of unpretentious but thorough professional attention. The Medical Department was employing an uncommonly large number of civilian doctors as consultants in 1948, and when General George Catlett Marshall, one-time Chief of Staff of the Army, Secretary of State and later Secretary of Defense, was admitted to Walter Reed for a kidney operation. Strictly ethical in all his relationships, "Big Jim" advised his patient that he could have any consultant, or all the consultants, to attend him. Interested eye witnesses reported that the astute General merely smiled and said quietly, "What's wrong with the Army?" What was good enough for his men was good enough for him.

The day selected for surgery found the individualistic Colonel Kimbrough in a more mellow mood than usual. His low moment came in the early morning hours, when he was shaving. As he looked at himself in the glass, meditating all the while on the surgical sequence of the next few hours, he said to himself, "Jim, you ugly old devil, you're taking a powerful chance operating on the greatest man in history. What if he dies on you?"

The so-called "ugly old devil" made no audible reply and so, sighing a bit over his responsibility to the nation, he stalked off to the hospital at his customary hour, 7:30 a.m. In his usual modest way and without special fanfare, he discharged his simple duty, supported only by his own skill and the homely philosophy of the Tennessee hill people – "The Lord despises a coward."[53]

References

1.   Jose Maria Sert.

2.   Interview with Maj. Gen. Robert U. Patterson, M.C. Ret., Aug. 24, 1950.

3.   *Ibid.*

4.   *Ibid.*

5.   Ltr from Albert E. Truby, Brig. Gen., Ret., to the writer, May 19, 1951.

6.   Interview with Col. Herbert N. Dean, MAC, Ret., Apr. 12, 1950.

7.   Promoted to Brigadier General May 24, 1933, date of rank retroactive to January 1933.

8.   Albert E. Truby, *Memoir of Walter Reed*... New York, Paul B. Hoeber, Inc. 1943, Chpt I, pg 1-13.

9.   Medical and Military Notes, *The Military Surgeon*, Vol. 73, 1933, pg 38-39.

10. Interview with Brig. Gen. Albert E. Truby, M.C., Ret., June 27-28, 1950.

11. Ltr from Truby to writer, *op cit.*

12. Patterson interview, *op cit.*

13. Personal knowledge of the writer.

14. Annual Rpt TSG... 1932, pg 261

15. *Ibid.*

16. *Ibid,* pg 262.

17. Annual Rpt WRGH, 1932.

18. *Ibid.*

19. *Ibid.*

20. *Ibid.*

21. *Ibid.*

22. *Ibid,* 1933.

23. Annual Rpt, 1931, U.S. Veterans Adm., GPO, pg 20.

24. *Ibid,* 1933, pg 11.

25. *Ibid.*

26. Annual Rpt WRGH, 1934.

27. *Ibid,* 1933.

28. *Ibid,* 1934.

29. *Ibid*, 1932.

30. *Ibid*, 1933.

31. Annual Rpt TSG... 1931, pg 37.

32. *Ibid*, pg 267.

33. Annual Rpt WRGH, 1933.

34. *Ibid*.

35. *Ibid*, 1934.

36. *Ibid*, 1934.

37. *Ibid*, 1933.

38. *Ibid*, 1932.

39. *Ibid*, 1934.

40. Annual Rpt TSG... 1932, pg 248.

41. AMB, No. 42, Oct. 1937, pg 40-41.

42. Reduced to 6.4 per 100 in 1939. Edgar Erskine Hume, *History of the Ass. of Military Surgeons of the U.S., 1891–1941*, pg 176.

43. SGO 391.1-2 (AMS) GG, War Rec. Div., Nat'l Archives.

44. Annual Rpt WRGH, 1932.

45. R.A. Kelser, "Mosquitoes as vectors of equine encephalomyelitis," in *Am. Vet. Med. Ass.*, May 1933, VS Vol. 35, No. 5. (quoted)

46. Annual Rpt, WRGH, 1934, pg 40.

47. As told to the writer in 1939.

48. Conversation with Col. James C. Kimbrough, 1941.

49. See Rpt, Urology Section, Annual Report WRGH, 1931–1934.

50. Conversation with Miss Mary E. Schick, 1941.

51. Personal knowledge of the writer.

52. Social conversation Colonel James C. Kimbrough, 1939.

53. Social conversation with Colonel James C. Kimbrough, MC, Ret., Sept. 20, 1950.

The Kingpin

1936–1939

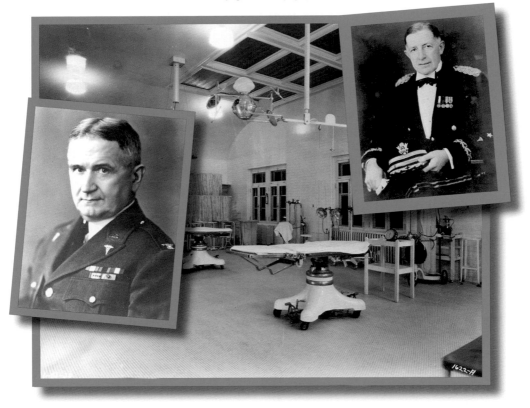

"And we should have only such men as are adapted to its peculiar requirements."[1]

The low year in Veterans' bed occupancy in Army hospitals came in the fiscal year 1934, when only 457 of the approximately 2,000 beds formerly allotted to veterans were occupied. This sudden drop brought a small reduction in personnel and operating costs, with the Surgeon General's Office reporting that the average cost per inpatient day for the Army's six largest hospitals was $4.60.[2] Passage of more liberalizing Veterans' legislation in March 1934 partially restored the old order. At Walter Reed, during 1934, 760 Veterans, 2,989 members of the Civilian Conservation Corps and 2,517 "others" were admitted in addition to the 2,080 officers, nurses and enlisted men.[3] Again, the inpatient cost rose, this time from $4.60 to $4.90 daily.[4]

On June 29, 1934, the President adopted the Federal Board of Hospitalization's resolution in regard to a uniform reciprocal rate of hospitalization, and during the fiscal year 1937, all but one of the Army hospitals received the flat rate of $3.75 a day for non-military patients[5], except dependents.[6] By 1938, with the depression beginning to wane, the inpatient costs averaged $5.09, although the reciprocal rate had not been raised.[7] Concurrently, as of June 1938, only 932 of the 1,225 authorized beds at Walter Reed were occupied,[8] and balancing the local budget was a difficult problem.

Folklore

Brigadier General Wallace C. De Witt succeeded General Truby as Post Commander in August 1935. The appointment was appropriate, for by popular acclamation he was accepted as the Medical Department's outstanding hospital commander. Sandy-haired, square-jawed and of ruddy complexion, energetic and thorough[9], his unbounded energy was occasionally curtailed by a temporary siege of gout. Once recovered, he appeared to compensate for lost time by moving even faster than usual. From his father, Colonel Calvin De Witt, one-time commandant of the Army Medical School and an Army doctor of the frontier period, he inherited a passionate love for military service. His early life was spent on Army posts, and "the line" influence showed in many small personal characteristics, such as the fact that he almost invariably carried a riding crop.

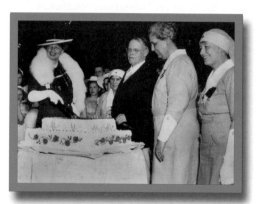

Red Cross Birthday Party, 1938; Mrs. Roosevelt, General De Witt and Miss Lower in foreground

Whereas some medical officers sniffed indignantly at the multitude of absorbing administrative duties that encroached on their professional time, Wallace De Witt apparently sought them out, enjoying the struggle to conquer or be conquered by a knotty problem in organization or medical economics. His previous assignments had been largely administrative, although his basic career as a hospital commander did not begin until after World War I. Then, at the Station Hospital, Fort Sam Houston, Texas[10], he demonstrated his ingenuity in stretching the budget. When patients were transferred to other hospitals, civilian or military, and required the attendance of a doctor, it was often the hospital commander rather than a ward doctor who made the trip.[11] In this way he managed to examine the construction of many new installations with great care, sometimes learning more of the defects than were known to the local management. He was a strict disciplinarian, was critical of wastage, liked graphs and kept accurate statistics on his own organization.[12]

He was long considered by younger Army doctors to be the model hospital administrator, and his free use of statistics enabled him to evaluate management costs with such ease that his admiring associates credited him with some occult ability to spot trouble. It is extremely doubtful that this busy and practical man wasted much of his valuable time indulging instincts, and it is more probable that his excellent system of record keeping concealed the answers to some anomalous administrative economies. In fact, he was so ingenious in the

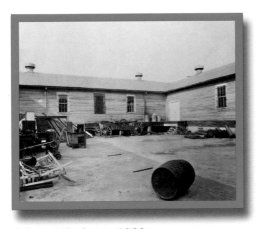

Salvage Warehouse, 1929

preparation of the budget that Surgeon General Reynolds believed that to have fully satisfied his financial demands would have pauperized the other general hospitals, for he began, considering the period of economic uncertainty, what appeared to be a lavish spending program, and he junked much allegedly serviceable property such as kitchen equipment and hospital furniture in order to provide more attractive items (ltrs G. R. Reynolds to writer 21 March 1952; A. E. Truby to writer 25 Apr 1952).

The latter predilection was not especially helpful, for the Medical Department budget then was in such a lean condition that economies were a necessity. In 1935, when he began the first half-year of his tenure at the Army Medical Center, one-third of the staff physicians at the hospital[13] were reserve officers. This group had been called to active duty in order to replace some of the young regulars forced to assume some of the administrative responsibilities of the CCC program, and to replace the unusually large number of World War doctors then being lost through retirements for physical disability.[14]

Personnel new to the institutional practice of medicine not only had less appreciation of the need for administrative economics, but, unlike the old regulars, some apparently shared the popular belief that government issue was free issue and took little note of the fact that in the end the taxpayer footed the bill. It was therefore during the De Witt administration that for the first time in the history of the hospital some of the professional services were required to re-use properly washed and sterilized gauze and economize on such seemingly small items as adhesive tape.[15] Salvaged cotton was even reissued as cleaning rags, accountable to the issue clerk before replacements could be obtained. Further General De Witt's enthusiasm for statistics was noticeable in the detailed table and graphs attached to the Annual Reports, such as the cost accounting reports rendered on the laundry service. For instance, 2,549,760 pieces of institutional linen were laundered at a cost of 0.047 cents per patient in 1935.[16]

In spite of his minor economies and exacting inspections, the General was as popular with the nurses and corpsmen as with the medical staff.[17] The Saturday morning inspection was still a customary routine in Army hospitals. Consequently on Friday

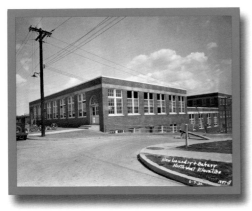

1932, Laundry and Bakery (Dogwood Street)

the entire menage was upset by the hum of electric floor waxers and the diligent "spit and polish" methods of custodial help, giving that last minute see-your-face-look to the floors before "the old man" arrived. Whereas former commanders had maintained a sedate military bearing and left the search for dust to the First Sergeant, usually in attendance, Wallace De Witt probed into dark corners for himself. Even more shocking, he formed the habit of arriving for unscheduled inspections on Tuesday as readily as Saturday. He occasionally climbed on a chair better to examine the top of the clothes cupboard, shifted bottles in the medicine cabinet to see how recently the glass shelves had been washed, or ran an exploring finger between the mattress and headboard of the bed, where he claimed, the corpsmen and maids invariably failed to dust. If the results were questionable he was apt to drop the riding crop and dart under the bed for a quick look at the springs and mechanical apparatus.[18] Peculiarly, for a man otherwise so tidy, he used the pencil slot in the top drawer of his desk as an ash tray, and woe to the office custodian who failed to dump the contents before 8 a.m.[19]

There was one personal problem that baffled him – his false teeth – which he kept conveniently in the right hand top drawer of his desk, if luxuriating in privacy, and which, protected by a large white handkerchief, he would hastily pop into place as official callers arrived. Now and then he roamed absentmindedly about the grounds on an inspection trip, or went to the Army Medical School to make a speech, having left the troublesome teeth in the drawer. Keeping owner and property together became a special responsibility of his secretary, who often sent the offending denture by special messenger.

In addition to the Keller and De Witt gardens, part of the area behind the Post Commander's quarters was subdivided into plots for younger members of the command. There the amateur gardeners met on summer afternoons, hailing each other in friendly fashion and competing for friendly praise of their produce. Finding himself alone in the area one afternoon, the General suddenly decided he could better discharge his horticultural duties if unencumbered by the troublesome teeth. A sturdy tomato plant offered safe concealment, and he promptly forgot about having removed them.

Army social calls are made at prescribed times: new members of the command call on the ranking officer within forty-eight hours after arrival; other calls are exchanged on Sunday from four until six or on week days from six until eight. Callers arrived unexpectedly during the evening, but the General was happily unaware of his appearance until his old dog came romping in the garden – and deposited the gleaming dentures at his feet![20]

The End of a Dynasty

The various professional activities at Walter Reed shared one thing in common from 1935 until 1939 – they expanded. One of the most noticeable changes concerned the Obstetrical Section, which occupied the building the Birmingham children once dubbed "The Pest House," but was by then known as Ward 21. An increasing number of women were seeking admission to the hospital, and whereas Ward 21 had a bed capacity of eighteen patients at a time, a total of 195 women were treated there during 1935,[21] and 222 during 1936. In May 1936, a remodeled medical ward, No. 29, was assigned to obstetrics, and the two upper floors of Ward 21 were remodeled for an acute infectious disease ward. The lower floor was occupied by the internes.[22]

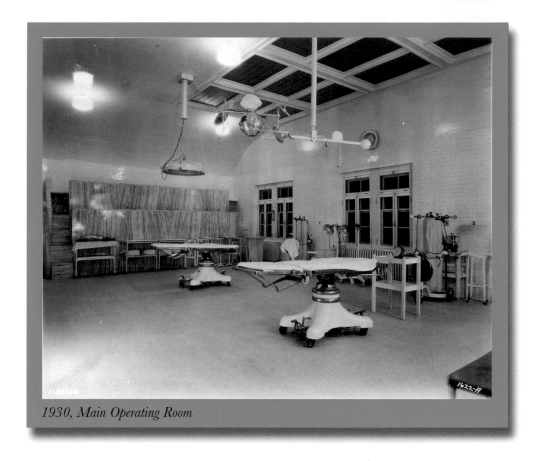

1930, Main Operating Room

The Medical Service made an analysis of the electrocardiograph records in 1934, discovering that approximately sixty-seven per cent of the films showed essentially normal findings.[23] About twenty-two per cent of the cases on the Officers' Section indicated cardiovascular diseases but only ten per cent of the female medical cases showed such deterioration. Of the 80.2 per cent of the 166 deaths autopsied in 1935, twenty-seven deaths were directly attributable to cancer.[24] A year later, when only 73.7 per cent of the total number of deaths were autopsied, as existing policy by then required family permission for postmortem examination of deceased retired officers, the findings were even more significant, for 22.1 per cent of the deaths were due to this cause. In 1939, almost half of the deaths in the Surgical Service were due to malignancy. Prior to this period all cases requiring radium treatment were sent to Johns Hopkins Hospital, Baltimore, Maryland, but, after the significant increase in neoplastic diseases, the hospital was provided with its own radium.

The Surgical Service authorized 243 blood transfusions in 1935, a total increase of sixty-two over the previous year. Of these, 107 were performed by the direct multiple syringe method and 136 by the indirect citrate gravity method. Of the 7,505 new admissions in 1936, almost one-third of the cases received an anesthetic, with the number of spinal anesthetics increasing by 225 over the previous year, and the gas oxygen, gas-oxygen-ether, and avertin decreasing proportionately.

Colonel Keller retired as Chief of the Surgical Service in June 1935. Young officers had quailed at his approach and older officers had deferred to his judgment with unequivocal respect. He was quiet, stern and hard-working, and so some of his staff members maintained that they had two vacations annually, their own and the month "the Chief" went fishing. A determined individualist, he ran his own show and that, a contemporary later said humorously, was probably why he was never investigated.[25]

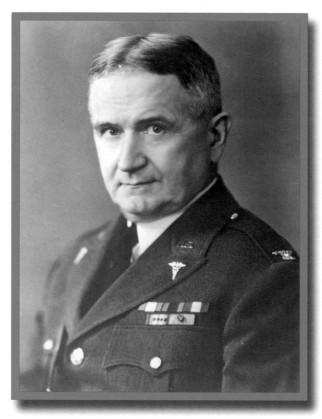

Colonel William L. Keller

Even the Congress recognized his merit by retiring him on full military pay as a lifetime consultant in surgery to the staff at Walter Reed. Thereafter he maintained a small but seldom used office in the library, where he retained the complete clinical and photographic files of his surgical exploits. Faithfully, he came to Walter Reed twice weekly for nearly fifteen years. Old friends who knew his regular visiting days called on him at the surgical office, or went to the library to add their cards to the graying collection in his desk drawer, where the aged rubber tubing on his old sphygomanometer was cracking and disintegrating, and a few long-since forgotten pathological specimens floated dismally in their sealed jars.[26] Empyema cases who were young men in 1919 and 1920 returned as old men to visit him, sure that they would be remembered as readily as before. Children on whom he had performed skin grafts in their youth returned with their children, asking only to be remembered by the master, and with unerring instinct he restored their past from the files.

When pain so wracked his arthritic joints that steel braces were required for support to his weary frame, he finally bowed to the inevitable and grudgingly entered a wheel chair at the hospital's portals, in order to make his routine visits or attend the physiotherapy clinic. Only the tranquil expression in his candid china-blue eyes and his compassion for the suffering of children seemed unchanged. The passing years had grayed "the stormy petrel" and shortened his flight, but no other Army surgeon had matched his long and distinguished career at Walter Reed.

Hospital Activities

The first twelve-month training course for physiotherapy aides was given in 1935. Approved by the American College of Physicians, the anatomy course was increased from 180 to 220 hours, and a course in bacteriology and pathology was added.[27] In 1935 alone, a total of 129,419 physiotherapy treatments were given, 53,454 of them to non-military patients. Obstetrics and Gynecology was normally a busy section of the Surgical Service, but after Colonel Raymond F. Metcalfe became Chief of the Surgical Service in 1935, a special clinic was established for examination of all female out-patients referred by the General Dispensary, Military District of Washington. Further, such cases were re-examined three weeks post-operatively. In fact, the Surgical Service was so busy that elective cases were listed for operation and admitted as beds became available.

Whereas Colonel Keller was known throughout the Medical Corps as professionally autocratic,[28] Raymond W. Metcalfe was the complete opposite. His reputation as a skilled surgeon, especially for women, was almost legendary. Soft-spoken, quiet and self-contained,[29] he was one of the twelve doctors who passed the Army Examining Board in 1902, without defensive championship from any of that exacting group of dignitaries.[30]

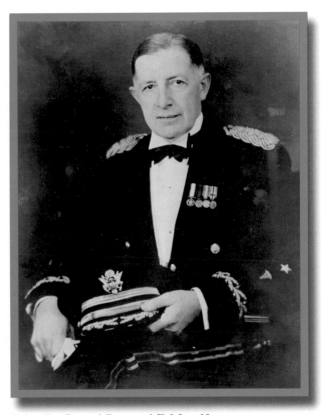

Brigadier General Raymond F. Metcalfe

A bachelor for many years, he never "traveled with the herd," and when with other single officers he went to theaters and concerts, he usually sat alone.[31] Friendly, but inarticulate, he appeared anxious to participate in the informal group activities of his contemporaries but "did not have the knack of being undignified."[32] At some early stage in his career he formed a close friendship with Malin Craig, Chief of Staff of the Army at the time he finally had the opportunity of serving at Walter Reed. Promoted to Brigadier General in March 1937, while serving in a professional rather than a command position, he broke the traditional Army promotion pattern of correlation between rank and organizational and manpower responsibility. Whereas many other officers played golf for a pastime, General Metcalfe studied the stock market with the same care and devotion that he lavished on surgery, and he appeared to be conspicuously successful in either role. Impeccably well groomed, abnormally shy but quietly humorous, he was popular with Army wives, some of whom vied with Irving S. Cobb in *Speaking of Operations*, if they happened to bear the seal of the Metcalfe technique. A few even traveled from West to East of these United States to secure his reassurance that physically all was well.

By 1939, the major part of the General Dispensary was moved to the Center, located in conjunction with Ward 30 and designated the Out-Patient Service, Walter Reed General Hospital.[33] Thus another step in Dr. Borden's plan for a medical center was complete, for it was he who had proposed affiliation of the city dispensary with the U.S. Army Hospital, Washington Barracks, DC. Only the Army Medical Library and Medical Museum now remained from under the administrative canopy.

Out-patients were referred from other posts, and residential calls were made on Army families residing in the District of Columbia, provided the patient was unable to attend the clinic. Former Dispensary personnel of the X-ray, Dental, EENT and Laboratory Sections transferred to these sections of the hospital, and the technical procedures of the two organizations became closely intertwined.[34] Eight doctors, five nurses, one stenographer and ten enlisted men were permanently assigned to the Out-Patient Service, where, in the first eight months, three-fourths of the treatments were given to civilian dependents.[35] The new arrangement created parking problems as well as food service problems, for many of the patients made the trip "out to Walter Reed" an all-day affair.

The overall quota of nurses assigned to Walter Reed during the closing years of the thirties was numerically adequate in proportion to the general average of six nurses per 1,000 men as established by the Troop Basis allowance of the War Department General Staff. The hospitalization rate of the troops was less than anticipated, and as Veterans' Bureau and CCC funds permitted the employment of civilian nurses and/or Red Cross reserve nurses, Captain Lyda M. Keener, who in May 1934 succeeded Mrs. Flikke as Principal Chief Nurse, had a pleasant assignment, one with few administrative problems. By and large the nurses then on duty at the hospital represented a mature group, settled women in their late twenties and early thirties. Therefore Miss Keener was seldom required to act as "matron," reputedly a time-consuming chore of many civilian nurse superintendents. She wisely believed that Army Nurses were as well able to manage their private affairs, without surveillance as were the male officers.

A tall, white-haired, kindly, gentle, slow-speaking woman, she performed her official duties with the minimum amount of physical exertion. Like her good friend Miss Molloy, she was "addicted" to frequent vacations, and in this way she pleasantly and at no personal

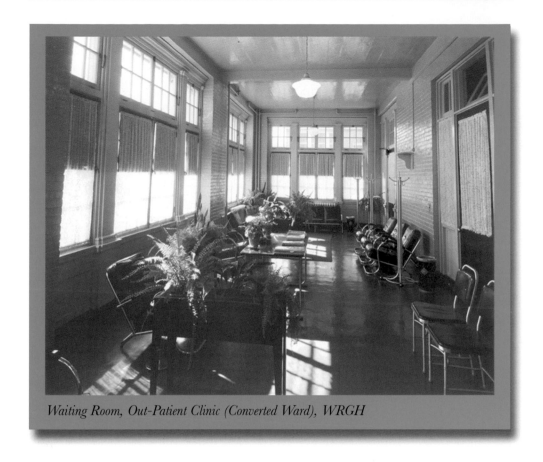

Waiting Room, Out-Patient Clinic (Converted Ward), WRGH

inconvenience solved many awkward situations, for by the time she returned, the administrative storm had spent itself.[36] Nurses rarely appeared in Class A (street) uniforms in those days, and the sudden appearance of the quiet, white-clad Chief Nurse, meandering through the wards on an informal inspection trip, was comforting as well as entertaining to some patients. Her impersonal conversation, unruffled calm and highly developed sense of humor invariably conveyed the impression that she was perpetually relaxed. She had, for the majority of her thirty-odd years in the Army Nurse Corps, been a Chief Nurse, and many of the older medical officers, including General De Witt, were her personal friends.

The professional staff was not large at that time and a four-year assignment in Washington was customary. Post social activities were popular. The nurses entertained in their beautiful ballroom at Delano Hall, the nurses' residence, which "was clean and well kept and (had) the appearance of a high-class modern hotel,"[37] and as a rule the doctors and their wives were invited. The Post had no organized Officers' Club as such, but the Sternberg auditorium was used for staff dances, with catering service provided by outside firms. These affairs, the dances at Delano Hall and the officers' "hops," after the Army adopted a blue dress uniform in 1939, were colorful as well as gay.

The Hospital Corpsmen

By 1936, the 576 men at the Army Medical Center had increased to 596, but there were always unfilled requirements. All new recruits were given a course in the duties of a soldier, and night classes in stenography, typing and general subjects were conducted by PWA teachers, under the general supervision of the Chaplain. A special course for ward attendants was planned but was abandoned because of insufficient instructors.[38] The hospital Laboratory Section apparently felt the deficiencies of the local training system more keenly than other services, for during the year all but one of the laboratory technicians received a discharge by purchase in order to secure better paying positions. A the end of December 1936, the enlisted men in that section consisted of thirteen Privates 1st Class, of whom seven had an average of only 2.5 months of training in laboratory procedures.[39]

The Medical Department Professional Service Schools were requiring more enlisted men, as the teaching, research and routine examinations were being constantly improved by the new methods. Moreover, the new equipment and delicate instruments required considerable expert care.[40] The morale of the School technicians was, however, higher than that of the men in the Walter Reed Detachment, where they performed twelve-hour duty rather than the eight-hour duty of the Medical Department Professional Service School group.[41]

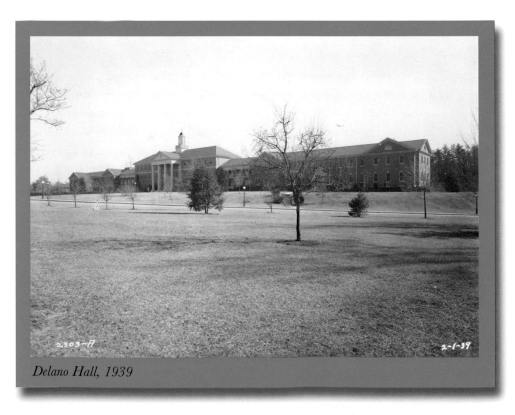

Delano Hall, 1939

About thirty per cent of the enlisted technicians were reasonably well educated. Thus they passed examinations for non-commissioned officer ratings, and many eventually passed the examination for officer rating in the Medical Administrative Corps.[42] This upgrading complicated the personnel situation, as well educated but excellent men, many with leadership qualifications, were unable to secure ratings enabling them to become group leaders. Still more unfortunate, the technicians competing for ratings were also the most employable in civilian fields and many were ultimately lost to the organization. Consequently, General De Witt urged an increase in the number of ratings for the first four grades,[43] as this might encourage the trained technicians to re-enlist,[44] a proposal which did not receive ready approval from overhead administrative agencies.

Since there appeared to be no satisfactory solution to the unstable technical personnel situation, on October 4, 1937, the Surgeon General authorized the employment of two trained civilian technicians.[45] The results were so satisfactory that School authorities urged all key technical positions be filled by civilians, preferably female, and urged that eight civilian employees be so employed.

The number of enlisted technicians trained at the various schools had increased steadily since 1935, and in 1939 the training course was lengthened from four to twelve months. Instruction in clinical medicine, for the doctors, was limited to neuropsychiatry during the 1939-40 session, although the two-to-four-year courses in the preparation of specialists continued.[46]

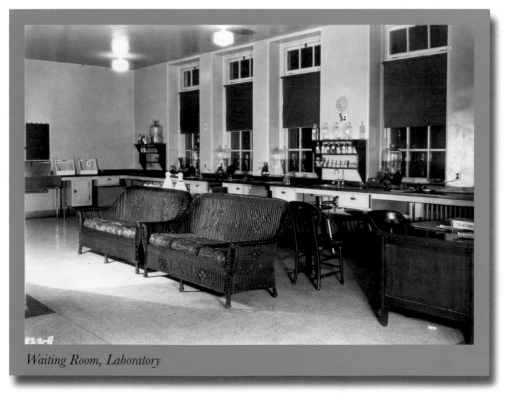

Waiting Room, Laboratory

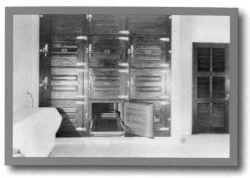 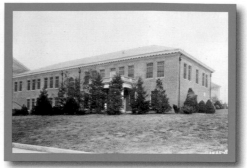

Morgue and Receiving Vault, WRGH

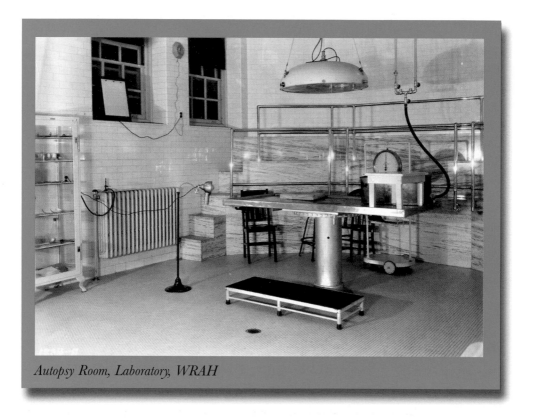

Autopsy Room, Laboratory, WRAH

Beginning in 1932, and then strictly as a source of supply for Walter Reed Hospital, the _Division of Biological Products_, Army Medical School, began preparing, at an approximate cost of twelve cents a bottle, 50 cc bottles of 50 per cent glucose for intravenous therapy. The distribution increased to provide for other Army hospitals in the United States, this division preparing, in 1936, a total of 16,324 bottles and by 1940, a total of 53,457 bottles.

The branch laboratory, at Walter Reed, was transferred to the administrative control of the Assistant Commandant, Medical Department Professional Service Schools, on January 1, 1938, but on May 19, 1939, it was returned to the jurisdiction of the hospital commander.[47]

Odds and Ends

During the mid-twenties, General Fred C. Ainsworth, famous as a controversial figure in the early history of the War Department General Staff, contemplated establishing some sort of hospital memorial to his wife, who had died at Walter Reed. Various suggestions were made, including the baseball grandstand so generously provided by the Senator from West Virginia, but neither decision nor funds took definite forms until after General Ainsworth's death. At that time the hospital authorities learned that a $10,000 bequest was available to the Post library, provided it bore the donor's name.[48]

The stipulation was not agreeable to the governing authorities, who finally agreed to Miss Schick's suggestion that the income from the endowment be devoted to the purchase of books on the history of medicine. There were neither procurable through medical supply channels nor allowable purchases from local welfare funds, which must be spent only on items of direct benefit to the patients. Consequently, in 1936, a small periodical room adjoining the Medical Library section was designated the *Fred C. Ainsworth Memorial Endowment Library*. The collection grew slowly but steadily and included not only a number of interesting and rare volumes on the history of military medicine but some of the papers prepared by Major Walter Reed. After Colonel Keller's retirement, he used this section of the library as his private domain.

In 1936, the east porches to Wards 33, 34 and 35 were enclosed in order to increase the bed capacity. A meat market and cold storage room was installed in the basement of the Quartermaster Building, as an addition to the Commissary. Air conditioning was installed in the main operating room and part of Ward 12, and all diet kitchens in the NP Section were made sound-proof. The center wing of the Post Exchange was enlarged to form a cafeteria, and two clay tennis courts were built for the nurses. Of especial interest to the Dietetic Department, an automatic dishwasher, with water, heat and duration controls was installed in Mess I. This was a sanitary as well as physical economy, for during the year the Diet Kitchen, Officers' Mess, served 31,813 special diets of forty-seven different types. Like the Laboratory, the Dental Clinic was having difficulty securing trained (prosthetic) technicians but during 1936 treated a total of 5,191 patients in 23,163 sittings.[49]

In 1937, the EENT clinic, which had long used the services of Dr. Robert H. Ivy of Philadelphia as a consultant in plastic surgery, reported its first use of the Wolfe-Schindler gastroscope.

Irrelevant from a professional standpoint but organizationally significant, the Commanding General reported that seven government horses, four mules and five private (officer) mounts[50] were stabled and that the government animals were needed and put to good use.

The Post Quartermaster had in service a number of the rugged Field Ambulances, or so-called Red Cross ambulances because of the identification, but only one Metropoli-

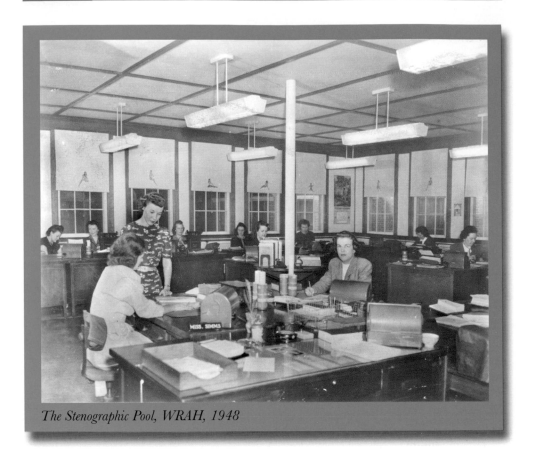

The Stenographic Pool, WRAH, 1948

tan Ambulance, of the type ordinarily used by civilian hospitals. As the Metropolitan Ambulance was originally consigned to Walter Reed for testing and had traveled some 44,308 miles and been in five accidents, General De Witt believed another was needed. Further, he recommended razing the remaining wooden barracks at the Center in a final effort to eliminate the last of the World War I buildings. Post Quartermasters at "line" stations usually carried adequate stocks of government issue furniture to equip the quarters, but General De Witt noted in 1937 that the Army Medical Center had not been so favored, and that such items had been requisitioned annually for twelve years.

Many young ward officers and internes, as well as the reserved officers assigned to duty at Walter Reed and other military hospitals, complained vociferously about the large amount of "paper work" required by the Army. The military record must at all times not only be complete but irreproachably correct for judiciary purposes as it represented vital evidence in establishing service connected disabilities and pension claims. However, to the professionally-minded and enthusiastic young doctor, this represented a time consuming chore.

Ward secretaries were not available at this time; consequently the physicians spent many laborious hours typing, usually in a highly individualistic "hunt and peck" manner,

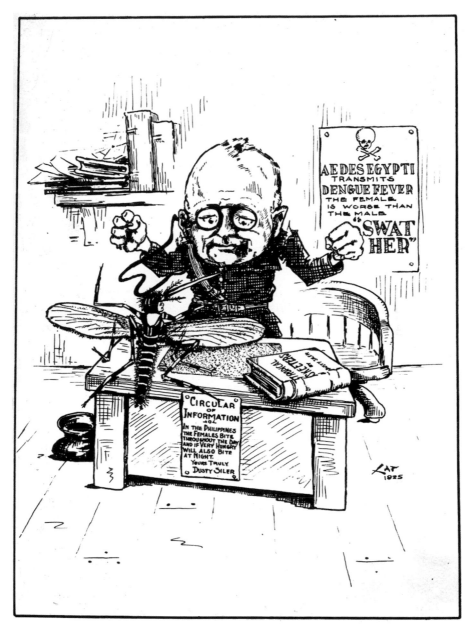

Cartoon of "Dusty" Siler

the case histories. As the appointment of internes was interrupted in 1938,[51] it is especially interesting that a year later General De Witt had procured the first ediphones for dictating clinical histories and had formed the rudiments of the present stenographic pool, by having the many case histories, reports of operation, etc., transcribed in a central office.

The Post Exchange sales served as business index to local spending, and the $10,602 in dividends, accumulated in 1939, was assigned to the Recreation Fund, Chaplains' Fund, Post Library and the Hospital Fund.

Research and Investigation

In addition to the teaching and routine investigative work at the Army Medical School, the Division of Laboratories initiated a comprehensive study of typhoid organisms. Some phases of the work perfected in other parts of the world were repeated in an effort not to overlook any possible improvement in the antityphoid vaccine produced for the Army, Navy and other governmental agencies. The work was begun in 1935 and reported in 1937, the faculty claiming that the new "Strain 58" typhoid bacillus, was distinctly superior to the Rawlings strain heretofore used.[52] In this connection Colonel Joseph F. Siler, Commandant of the School, and his deputy, Lt. Colonel George C. Dunham, two of the Medical Department's outstanding specialists in public health and preventative medicine, were commended for their significant work.[53]

Whereas the investigative branch of the medical and allied health functions were customarily identified under the general title of "The Army Medical School," by 1935 the auxiliary corps were anxious for more independent recognition. Thereafter the combined group activities were known as the Medical Department Professional Services Schools. Historically, the program for the 1935 graduation exercises was the last announcement of "The Graduation Exercises of the Army Medical School."[54] The Professional Schools graduated, in 1937,

55	*Officers and 101 Enlisted Men*	(Medical Corps)
10	*Officers and 25 Enlisted Men*	(Dental Corps)
11	*Officers and 12 Enlisted Men*	(Veterinary Corps)
5	*Nurse Anesthetists (at Walter Reed)*	(Army Nurse Corps)
10	*Dieticians* " " "	(Civilian)
8	*Physiotherapists* " " "	(Civilian)[55]

A great deal of laboratory work, such as Wasserman, Kahn, Colloidal Tests and autogenous vaccines, was done at the laboratories of the Medical Department Professional Services Schools, with the hospital laboratory service performing only routine work. This relationship apparently satisfied all concerned, for it reduced the duplication of effort and economized on personnel, equipment and supplies.[56]

The functional organization of the Medical Department Professional Services Schools provided each director with administrative access to the Commanding General, Army Medical Center, through the Secretary of the School. The Secretary's functions were comparable to the usual functions of the military executive officer. Functionally, school activities channeled from this office through the Assistant Commandant of the Post, a position later called Deputy Post Commander. Each School had its own Assistant Secretary and section chiefs for the various specialized courses. The sponsors of the Aide, Dietetic, Internes and the Anesthesia training courses for nurses reported through the same administrative channels, the Secretary and Assistant Commandant. The Director of Laboratories, more independent than the others, functioned directly under the Assistant Commandant.[57]

The European war clouds were darkening perceptibly by 1938. Although the Medical Department had established the field medical service in 1920, to insure departmental readiness for mobilization, General De Witt's philosophical comment on the functions of medical officers reflected the growing tension of Army planners.

> *Unlike his conferee in the line of the Army, the newly appointed officer of the Medical Department is unfamiliar with the operation of military forces and with military life. He is not ready to apply his professional knowledge to the best advantage of all concerned. He must be taught the organization and employment of armed forces, the most satisfactory procedure for evacuation of battle casualties, and the principles and methods of field sanitation.[58]*

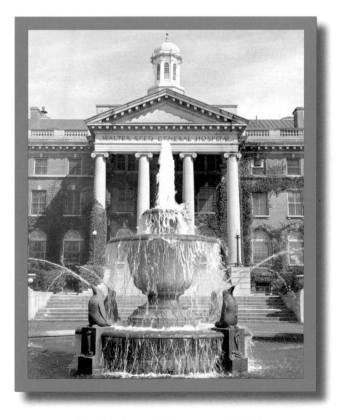

Hoff Memorial Fountain, 1934*
*Reviewers have noted the absence of the flag pole. See text, page 290.

The Hoff Memorial

With the completion of the Army Medical School Building in 1932, the administrative offices of the Commanding General and his executive staff were moved to this location. Thus the Executive Officer, Army Medical Center, and the Adjutant, the Provost Marshall, the Recruiting Officer, the Finance Officer, the Signal Officer etc., and the telephone exchange for the Center, were located in part of the new building. [59] As the American flag invariably marks the headquarters of a military installation, the flag was moved from the circle in front of the main hospital building in 1935. A year later the space was filled by the Hoff Memorial Fountain, in part a gift of the widow of John Van Rensselear Hoff, 1848–1920. [60]

General Arthur, by then an aged man but apparently jealous of his one-time position as Commanding Officer of the hospital, questioned the appropriateness of erecting the four-penguin fountain at Walter Reed. He may have forgotten, or merely preferred to ignore, the intimate association of John Van Rensselear Hoff with many of the Medical Department's milestones of progress. It was he who organized the first detachment of the Hospital Corps, prepared the first drill manual for the Hospital Corps, organized the first Company of Instruction, at Fort Riley, Kansas, and was the first instructor in sanitation in the General Service School at Fort Leavenworth, Kansas. It was Colonel Hoff, in 1901, who first assembled emergency field medical supplies in a basement room of the old Museum, from which Darnall later began the Field Medical Supply Depot, so important in World War I. It was Colonel Hoff who, in 1902, first proposed a school of nursing. He was the instructor in the Army Medical School, after the Spanish-American War, and he was not only a member of the board that selected the site of Walter Reed General Hospital, but he brought the members of the board to the grounds for their last official conference. [61]

Colonel Hoff was an enthusiastic field medical officer rather than internist or surgeon, and to him it was axiomatic that "to sustain medical morale was to sustain military morale." [62] He, more than most, had influenced the militarization of the medical soldier, for which he was cheerfully ridiculed by many of his contemporaries. [63] While still a Captain and Assistant Surgeon he drilled his Company of Instruction diligently, insisted on a military title for himself, and worked zealously to make the untrained recruits into self-respecting soldiers instead of mere attendants of the sick. [64]

Son of a distinguished medical officer, in 1897 he founded, in memory of his father, the Alexander H. Hoff memorial prize, awarded annually to the Army Medical School graduate having the highest class standing. [65] The Spanish-American War prevented bestowal of the medal until the School reopened for the 1901-1902 session. It set a pattern for bestowal of the Sternberg Medal, awarded after the 1920-21 session of the School, to the graduate attaining the highest class standing in Preventive Medicine; [66] the Dental Corps Medal, awarded by the Dental Corps, after 1924, to the Dental Officer having the highest average class standing in the basic course, Army Dental School; [67] and similarly the Hoskins Medal, first awarded in 1924, by the American Veterinary Medical Association, for excellence in the Army Veterinary School. [68]

Colonel Hoff wrote energetically on such subjects as Medical Department history, observations of the Russo-Japanese War and small pox vaccination as a prophylactic. Although Dr. Welch had long resented the emphasis of American doctors on the two-serpent emblem on the Staff Aesculapius rather than the single serpent, a practice he thought "both ludicrous and tragic, for it belongs to Mercury, who was the God and patron of merchants and thieves and was charged with conducting souls to another world," it was Colonel Hoff who influenced the adoption of the caduceus for the Medical Corps, for he viewed it as an emblem of neutrality rather than medicine.[69] He was retired in 1912, but by 1917 he was again on active duty, as editor of *The Military Surgeon*, which then was essentially a medical service bulletin. As the European war clouds moved closer home, in 1917, Colonel Hoff, like many of the older Regular Army officers, may have become uneasy over the state of national preparedness. In July 1918, his apprehensions were expressed in a poorly named editorial, "The Passing of the General Staff," in which he lamented the nomination of medical reservists rather than more experienced policy-minded members of the regular corps, for duty with the War Department General Staff.[70]

Reprisals from the War Department followed; Colonel Hoff was relieved from active duty and resigned his position. A year later the Secretary of War "re-examined the whole question afresh and in the light of the more composed situation" withdrew the reprimand and "restored" Colonel Hoff's military record.[71] As *The Military Surgeon* noted in January 1920, this was an "act of justice to an old and faithful soldier." John Van Rensselear Hoff was one of a now rapidly passing generation of medical officers rather than professionally limited Army doctor. Thus the tribute is not only in "addition to those which already stand in the record of his long and honorable, and useful life,"[72] but is in its way a tribute to a Medical Corps that could inspire such men to a lifetime of faithful and often unrewarded service.

References

1. Annual Rpt TSG... pg 109.

2. *Ibid*, 1934, pg 139.

3. *Ibid*, 1935, pg 186.

4. *Ibid*, 1935, pg 132.

5. *Ibid*, 1937, pg 151.

6. A charge of $4.00 daily was made at Fitzsimons, for tuberculous patients.

7. Annual Rpt TSG... 1938, pg 159.

8. *Ibid*, pg 160.

9. Interview with Major General Shelly U. Marietta, M.C., Ret., April 25, 1950.

10. Station Hospital in name only as it served as a general hospital; later renamed Brooke General Hospital.

11. Interview with Col. Herbert N. Dean, M.C., Ret., April 12, 1950; Interview with Miss Dora E. Thompson, June 26, 1950 and others.

12. *Ibid.*

13. Annual Rpt WRGH, 1935.

14. Annual Rpt TSG... 1935, pg 136.

15. Annual Rpt, WRGH, 1937.

16. *Ibid*, 1935.

17. Interviews: Jessie M. Braden, Sallie Shoenberger, Dora E. Thompson, retired members of the Army Nurse Corps, June 25, 26, 1950.

18. Conversation 2nd Lt. Katherine V. Young, Chg. Nurse, Wd 11A, 1938.

19. M/Sgt. Franklin F. Houston, April 1950.

20. Conversation, Miss Margaret Sims, July 11, 1947.

21. Annual Rpt, WRGH, 1935; approximately 15 days hospitalization was expected of obstetrical cases at that time.

22. *Ibid*, 1936.

23. *Ibid*, 1935.

24. *Ibid.*

25. Conversation, Col. Arden Freer, M.C., Ret., Feb. 7, 1951.

26. The writer shared Colonel Keller's desk for nearly two years.

27. Annual Rpt WRGH, 1935.

28. Thompson interview, *op cit.*

29. Col. James M. Phalen, M.C., Ret., April 19, 1950.

30. *Ibid.*

31. Interview with Col. James F. Hall, M.C., Ret., April 17, 1950, Aug. 8, 1951.

32. Marietta interview, *op cit.*

33. AG 029.21 (4-25-39) April 25, 1939, misc.

34. Annual Rpt., WRGH, 1939.

35. *Ibid*, 1939.

36. Braden interview, *op cit*; Thompson interview, *op cit*; Interview with Miss Jane Molloy, RN, June 30, 1950.

37. IG Report attached to Annual Rpt, WRGH, 1937.

38. Annual Rpt WRGH, 1936.

39. *Ibid*.

40. *Ibid*.

41. *Ibid*, 1937.

42. The Sanitary Corps Reserve was established under the provisions of Section 37, Act of 4 June 1920 (41 Stat. 775). The Medical Administrative Corps was made a part of the Medical Department in order to provide auxiliary service to the doctors and obviate their assignment to many administrative duties. Corps strength was first limited to 140 officers, to be obtained by giving permanent commissions to enlisted men commissioned in the Sanitary Corps during the war. The vacancies were filled through promotion by examination of non-commissioned officers.

43. M/Sgt; Tech. Sgt; Staff Sgt; Sgt.

44. Annual Rpt WRGH, 1937.

45. Annual Rpt, MD PSS, 1939, on file, Office of the Commandant, AMS.

46. Lack of barracks space limited the number to 100; slightly more than half this number was trained during the last few years before the war.

47. Annual Rpt, MD PSS, *op cit*.

48. Conversation, Miss Mary E. Schick, Librarian, WRGH, 1941.

49. Annual Rpt, WRGH, 1936.

50. Medical officers were considered as "mounted officers" and drew a forage ration if owning a private mount.

51. Resumed in 1939.

52. Annual Rpt TSG... 1937, pg 229.

53. Annual Rpt WRGH, 1937.

54. See AMS program file, Office of Commandant, AMS, AMC.

55. Annual Rpt WRGH, 1937.

56. *Ibid*, 1938.

57. Annual Rpt...TSG, 1937, pg 228.

58. *Ibid*, 1938, pg 241.

59. *Ibid*, 1937, pg 227.

60. Died at Walter Reed April 19, 1936.

61. Address by General Ireland in Presenting Portrait of Colonel John Van Renssalear Hoff to AMS, May 30, 1930. Copy from General Truby's files.

62. Ltr. Garrison to Welch, April 29, 1927, Collection of the Institute of the History of Medicine, Welch Memorial Library, John Hopkins University, Baltimore, Md.

63. Edgar Erskine Hume, *History of the Ass. Mil. Surgeons of the U.S. 1891-1941*, Boston and NY, Houghton & Mifflin, 1929, pg 13.

64. *Ibid*, Interview with Brig. Gen. Frank Keefer, M.C., Ret., Apr. 20, 1950.

65. Records of the AMS, Vol. III, Session 24-26, August 1, 1919-February 13, 1932, pg 269.

66. *Ibid*.

67. *Ibid*.

68. *Ibid*.

69. Welch to F. F. Russell, Aug. 15, 1920; Russell to Welch, Sept. 22, 1920. Collection, *op cit*.

70. Hume, *op cit*, pg 70-74.

71. Memorandum from Baker, S/W to C/S, Dec. 20, 1919 quoted from Hume, *op cit,* pg 75.

72. Hume, *op cit*, pg 75.

With the Suddenness of War

1940–1943

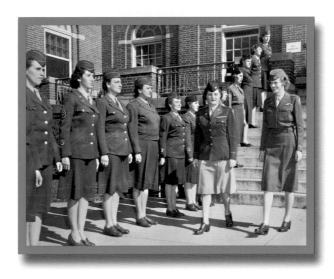

"But only through the agency of competent medical administrators will these medical practitioners be able to work to proper advantage in the new conditions created by war."[1]

The President declared a state of limited national emergency on September 8, 1939, less than four months before General Metcalfe succeeded General De Witt as Post Commander.[2] The international situation steadily became more alarming, and on September 19, 1940, the American Army began calling reserve officers and nurses to active duty and increasing the troop strength. On October 1, the Out-Patient Service[3] at Walter Reed opened a *Physical Examining Section* to examine retired, reserve and National Guard officers prior to assignment or reassignment to active duty.

It was not only impractical but impossible that some old customs and strict procedures be maintained. As a result of the Act of November 29, 1940 (P.L. 884, 76th Congress), the Secretary of War was authorized to dispense with any part of the examination for promotion of Regular Army Medical, Dental and Veterinary officers *except* the physical examination.

Thereafter, with rapidity which was often confusing to interested bystanders, junior officers became field officers and hospital commanders, although the majority were without the prior leavening of experience which had formerly marked the transition in the Regular Army Medical Corps from ward doctor, section chief, chief of a service and, in time and if the position was desired, hospital commander. Their staffs were, by and large, Reserve Officers on extended active duty or Army of United States personnel, men who may have practiced their profession in civilian institutions but who had rarely been attached permanently to an organization complete with regulations and insigne and where military rank rather than ingenuity governed their income. There would be adjustment problems for some, with the personal struggle of the individual reluctant to meet the organizational code reminiscent of the axiomatic proverb concerning immovable objects and irresistible forces. As a consequence, perhaps, a whole new era of military medicine was in the making.

Any appreciable increase in manpower affected the hospital system, which at best provided only a fifteen per cent emergency expansion in fixed beds. As the number of dependents likewise increased, at a time when the professional personnel situation was critical, the Secretary of War found it necessary to limit the medical care of dependents during the national emergency.[4] By May 27, 1941, the President had declared a state of unlimited national emergency, and personnel and training became ever-present problems to all types of Regular Army commanders, most of whom appeared to realize that war was almost inevitable. At the Army Medical Center, during 1940, the number of fixed

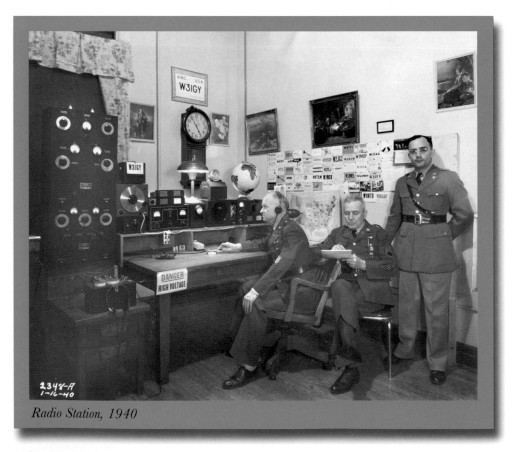

Radio Station, 1940

beds increased from 1,250 to 1,440. The area behind the old gymnasium, still used as a plant propagation field for the greenhouse, was selected as the site for new barracks and bachelor officers' quarters for additional reserve officers and Medical Department Professional Service School students.[5]

Within the hospital organization, the latent and usually unacknowledged morale problem of military service versus civilian personnel emerged clearly at the ward level. The difference in cash or take-home pay and hours of work for military and civilian personnel caused more than the usual dissatisfaction in the former group. Whereas an enlisted ward attendant received a cash salary of $360 annually for twelve-hour duty, and all of the amenities such as food and clothing, shelter, medical care, including indefinite absence from duty, the civilian employee received $780 annually, none of the amenities and a restricted fifteen-day sick leave. Some of the basic dissatisfactions would in time be reconciled somewhat through Congressionally authorized increases in military pay, but the psychology of group identification, i.e., the man in uniform versus the civilian, was deeper than the dollar value placed on service.

Judging from the early recommendations for meeting personnel shortages, General Metcalfe was in complete sympathy with the expressed sentiments of national policy groups, including medical, that all able-bodied men must train for combat. In fact, he went one step farther and openly advocated replacing all enlisted personnel with civilian employees. A year later, however, under the pressure of the expansion, he realized that a fluid civilian staff presented even more complications than a fluid military staff. Wages, hours, availability and preference for hospital employment affected the civilian group significantly. As both industry and the Army were competing for skilled as well as adaptable trainee personnel, hospitals, civilian and military, were compelled to be less selective in their employment practice than was desirable in the interest of economic management.

By 1941, a soldier-assistant appeared even more preferable than usual to the hospital commander, who noted in the Annual Report that "the enlisted men in surgical clinics and wards, to a great extent, have been replaced by civilian personnel, which on the whole has been a poor substitute, and valuable training for enlisted technicians has been lost."[6] Training, the ever-present responsibility of the military hospital commander, was not incidental to the care of the sick but inseparable from that care.

Preparing for Mobilization

Recruits newly arrived at the Army Medical Center were assigned to the *Recruit Training Section* of the Headquarters and Service Detachment for three to four weeks of basic training. Following such training the more adaptable men were detailed to the Medical Department Professional Service Schools and to form a pool of qualified technicians, cooks, etc., for other Post activities and for stations in the field. Whereas the hospital and the School had long provided an indirect but steady flow of training technicians for other Army medical installations, the training program now had a three-fold objective: (1) maintaining the usual hospital activities; (2) maintaining the usual School activities; (3) providing men trained in administration and general service (Headquarters and Service Section) for ultimate reassignment to holding or inactive units in the Troop Basis.[7] The third requirement created an especially difficult problem, for the current lack of Post housing and food service facilities did not then permit the training of a large number of men, while the overall demand for such personnel was mounting.[8]

All of the non-commissioned officers in the Walter Reed Detachment, men assigned to the hospital, were qualified to operate iron lungs and oxygen tents, and all wardmasters were trained in the latter technique. By and large, however, the general spread of Medical Department activities was so broad that it was necessary to have the men specialize in some aspect of the professional program. By November 11, 1940, a special training course was initiated which would prepare corpsmen for duty as assistants to surgeons in small hospitals. On December 1, fifteen corpsmen began a course in instruction in the duties of wardmaster and ward attendant.[9]

The Medical Service then controlled 807 beds and five cribs and conducted the usual specialty clinics. The number of consultations was increasing rapidly, for the military population of the District of Columbia had increased 400 per cent in 1940 and 1941. This placed an extremely heavy burden on the staff of the Out-Patient Service, which in 1941 attended 3,449 military personnel and 38,099 dependents.[10]

With one exception, the chiefs of the medical sections were still Regular Army

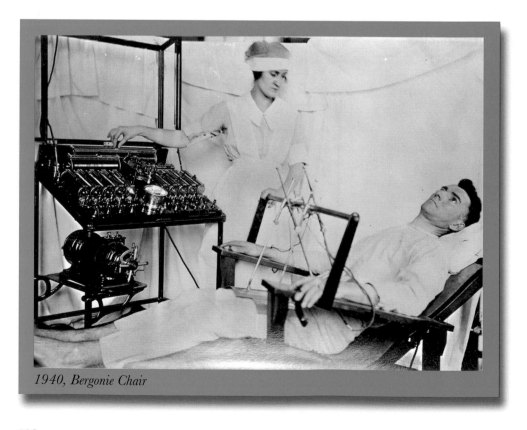

1940, Bergonie Chair

doctors, but Reserve officers were beginning to replace the ward doctors. Although they were well trained and conscientious "as would be expected, a certain amount of time (was) necessary for training them in the peculiarities of military medicine and government hospital administration."[11] By 1941, an attempt was made to correct such drawbacks by accepting fifty officers for one to three months of professional and administrative training at Walter Reed, prior to reassignment as directed by the Surgeon General's Office.

The Neuropsychiatric Section, perhaps even more than some other medical sections, was pressed for space and expanded to eight wards and 311 beds. Further, through a temporary arrangement with St. Elizabeth's Hospital, military patients could be transferred to that institution but remain under the administrative authority of Walter Reed. In order to expedite the professional care, two doctors, ten civilian nurses and three stenographers were assigned to St. Elizabeth's for temporary duty. The ten patients present on January 21, 1941, increased to 144 by July 31, but thereafter the number declined steadily until the program was terminated on December 31, 1941.[12] There were more than 400 fewer inpatients at Walter Reed in 1941 than in 1940; still, the administrative operations increased. The United States Government had already sent military observers' groups to many strategic areas, but the later large overseas hospitalization program had not developed, and so 413 patients were transferred from Panama, Puerto Rico, Bermuda, Trinidad, Greenland, Iceland and Newfoundland to Walter Reed during this year. The work of the *Disposition and of the Line of Duty Board* in this and other Army hospitals increased so rapidly that, as a further effort to economize on time and personnel, War Department Circular No. 217, October 15, 1941, permitted the former board to perform both functions.

Some other organizational changes were incidental to the mobilization program. For instance, in the spring of 1941, a sub-section of maxillo-facial surgery was established at the hospital, under the direction of the chief of the EENT Section. In August a joint course of instruction was inaugurated for medical and dental officers, with Colonel Roy Stout, Dental Corps, representing the latter service. A one-to-three month course in Orthopedic and Traumatic Surgery was given forty Reserve Officers with prior experience in this field, the course including ward administration and military routine. Further, five enlisted men were given a four-to-six month course in shop training, thereby becoming qualified brace-makers and fitters of prosthetic appliances. Although blood substitutes were still not in general use, both the liquid and dried type were provided by the Army Medical School, for use in the operating room at the hospital. Such substitutes, the professional staff decreed, not only had no ill effects on the patient, but they were more readily available for transfusions than the former system of individual typing or cross-matching with donor. As a further concession to time saving factors, the hospital staff began using commercially prepared intravenous fluids, purchased through medical supply channels rather than made entirely at the laboratories of the School, with their depleted personnel.

Of the 22,355 patients examined in the various surgical clinics of the Walter Reed General Hospital during the year, 1,175 were gynecological. The increasing size of the Army was not confined to uniformed manpower, for 3,015 female patients attended the pre-natal clinic in contrast to the 1,182 of 1940, and 302 infants were delivered, in contrast to the 175 of the year before. It was necessary, therefore, not only to establish an appointment system for the pre-natal clinic, but as a matter of War Department policy, Army hospitals were allowed to admit female dependents on the Surgical Service for emergency work only.[13]

The demands for additional personnel and services were not confined to doctors, nurses and corpsmen, but included dieticians and physiotherapy and occupational sides. In an effort to cooperate with the Army training program, the *American Medical Association Council on Medical Education and Hospitals* reduced the usual one-year physiotherapy aide-training to six months, provided the half-year in theory and practice was supplemented by a six-month supervised practice period in an Army hospital.[14]

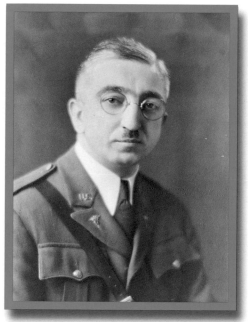

Civil defense preparations brought a large-scale redraping of many of the hospital windows with blackout curtains, including six rooms in the Obstetrical Section. An air conditioner was provided for the delivery room. Further, as there was always a possibility that the power system would fail during a bombardment, a new Army field X-ray machine, with film processing and drying units, was acquired for accessory and reserve (emergency hospital) functions. Corpsmen and civilian personnel were instructed in air raid precautions and fire fighting, and all wards and services were issued flashlights and other paraphernalia needed during such an occurrence.

Colonel Roy Stout, Dental Corps, Oral and Maxillo-facial Surgeon

Increasing the Tempo

Brigadier General Shelley U. Marietta succeeded Brigadier General Raymond F. Metcalfe on February 1, 1941, and the Army Medical Center had for the third time in its history a former staff member and chief of a professional service as Post Commander.[15] As noted elsewhere, General Marietta's professional reputation required no enhancing.

Following the declaration of war with Japan, December 8, 1941, the tempo of hospital activities increased rapidly. Single rooms became two-bed rooms. Double rooms became three-bed rooms, and cubicles and wards were crowded to capacity as stand-by beds were set up. The 8,025 admissions for 1941 increased to 10, 818 during 1942, and providing satisfactory hospital service for such a number presented many difficulties. The patients were restless, apprehensive over the mobilization objective, duration of emergency service and their families, in many instances still residing in the home communities. Hospital activities were influenced by an atmosphere of tension which had not characterized the World War I expansion period. In the former emergency, of short duration, evacuation of the wounded was not only a longer process, but the war was practically over before the peak load of evacuees began arriving in the United States, and few if any were returned to active combat. By the spring of 1942, however, when the convoys began arriving from North Africa, a global war had become almost a front-yard affair. Later, some patients followed the order of battle so closely that on occasion, as they underwent anesthesia, their last comprehensible mumblings were pleas for information on siege of Bizerte.[16]

Regular Army service or maintenance personnel was not only in short supply, but the demands of the civilian labor market, supported by increasingly tempting salaries, created such a grave civilian personnel situation that by September 1942, General Marietta was compelled to replace some civilian ward mess attendants with enlisted personnel in order to maintain the necessary services to the sick. There were no major changes in the hospital organization during the year. On the other hand, the changing type of cases admitted, such as an increasing number of burns, maxillo-facial injuries, orthopedic, paraplegic, infectious hepatitis and neuropsychiatric cases, required more medical and nursing care than usual. The principal interruption of professional activities arose from the requirements for training a large proportion of reserve officers, the majority of whom apparently had no prior service,

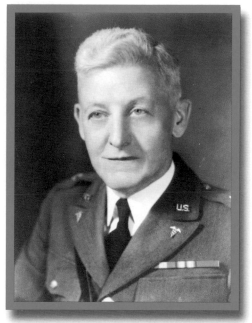

*Major General Shelley U. Marietta,
February 1, 1941–February 9, 1946*

while maintaining the usual high quality of medical care afforded the sick. Such an arrangement, while necessary to the war effort, placed a heavy burden on the staff and probably prolonged the hospitalization of some patients. Many patients objected to the rapid change in staff members as this interrupted the doctor-patient relationship so important in maintaining confidence and a sense of professional security, the lack of which retard physical and mental recovery in some types of cases. The Medical Service, with an authorized allowance of forty-three duty officers, had only thirty-three regularly assigned, who must also supervise 152 trainees and six internes on rotating assignments.

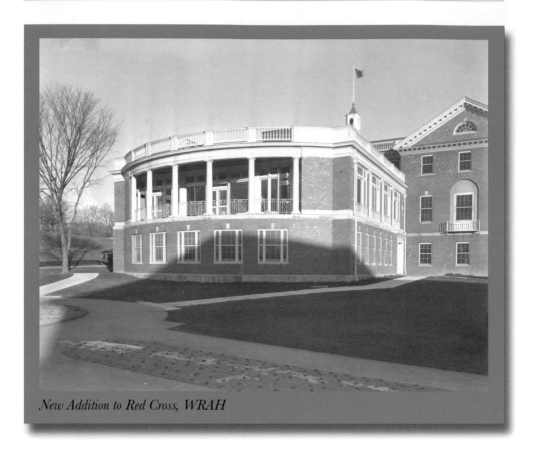

New Addition to Red Cross, WRAH

The enrollment of physiotherapy students not only increased, but four doctors from the Medical Department Replacement Pool[17] were given brief courses in this department during 1942. A Dieticians' Pool was organized in June 1942, to train in Army methods and procedures, and with a view to future foreign service assignments, dieticians admitted from civilian hospitals. The regular student training course was, like the course for aides, shortened from one year to six months. Regularly scheduled courses were conducted for mess officers, sanitary officers, enlisted cooks and mess stewards. Large numbers of officers from the Adjutant General's Departmental (nutrition) School made "field trips" to the hospital kitchens, messes and ward kitchens during the year. Further, the director of the Dietetic Department lectured monthly to the Medical Department Replacement Pool officers then being trained for unit assignment, and to newly assigned duty officers at the hospital.[18]

As a result of some defective commercially prepared yellow fever vaccine, the Army experienced an outbreak of toxic hepatitis in late 1942, with 116 cases admitted to Walter Reed from the United States and overseas stations. This unfortunate circumstance encouraged intensive study of this condition both at the Army Medical School and in other military medical installations. As was to be expected during a period when personnel faced

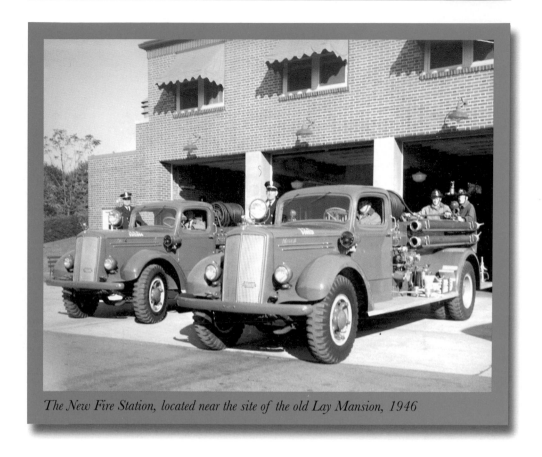

The New Fire Station, located near the site of the old Lay Mansion, 1946

increased exposure to the elements, there was an unusually large number of admissions for atypical pneumonia. Further, the doctors at Walter Reed noted that "a new drug, Penicillin, was tried for the subacute bacterial endocarditis."

The Surgical Service met many of the expansion problems which characterized the World War I period. Orthopedic surgery increased, and all of the attendant functions, such as plaster, X-ray and dressing rooms were concentrated on Ward 11, in the Main Building. Moreover, the brace shop began training additional brace-makers for overseas stations. An Orthopedic Branch of the occupational therapy program began functioning in February 1942 with diversional work carried on with bed patients. In December the entire Occupational Therapy Department was placed under the supervision of the Orthopedic Section. The Surgical Service likewise experimented with Penicillin, finding it especially helpful in treating osteomyelitis.

From May 16, 1942, until the end of December, 105 major neurosurgical operations were performed at Walter Reed, the work becoming so heavy that a separate section was established on December 26, under the direction of highly a trained civilian doctor, commissioned to and assigned to duty. The majority of the patients were directly or indirectly under treatment because of trauma, although the usual percentages of neo-

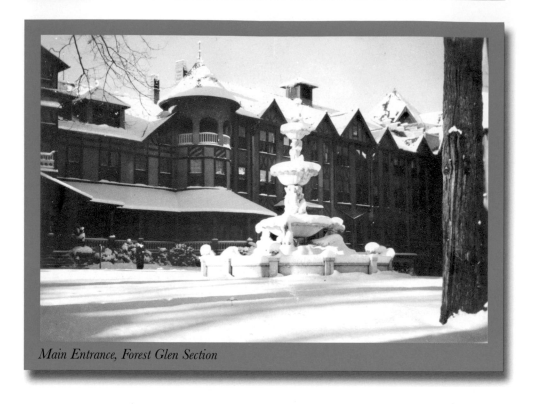

Main Entrance, Forest Glen Section

plasms, intractable painful maladies and congenital anomalies appeared. Of especial interest to the military service, thirty-nine patients were treated for intervertebral discs. As the war progressed and complaints of low back pain increased, distinction between discs, traumatic injuries of temporary nature and the fancied injuries of the neuropsychiatric casualty was a time-consuming process for doctors in the classified stations as well as those in the hospitals.[19]

The EENT and Maxillo-Facial subsection trained forty-one Medical Department Replacement Pool officers, in connection with a four-week course at the Army Medical School. In addition to the regular staff, a special detail of instructors was assigned which included Doctor John B. Davis of Baltimore and Doctors Robert H. Ivy and A.B. Batson of Philadelphia. Lectures, demonstrations, applications and visual aids were used in instructing the eighty-eight Dental and forty-seven Medical Officers so trained.

Pressed by bed shortages and too many patients, the Obstetrical Section, which had appeared busy when receiving thirty patients a month, was able to accommodate ninety by reducing the number of hospital days per patient. Thus, as a result of emergency economies, American women again adopted some post-partum habits of remote ancestors. The practice of early ambulation of the patient and early discharge from the hospital became so commonplace that by 1949 it was accepted therapy. In this, as in other sections of the hospital, able civilian doctors were in charge.

The Anesthesia Section (General Surgery) was especially busy, for in addition to the increased case load for surgery, the newly activated units required both doctor and nurse anesthetists. Some fifty-four one-hour lectures were given during the year. On October 1, 1942, six officers arrived for a three-month course in Anesthesia.[20] Replacement Pool officers assigned to temporary duty in this section were required to follow the established training program provided by the Surgeon General's Office. Twenty-one officers were so trained, all of whom received anesthesia assignments on departure from Washington.[21]

As the number of ward patients increased, the entire Red Cross welfare program expanded, and the Gray Ladies came into their own again. The Radiologic Section accepted Gray Ladies as chaperones for female patients, thus economizing on the services of nurses, for, like other sections of the hospital, the radiology work increased phenomenally. From 23,001 X-ray examinations in 1941, the number increased to 32,826 in 1942, with 720 consultations by mail. Further, an increasing number of diagnostic time-consuming procedures such as myelography, encephalography, venography and arteriography were performed in this department, directed by Colonel Aubrey Otis Hampton, a reserve officer on active duty, formerly Chief of Roentgenology, Massachusetts General Hospital, Boston.

In view of the steadily increasing number of carcinomas diagnosed at the Walter Reed General Hospital in the last ten-year period, formation of the *Tumor Board*, in 1942, is of special interest. This was encouraged by Major Milton Freidman, likewise a reserve officer on active duty. The board, composed of the chiefs of Medicine, Surgery, Radium Therapy, the pathologist and the senior roentgenologist, met weekly for discussion of all tumor cases with the ward doctors prior to adoption of specific therapy.

Expanding the Army Medical Center

Neither time nor costs permitted construction of a significant number of permanent-type general hospitals during this period, and some military authorities believed it more practicable to convert existing structures to emergency use. The building program was not without complications and misunderstandings,[22] for in March 1942 the War Department formed a new overhead agency called the Services of Supply, a year later renamed Army Service Forces, for coordinating and streamlining emergency activities. The Army Ground Forces, Army Air Forces and the Army Services of Supply were established, and the geographically divided administrative areas of the Army, once known as *Departments*, then as *Corps Areas*, in 1943 became *Service Commands*. Further, and unfortunately from the Surgeon General's viewpoint, the general and station hospitals were transferred from the direct control of his office to the Service Commands, each of which, however, had a senior ranking medical officer in charge of Medical Department activities. Thereafter, in the case of the Army Medical Center, an "exempted" station, some administrative affairs were under the jurisdiction of the Third Service Command, Baltimore, Maryland, and some were under the Military District of Washington.

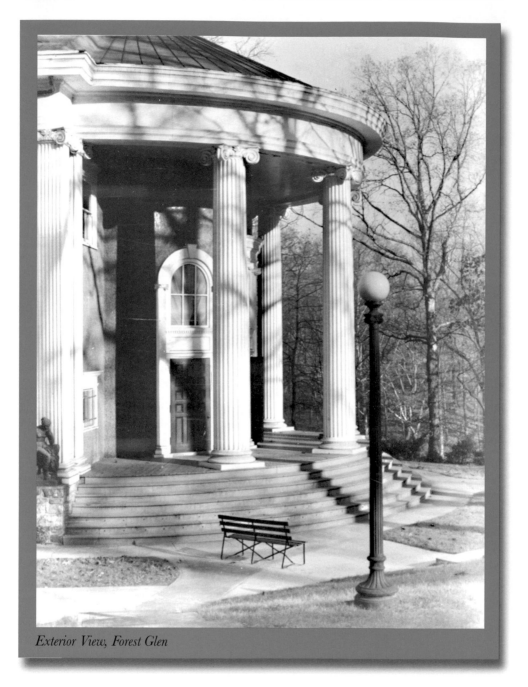

Exterior View, Forest Glen

During the summer of 1942, the Surgeon General's Office was directed by the *Services of Supply* organization to plan for emergency expansion by surveying hotels, hospitals and other buildings suitable for conversion to immediate use in the event of enemy action. In the meantime, a construction program was under way which would enable the Medical Department to provide increased hospitalization for troops in the Zone of Interior, the continental United States, and for long-term cases evacuated from overseas stations.

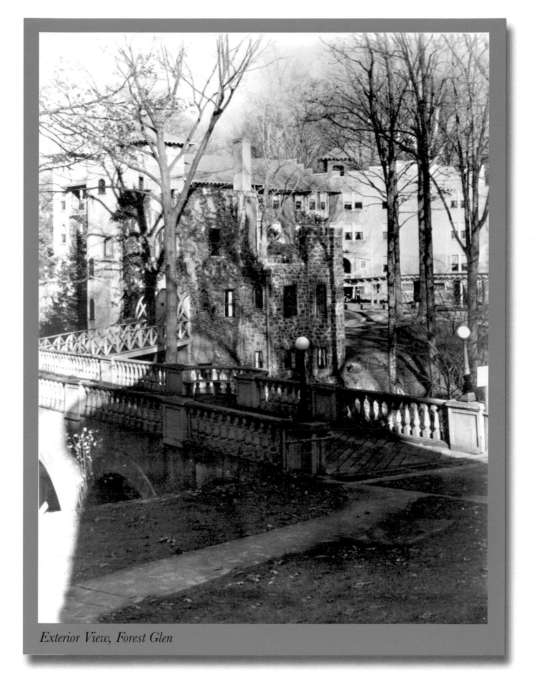

Exterior View, Forest Glen

In Washington and at Walter Reed, hospital authorities surveyed the adjacent neighborhoods of Takoma Park and Shepherd Park, apparently with some idea of adapting one of the larger apartment houses in the vicinity to convalescent use or as officers' quarters. In this as in other communities where civilian housing was to be affected, the proposal was unpopular. The Army Medical Center expansion problem was met through purchase, on September 1, 1942, of the National Park Seminary, a girls' school at Forest

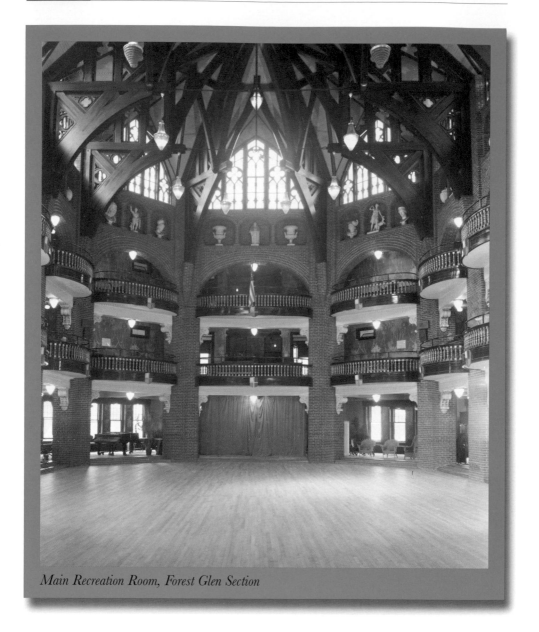

Main Recreation Room, Forest Glen Section

Glen, Maryland. The buildings were heterogeneous, old and in poor repair, but the 185-acre tract was only four miles from the Center, and valuable. On one side it adjoined property of the Baltimore and Ohio Railroad, which afforded a way station, and excellent paved roads connected the tract with Washington and Silver Spring, Maryland.

The restoration and adaptation of the school structure was both more extensive and more costly than at first contemplated. By December 31, 1942, when the first patients arrived, 1500 people could be fed there, regardless of the fact that the principal features of the plant were incomplete. Called *The New Section, Convalescent Section* and finally the *Forest Glen Section,* the addition was used for the extended care of convalescents. Occupational Therapy and

Physiotherapy rooms were provided, and the Post Exchange and Library maintained branch services. In fact, except for the professional care of bed cases, administration at the Forest Glen Section emulated the usual Post functions so familiar at the Army Medical Center.

A Distaff Branch

The National Capital Parks donated two greenhouses to the Army Medical Center in 1943. One was located, rather conspicuously, on the Georgia Avenue side of the reservation rather than behind the formal garden area with other greenhouses. The structure was dismantled by the Post Engineer, who salvaged eighty per cent of the wood and forty-five per cent of the glass. Half of the building was redesigned as a moving picture theater, and all of the equipment, including the picture screen, was furnished by the Army Motion Picture Service. General Marietta had long considered more extensive recreation facilities a necessity for enlisted men of the Post, but because of nearby community facilities, the movie project was not authorized by the Military District of Washington. Movies were shown only on the wards and in the Red Cross house, for patients; therefore, the makeshift "greenhouse theater" was a welcome addition to the recreational facilities of the command. The remaining half of the building was converted into a recreation room for the enlisted men. One company of service troops was assigned to the Center during the year, quartered at Forest Glen, and provided with appropriate recreation facilities in that area.[23] The remaining greenhouse was erected adjacent to other greenhouses under the jurisdiction of the head gardener.

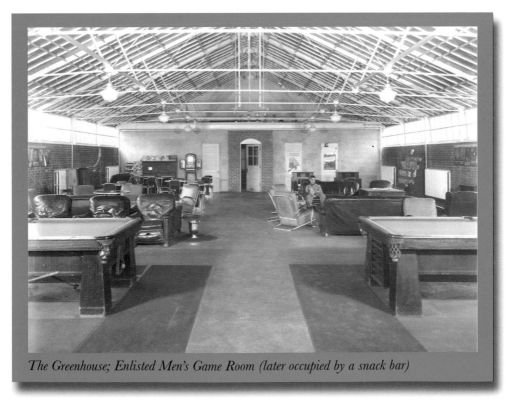

The Greenhouse; Enlisted Men's Game Room (later occupied by a snack bar)

Lumber from a dismantled chicken house was used to convert an old granary into a rabbetry, for the hard-pressed Army Medical School. About 200 shrubs were replaced, and at Forest Glen, some 1,000 pieces of mixed trees, shrubs and evergreens were added. The plant heating facilities of the Center were expanded; a second story was added to the Guard House, and in the Main Building the air conditioning apparatus, installed in 1934, was removed to the attic in order to provide additional space for hospital activities. A radiation therapy extension was completed in October 1943, and a 100,000-volt, a 200,000-volt and a 1,000,000-volt therapy room were installed. In July 1943, facilities were prepared for housing a forty-piece band at Forest Glen.[24] New tennis courts were constructed as the personnel increased, and schedules at the Rea swimming pool were modified to accommodate the increased members. Road maintenance and upkeep was constant throughout the Post, and the usual repair, utilities and enlargements were made as required in a rapidly expanding organization.

Lt. Colonel Gertrude L. Thompson, Principal Chief Nurse at Walter Reed following Miss Keener's retirement in the summer of 1943, faced a hard four-year period during which demands for nursing service increased rapidly. Supervision of the auxiliary training program for WAC's, nurses and corpsmen was a function of her office, as well as increased responsibilities which came at a time when she had fewer Regular Army nurses as assistants. Petite, agreeable and scholarly, Colonel Thompson had a quietly expressed preference for being addressed as "Miss," and she seldom invoked the "official" title of her office.

The Women's Army Auxiliary Corps was authorized on May 14, 1942 (Public Law 554, 77th Congress) without full military status or the corresponding military grades afforded the Regular Army, inequalities which were corrected in the reorganization of the Women's Army Corps a year later. The pre-authorization public relations material featured the Auxiliaries as numerical replacements for able-bodied enlisted men required by the combat forces, and this idea became firmly fixed in the minds of some military authorities, including key personnel in the Surgeon General's Office.

Organization of such a Corps had strong Congressional support from Congressman Edith Nourse Rogers, of Massachusetts, a Gray Lady at Walter Reed during World War I, and from influential military leaders such as the Chief of Staff, General George Catlett Marshall.

At the time of organization, the Surgeon General and the Superintendent of the Army Nurse Corps objected to using WAC's as hospital attendants. The Surgeon General believed such a policy would result in dismissal of faithful civilian employees, as well as creating a housing problem. The Superintendent of the Army Nurse Corps disapproved on the general principle that non-professional personnel, including nurses' aides, should not care for patients.[25] As personnel shortages became acute, circumstances forced a reevaluation of Medical Department policy. Because of an already critical housing situation for the Troop Command, as well as the inherent problems of administering two classes of enlisted personnel, both General Marietta and his executive officer, Colonel Thomas Hester, MAC, resisted the assignment of WACs as long as possible.[26] However, as Walter Reed was in the spotlight of national affairs, in proximity to WAC (policy) headquarters, it afforded an excellent background for public relations and recruiting media featuring the WAC. It was, therefore, a foregone conclusion that Walter Reed, as the Army's best-known general hospital, would have a detachment of women.[27]

> *On June 1, 1943, a group of enlisted members of the WAC were assigned to duty in ward kitchens, replacing a like number of soldiers, and, with additional WACs arriving periodically, their total strength in the Dietetic Department (was) forty-six, thus relieving an equivalent number of men. Two WACs (were) Staff Sergeants serving as assistant stewards and two (were) corporals.[28]*

An old landmark lost part of its identity in December 1943 when Building No.7, the enlisted men's barracks, underwent modest transformation into barracks for female enlisted personnel. A beauty shop, laundry tubs and ironing boards were installed in the basement, with clothes lines in the basement and on the second floor porches. The former recreation and lounge rooms were expanded and equipped for women.

The early public relations media claiming that women could serve as numerical replacements for men created problems for the Director of the WAC as well as for some hospital commanders. The former, responsible for the morale and efficiency of the women only, and the latter, responsible for the morale and efficiency of an entire organization, thereafter including women, plus his primary mission – care of the sick – sometimes found their mutual problem difficult to solve. As a result, the Medical Department, including the Commanding General of the Army Medical Center, was criticized for showing a lack of understanding of the problems of women, poor utilization and the misuse of enlisted women beyond the limits of their physical endurance. In fact, in the opinion of some WAC officers,[29] the Medical Department was an organizational "Simon Legree" of the worst order.

For a time some Army nurses allegedly resented the assignment of WACs to ward duty, viewing them only as female orderlies or manpower replacements as promised by recruiting propaganda and not as equally fragile members of the reputedly weaker sex. Some enlisted men resented the arrival of the enlisted women; and many believed the women were favored in the matter of ratings. The situation was in some respects like the earlier objection of the hospital stewards and corpsmen to the Army's use of graduate nurses. Although the WACs had basic training, drill, were instructed in social hygiene, gas-mask drill and, after conversion to the WAC in August 1943, attended many of the same orientation lectures, they were for at least two years something of a public curiosity. Unavoidably, since progress is ever painful, some civilian and military staff members accepted them as such. Some of the early job-placement difficulties developed from the too literal interpretation of "the law," for insofar as heavy work was concerned, the women were not one-for-one replacements for men. By the end of 1943, it was obvious to administrative officers and Walter Reed that

> *In the progressive replacement of male by female technicians, a minimum of men is necessary for certain work, such as heavy lifting, unpleasant clean-up duties, morgue or veneral work.[30]*

The Laboratory Service, whose procedures increased in proportion to the 18,046 inpatient admissions for the year and which had voiced longstanding complaints over both the quality and inconstancy of technical personnel, apparently welcomed the WACs more enthusiastically than some of the other hospital sections. The first WACs were assigned to the Laboratory in July, and by the end of December, twelve were on duty in this section, the Laboratory officer noting that his problem was minimal, for

> *As a whole they were professional medical technicians before entry into military service and hence, they were rapidly assimilated.*

As was to be expected, the fact that both male and female personnel believed themselves appreciated and necessary to the war effort contributed to harmonious working conditions. In fact, the Laboratory officer wanted at least twenty-five to thirty-three per cent of the staff to be in this category. With the change from WAAC to WAC, only twenty per cent of the auxiliaries at the Army Medical Center requested release in comparison to twenty-five per cent at other stations.

During the first year of their assignment the days lost by women on furlough never exceeded ten per cent; no days were lost for *Absence Without Leave*, arrest or confine-

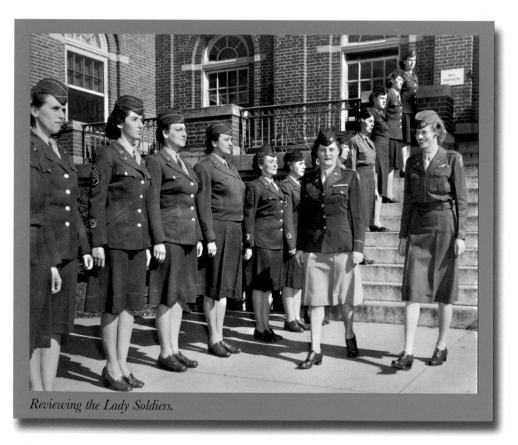

Reviewing the Lady Soldiers.

ment in the guardhouse. The average duty strength from July to December, 1943, was 141.15; the women had so proved their abilities that General Marietta noted cautiously in the Annual Report that "the arrival of WAC personnel entailed considerable office work at the outset; however, their efficiency as soldiers had greatly overshadowed the problems first encountered."

Associate Activities

The 28th Portable Surgical Hospital was activated at Fort George C. Meade, Maryland, on June 14, 1943, and transferred to the Army Medical Center on September 6. The Commanding Officer and a cadre of six enlisted men were present for duty, and two surgeons and one internist joined later.

The transient unit personnel had almost doubled by September, and activities transferred to the Military District of Washington required the maintenance of new files and the initiation of new procedures. Essentially a responsibility and a function of the Medical Service of the Army Ground Forces, the portable surgical unit was developed to create a self-sustaining portable hospital capable of portage over terrain inaccessible to motor transportation. The training emphasis was placed on emergency nursing and surgical procedures and individual protective measures against the enemy. Although the unit had not actual maneuver experience, its activities formed the basis for preparing experimental work reports to the Surgeon General's Office. The unit headquarters, for organization and personnel, was established at the Army Medical Center, but the unit supply depot was at the Forest Glen Section. The men lived a life of simulated field activity, housed in pyramidal tents erected on the old playing field, on the north side of the reservation.

In preparing the final report of this experiment for the Surgeon General's Office, military medical authorities agreed that both officers and men should be general service personnel (rather than specialists), the former as graduates of the Medical Field Service Training Course at Carlisle Barracks, and that the unit should have maneuver experience, with all of the supplies and equipment functionally marked at supply depots prior to issue.[31]

The presence of this unit did not directly affect the hospital staff or the inpatient care, but its location and association with the organizational set-up of the Army Medical Center was reminiscent of the early post-Spanish-American War plans. At that time the Companies of Instruction formed the basis of determining the training and equipment required by the medical components of a field medical Army; and because of this a Field Hospital was assigned in conjunction with the Walter Reed General Hospital when it was opened for service in 1909.

References

1. Editorial: *Military Surgeon*, Vol. XLI, 1917, pg 721.

2. From December 26, 1939 to January 31, 1941.

3. Called Service rather than Clinic in order to agree with later designations.

4. AG 702 (11-28-40) M-A-M (Ltr of Dec. 18, 1940).

5. Annual Report, WRGH, 1940.

6. *Ibid*, 1941.

7. The overall planning program for present and future military activities. The Troop Basis is ordinarily forecast a year or more in advance, but in periods of military activity it is under constant study and revision.

8. Annual Rpt. WRGH, 1940.

9. *Ibid*, In evaluating Medical Department training activities at the Army Medical Center, it should be recalled that the medical doctrine is prescribed by the Surgeon General's Office.

10. In terms of visits, or treatments.

11. Annual Rpt. WRGH, 1940.

12. *Ibid*, 1941.

13. AG Ltr. 18 Dec. 1940. As the war progressed all regulations governing the medical treatment of dependents were tightened, and dental care was eliminated for all cases except extractions and actual emergency work.

14. Annual Rpt. WRGH, 1941.

15. Percy M. Ashburn, CO from Sept. 19, 1915-October 5, 1916, was Chief of the Medical Service and Adjutant.

16. Personal knowledge of the writer.

17. Pools were established for all classes of personnel, in order to provide ready assignment or replacement.

18. Annual Rpt. WRGH, 1942.

19. *Ibid*.

20. One additional student joined later.

21. Annual Rpt., WRGH, 1942.

22. Blanchfield, *Organized Nursing and the Army*, *op cit*.

23. Annual Rpt. WRGH, 1943. In this case the service troops were Negro.

24. The hospital had a band for a short time during World War I, and during the early twenties, an orchestra.

25. Blanchfield, *op cit*.

26. Conversation, Col. Thomas Hester, MAC, 1943.

27. Interview, Miss Mattie Treadwell, WAC Historian, 1946-1950.

28. *Ibid*, and informal review of the official history of the WAC organization.

29 *Ibid*.

30. Annual Rpt. WRGH, 1943.

31. *Ibid*.

Wartime Readjustments
1944–1945

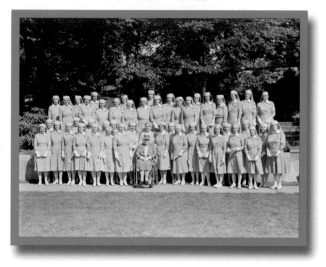

"The ordinary practice of medicine (is not) evidence of qualification to formulate sanitary plans and conduct intensive operations in time of war."[1]

General Training

The military personnel problems of the Army Medical Center command multiplied rapidly as many medical officers and enlisted men received objective training for overseas assignments. In September 1943, the enlisted personnel of the *Medical Department Professional Service Schools Company* (Army Medical Center) and the *Headquarters and Service Company* were consolidated into a *Detachment*, Medical Department, Army Medical Center.[2]

All men receiving basic training in the *Plans and Training Unit* were given instruction in the operation of oxygen tents and masks, lectures on anatomy, physiology, nursing and chemical warfare. Technicians trained in the X-ray, Dental and Pharmacy Schools and at the Cooks and Bakers School were primarily for overseas assignments. All changes in military regulations were posted on bulletin boards and read at military formations. The *Articles of War* were read periodically, and orientation lectures and training films were shown regularly, as part of the general War Department training program. All local stations at the Army Medical Center were covered by squads trained in fire fighting, disposal of incendiary bombs, and in first aid. As noted, practice raids and black-out drills were held at frequent intervals.[3]

Mobilization and expansion of the Army affected the female auxiliary services of nursing, physiotherapy and occupational therapy advantageously. In 1942, as a result

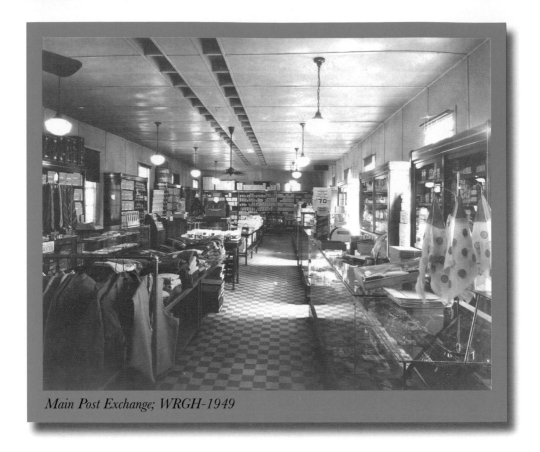

Main Post Exchange; WRGH-1949

of Public Law 828, 77th Congress, December 22, 1942, Army nurses, granted relative rank but unequal pay with male officers in 1920, received temporary actual rank and equal pay for the duration of the emergency and six months thereafter. The matter of salute and address by title was provided in 1920, but neither privilege was invoked to any great extent, as members of the Army Nurse Corps seldom appeared in military (field) uniform; further, the majority of them apparently preferred to be addressed by the more feminine title of "Miss."

In 1940, at the beginning of the military expansion period, the War Department General Staff noted that it was improper to address nurses and chaplains by military title, and received an immediate protest from the nurses. Encouraged by Major Julia C. Stimson, Army Nurse Corps, Retired, then President of the American Nurses' Association, the national organization adopted a firm stand in the matter of address by military title and the salute.[4] As Public Law 828 likewise incorporated into the military organization the physiotherapists and dieticians, with the emergency concessions accorded the nurses, persons making inquiries by telephone at Walter Reed and other Army hospitals were for a time nonplussed at the range and medley of voices answering the telephone to the unaccustomed title of "Lieutenant."

By August 22, 1943, qualified WAC enlisted personnel became eligible for a six-month intensive training course in physiotherapy, on completion of which, with an added three-month practical course in a selected Army hospital, such students were eligible for commission as second lieutenants.[5]

Whereas: The Civilian

There is no one quite so much outside the group activity during wartime as the civilian employee who works on a military post. For many of their "buddies" of last week or last month, having donned "pink" pants or earned sergeants stripes have thus gained entry into the brave new world in the making. Flippantly, perhaps, as some newly militarized personnel adopted a patronizing attitude, many simple and unclassified procedures of the daily routine assumed an unwarranted importance, and the term "Military Secret" was used in badinage. As a result of nation-wide commodity shortages and rationing, Post commissary cards were genuinely treasured. Thus the privilege of shopping at a Post Exchange well stocked with Kleenex, cigarettes, and even baggy rayon stockings made a vast difference in the comfort and ease with which two associated groups discharged their mutual domestic responsibilities. Thus, morale was, as always, an uncurrent problem, for each group believed the other favored in certain conspicuous ways.

Once in uniform, many civilians of a few weeks before resented the eight-hour-by-the-clock duty accorded their former associates. Some resented what they considered the unjustifiably authoritarian manner adopted by some minor military authorities, the objectionable "red tape" which so often characterizes management of any large organization, and the extra leave, in the form of "passes," accorded the enlisted military group. Many criticized the military tax exemptions, reduced train and movie fare and the postage-free mail which benefited military personnel on garrison duty in the United States as readily as combat personnel. Some believed there should have been some distinction in the privileges accorded personnel on overseas and domestic duty. Some of the military group resented the fact that of the many civilians who remained at home, many received cost-of-living raises and that their way of life was less interrupted by war. Class distinction had not been especially noticeable when employees rubbed "shoulder to shoulder" as civilians; on the other hand, the mere donning of a military uniform created an artificial condition for some, for in the majority of military agencies, officer-status governs job control.

Many soldiers, in the beginning, resented the WAC; some nurses resented the WAC; and after their acceptance in Army Hospitals, some enlisted WACs resented the paid nurse's aide,[6] who in a sense was a technical associate but had better working hours.

Disciplinary measures were less effective with civilians than with the military, for they could resign or transfer but, because of restrictive Civil Service Regulations, were difficult to fire. Hospital authorities, with ever increasing responsibilities for patient care, were at the mercy of unskilled employees, some of whom would have been considered unemployable in a less competitive labor market. This was especially true of mess attendants and custodial help, for many substandard and racial groups descended on Washington, where Government employment became a financial Mecca for many of the formerly underprivileged. Prior to the war and in addition to the soldiers' help, men were usually employed as mess attendants, cooks, janitors, laborers and ward attendants, but the personnel shortages of World War II soon caused the use of women. Many had never worked before, others accepted their jobs casually; thus job turnover was frequent and absenteeism was extremely high.[7]

The increased number of civilians employed at the Army Medical Center, and the hospital in particular, brought a reorganization and expansion of the Civilian Personnel Section of the headquarters, on November 1, 1942. Thereafter, all personnel actions for civilians were consolidated in the *Central Civilian Personnel Section*, where they were administered in compliance with Civil Service, War Department, Military District of Washington and Surgeon General's Office directives. This was obviously a complicated procedure, and sub-section personnel offices were established to manage group activities, such as the hospital employees, Quartermaster, School, etc.

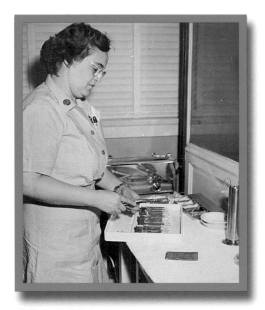

WAC Technician

On February 23, 1943, the Surgeon General's Office delegated certain of its functions to the station, these including immediate employment action on certain appointments below the CAF-6 Grade, or its equivalent, and upgraded employees paid by Medical Department and Hospital funds or funds from the Military District of Washington.[8] The *Central Civilian Personnel Section*, Army Medical Center, had a director and appropriate section supervisors for *Training, Classification, Correspondence, Position Control and Reports, File and Messenger Service*. These activities had made significant interval increases, for when the hospital was opened in 1909 four civilians[9] were employed, and by 1925, when Charles J. Considine came to the Post as Chief Clerk, 300 civilians were employed. By 1948, the number had reached 1,859.[10]

In Line of Duty

The year 1940, at the Army Medical School, was not unusually significant from any single aspect of the School's four-fold purpose of education, routine laboratory work, production of biological products or conduct of research studies.

Insofar as the first was concerned, the advanced graduate course for doctors was not offered after 1939; the time allotted to the basic course was curtailed thirty-one per cent in 1940 and eliminated entirely in 1941. The *Professional Specialists* course was still functioning, presumably on a two-to-four-year basis, depending on the background of the trainees. Thus the actual time required for completion of this course was not fixed.[11] Instruction in the Army Medical School course in *Clinical Medicine* was, at that time, limited to neuropsychiatry. At the beginning of the war about seven per cent[12] of all Regular Army doctors were listed as specialists, the greater majority of them serving in the general hospitals, and this percentage was considered adequate for the peacetime teaching and staffing program. These men were not only reputable and able but they were in some cases nationally known in their own field. The requirements for professional specialization, of increasing financial and prestige significance to civilian doctors, had not then resulted in the great stampede toward post-graduate training and Board certification which was to affect the Medical Corps some six years later. This was perhaps primarily the result of a difference in professional perspective. The income of the Army doctor was unaffected by competitive bidding for patients. The Army was, as one retired nose and throat specialist remarked wistfully, a place where the doctor could practice medicine honestly.[13]

The constantly expanding requirements for trained enlisted men, especially technicians, posed a hardship on the School authorities, for only one hundred men could be accommodated in the barracks space then provided for enlisted personnel. It was necessary, however, as part of the Medical Department training program, to inaugurate

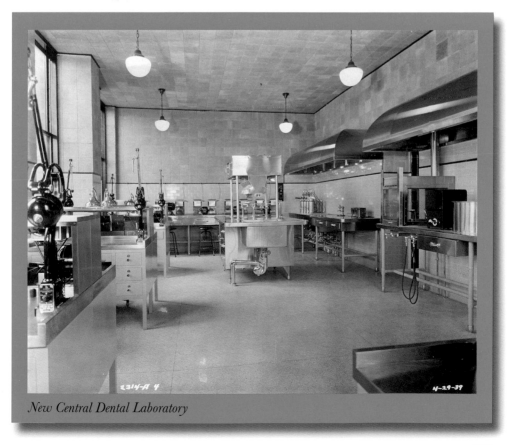

New Central Dental Laboratory

a course for hospital cooks on July 1, 1940. In regard to equipment-testing, two series of tests were made on the new Army Field Range, M-1937, to evaluate the possibilities of lead poisoning in the food or by the fumes therefrom. Gasoline, with varying lead contents, was used for fuel, and as a result of the findings some commercial producers of reagents became interested in the development of new products.

The production of routine biological products mounted in accordance with the increasing needs of the Army hospitalization program and of allied federal medical programs dependent on the School vaccine laboratory for supplies. Blood banks and studies of dried and fluid blood products, as noted, excited considerable interest at this time, with both the products and the subsequent clinical therapy of prime concern to Army doctors.

The *Central Dental Laboratory*, operating as a separate organizational unit for the first time during the fiscal year 1940– that is, July 1, 1939, to June 30, 1940-performed work which had heretofore been essentially a function of the Army Dental School. Thereafter it served as a group laboratory for Army areas in the East and as a prostheses laboratory for the Army Dental School. Nevertheless, recognition as a functional entity, with a separate director, but with administrative and fiscal accountability to the Army Medical Center, further complicated the organizational structure of this, the most complicated of all the Medical Department's installation activities.[14]

As noted, seventeen barracks buildings, each with an approximate capacity of sixty-three men, two bachelor officers' dormitories, with a capacity of thirty-eight men each, and a dining hall, with a seating capacity of 750 men, were constructed during 1941 to care for the expanding requirements of the Medical Department Professional Service Schools. Further, two of the semi-permanent buildings erected in 1918 were converted into school rooms. There were no changes in the basic functions of the Schools, whose activities increased approximately 700 per cent during the year.

Condensed Basic Graduate Courses, Professional Specialists' Courses and *Refresher Courses* were provided for reserved officers after 1941. Instruction courses for Regular Army officers were terminated in April 1941. The courses for enlisted men included the usual X-ray, Laboratory, Pharmacy, Orthopedic Appliances, Medical Technicians, Surgical Technicians and the course for hospital cooks, as well as a special course of instruction in photoroentgenology for both officers and enlisted men. Enlisted men were being drawn off to fill cadres for the newly activated medical units and for new stations in the Zone of Interior. As a consequence of this situation, the number of civilian employees at the School was increased to ninety-eight. Nevertheless, in spite of strenuous attempts to maintain the status quo, the depletion of trained personnel adversely affected the teaching program to some extent.[15] Colonel George R. Callender, the Army's well known wound ballistics expert and pathologist, was director of the Army Medical School at this time, a position he continued to hold during the war years. As a result of his magnificent effort in training many of the young reserve and Army of the United States officers during World War II, he was promoted to the temporary grade of Brigadier General, Medical Corps, in 1945.

The production of Triple Typhoid Vaccine exceeded that of 1941 by 164 per cent and the production of the combined years of 1937-41 by 20.4 per cent. The production of glucose exceeded the previous year by 17.9 per cent and the combined years of 1937-41 by 31.39 per cent. Production of Allergenic Protein Extracts and Pneumonia Vaccine was discontinued, and the Army Veterinary School was provided with the additional space for production of encephalomyelitis vaccine for humans. As in the past, however, the *Division of Biologic Products* prepared the hypodermic solution of codeine sulfate and some other biological products used at the Walter Reed General Hospital.[16]

By May 1941, the War Department had established a policy of bloodgrouping all members of the Armed Forces, with their identification tags properly stamped to show the (Landsteiner) International Classification System. This policy was economical from the administrative standpoint, and it doubtless saved thousands of lives by permitting immediate transfusion in emergency cases. Army Medical School personnel made the determinations on all military personnel reporting to the Post for active military service. Further, the *Division of Blood Research* made a study of human serum albumin, in an attempt to standardize a package of suitable transportable size yet one which would furnish adequate fluid and protein for the treatment of shock, hemorrhage, burns and other hypoproteinemic states. Courses in shock, surgical physiology and the treatment of war wounds were given to Medical and Dental officers stationed temporarily at the Army Medical Department Professional Schools, and in January, March and June, lectures on shock and the use of plasma by the Armed Forces were delivered at the Medical Field Service School at Carlisle. The blood program endorsed by the Medical Department was much too extensive to enable the School to act as purveyor of all blood products. During 1942, therefore, contracts were let to eight commercial laboratories for the preparation of dried plasma for use by the Armed Forces.[17]

The *Division of Chemistry and Physics* continued to perform nearly all the toxicological examinations for the entire Army. Further, it functioned as the Chemistry Section of the Third Corps Area Laboratory, thus doing considerable routine work. Similar work performed for Walter Reed increased during the year, for after a rather generalized outbreak of jaundice a medical survey was initiated, and the determinations placed a heavy load on the depleted staff of this section. Further, during 1942, the Divisions of *Food and Nutrition* and *Industrial Hygiene* were added to the School activities, and during the last three months of the fiscal year 1943, some basic research in food was begun in relation to the Army ration.

The *Division of Virus and Rickettsial Diseases* was especially busy, as infectious material received from Labrador, Iceland, Jamaica, Puerto Rico, Hawaii and many domestic stations in the United States, included material from cases of neurotropic virus diseases. The Virus Laboratory at the Army Medical School was the first of its kind in that diagnostic methods were employed *routinely* in the diagnosis of virus and rickettsial diseases. Like the Rockefeller Foundation, the School was sponsoring extensive research on typhus, work which could not then be published for military reasons but which had

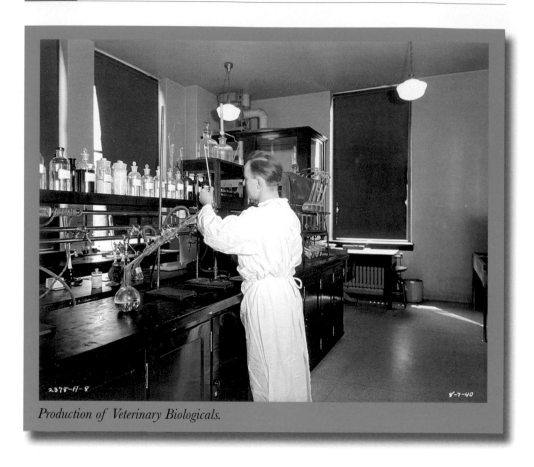

Production of Veterinary Biologicals.

far-reaching effects as an international public health measure. Some of this work was later evidenced in the Army's typhus-control program in Naples, Italy.

Concurrently, intensive four-week courses were given in *Tropical Medicine*, to prepare doctors for tropical service; an eight-week course in *Tropical and Military Medicine, 1942* was designed to prepare junior officers for service as assistants in the medical service of Army post hospitals in the United States and abroad, with the particular object of teaching the application of knowledge already acquired. An intensive four-week course in *Plastic and Maxillo-facial Surgery* was given, as noted, to instruct medical and dental officers of the Army of the United States in the principles and standard procedures applicable to this subject and to serve as "teams" in the Medical Department installations at home and abroad. The staff was selected from the Army Medical School faculty, the Army Dental School faculty and the hospital staff. Further, an intensive course in roentgenology was offered and a six-week refresher course for Sanitary Reserve officers.

In addition to the very special work in animal biologicals, the Army Veterinary School found it necessary to train an increasing number of men in meat and dairy inspection, and the Army Dental School, whose demands increased over 300 per

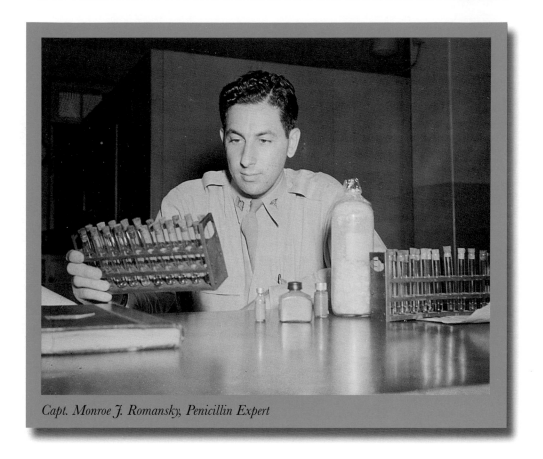

Capt. Monroe J. Romansky, Penicillin Expert

cent in the first six months of 1942, needed more men and more space. Enabled by funds transferred to the Army Medical Center from the *Office of Emergency Management*, on February 1, 1942, the maxillo-facial group was still experimenting with vitallium implants as replacements of mutilated parts of the body.[18]

An *Army Specialist Corps* was established by Executive Order No. 9078, February 26, 1942, with Section V providing for Medical Service. By November 4, however, all officers in the Corps were required to apply for commissions in the Army of the United States by December 1, or be discharged on December 31, 1942. Six months later, passage of Public Law 130, 78th Congress, Act of July 12, 1943, required the transfer to the newly created Pharmacy Corps, of Medical Administrative Officers of the Regular Army, this number in addition to the seventy-two officers authorized by law. Inasmuch as the top military grade for this Corps was raised from Major, as allowed for the Medical Administrative Corps, to Colonel, the Medical Department was destined to undergo some policy changes and effect more responsible administrative assignments for the Corps. Ultimately, the Pharmacy Corps provided opportunities for many qualified health workers other than exclusively graduate pharmacists, and some became deeply interested in hospital administration at Walter Reed and elsewhere.

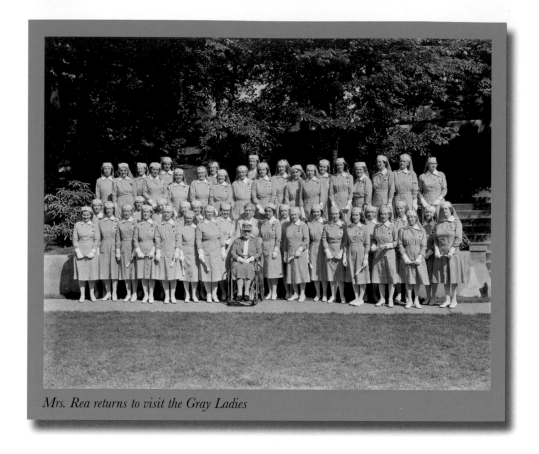

Mrs. Rea returns to visit the Gray Ladies

School for MD PSS Technicians

The manpower allotment of enlisted men for special training programs varied from time to time, depending on the size of the Army and the consequent number of medical installations. The enlarged classes at the Army Medical Department Professional Services Schools began on April 2, 1941. Under authority of an Adjutant General's letter of January 15, 1942, nearly one-half of the trainees were assigned from the *Medical Department Replacement Training Center* at Camp Lee, Virginia, later called Camp Pickett. Men from the Replacement Center often had some background in the specialties, rather than, as formerly, only basic military training. Part of the personnel for the early courses came from the Army Medical Center Detachment, but after the first few courses, the permanent personnel was so depleted as a result of providing cadres for new units that the Detachment could no longer provide replacements.

There was, especially in the early days of the training program, a wide variation in the quality of personnel provided for technical training. Directives established by the Surgeon General's Office required a high school education as preliminary to the Laboratory, Pharmacy and X-ray training, but Army Medical School authorities sometimes believed that classification specialists were more concerned with producing numbers of recruits than quality. In questioning some of the 1942 assignees, reclassification officers learned that above one-third of the men were not only unsuited for technical assignments but did not want such courses, factors which necessitated many transfers and adjustments. Further, many could not qualify as Grade 5 technicians, even after several attempts at training. Thus it was not only costly and wasteful to attempt to train such material but it was definitely dangerous to use substandard men, as the lives of patients were involved. Unfortunately, the frequently changing War Department policies governing the release of personnel made maintenance of a technically qualified and numerically adequate staff extremely difficult. Colonel Callender was unsympathetic with what he believed to be a prevalent but erroneous idea of classification experts that any available doctor could serve as instructor, especially in teaching tropical diseases. Further, he believed that many distinguished civilian doctors were prevented from seeking military appointment because of lack of suitable military grades.[19]

The medical and surgical courses were the only ones in which the staff at Walter Reed participated. The third month of this training was given at the hospital and the Army Medical School; the fourth, fifth and sixth months were given at Gallinger Municipal Hospital, Emergency Hospital and Providence Hospital, all in Washington, District of Columbia.

Actual management of the Technicians' School, where the enrollees increased from less than sixty in a session in pre-war days to more than 500 a session in the mid-war years, was not solely an academic responsibility, for a total military management problem was involved which included reception, classification, housing, feeding, training, discipline, physical examination, payment and the ultimate re-transfer of men to units.

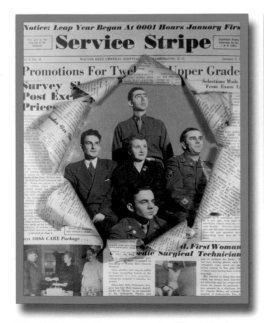

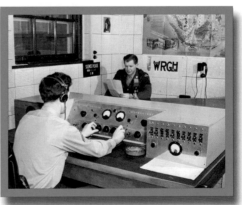

Mark Austed of Station WRGH, better known as Mark Evans of Station WTOP

World War II; Successor to the Come Back

Continued Expansion

The outstanding activities of the Medical Department Professional Services Schools group for the fiscal year 1943, the first complete year since the war, included not only increased production of biologicals but an unavoidable increase in the teaching load. The *Tropical and Military Medicine Class*, at first a mere thirty students, increased to 230. All of the other departments and courses at the School were similarly crowded, and some relief to the physical plant was effected through transfer of the roentgenology courses to Memphis, Tennessee, and cessation of the pharmacy classes, Medical Department Professional Services Schools. As a precautionary or security measure, a subsidiary laboratory was established in Lansing, Michigan, which by the end of the fiscal year was almost ninety-five per cent complete.[20]

Reserves in the diagnostic biologicals were built up, but this made further inroads on the already depleted supply of small laboratory animals so necessary to the investigative program. Studies and developments in the field X-ray, the processing and packaging of plasma and the development of byproducts of serum albumin production continued. Army Medical School research experts cooperated with contemporaries at Harvard and with the Typhus Commission.

Insofar as organization was concerned, the *Department of Tropical Medicine*, under the direction of the internationally famous Doctor Richard P. Strong, a reserve officer on active duty, replaced the former departments of *Clinical Medicine* and *Preventative Medicine*; the departments of *Military Medicine* and *Military Surgery* encompassed the

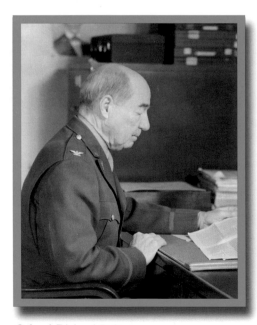

Colonel Richard P. Strong

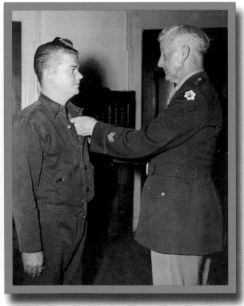

Major General Shelley U. Marietta decorating a patient with the Purple Heart.

former specialized and related subjects in these respective fields. In the case of *Military Surgery*, the courses in anesthesia and neurosurgery were modified as well as approved by the appropriate national professional groups. The *Division of Industrial Hygiene* was transferred to Baltimore, Maryland, in 1943, but remained under the direction of the Army Medical School. The *Division of Pathology* was, as in the past, largely operated by the Army Medical Museum.

The fiscal costs of operating the School unit, through local procurement and standard issue, without salaries and maintenance, approximated $700,000. The cash return to the Treasury of the United States, primarily for typhoid vaccines purveyed to other Federal agencies, equaled $212,422.[21] Measured in terms of manpower and the saving in human lives, these costs were incalculably small. The personnel, officers, enlisted men and civilians employed in the Medical Department Professional Services Schools' activities had increased three times over the numbers assigned in 1938. The training program produced about thirty-five times as many graduates and approximately thirty times as many biologicals.

More than eighty years had passed since the Civil War, when "country practitioners in green sashes (became acquainted) with hygiene and vaccinations" and since Surgeon General Hammond had proposed establishing a general hospital in Washington City; forty years had passed since Dr. Borden began talking to conferees of his plans for grouping the associated activities of hospital, school, museum and library in one location. Only twenty years had passed since the Army Medical School became part of the Army Medical Center. A war had cemented the organizational and functional relationship of these two great institutions and shown clearly that medically as well as tactically, "Training too was needed to make an Army."[22]

References

1. Major Paul F. Straub, "The Training of Sanitary Troops," *The Military Surgeon*, Vol XVIII, No.4, April 1911, pg 362.

2. General Orders No. 33, Hdq. AMC.

3. Annual Rpt., WRGH, 1943.

4. Memo to TSG from E.S. Adams, Maj. Gen., TAG, Sub: Military Titles for Members of the Army Nurse Corps, June 21, 1940. File 322.5-2 (Op.Sv.) Hist. Div., SGO; Ltr from Alta E. Dines to Miss Mary Beard, ARC, July 20, 1940, File 052.3, Archives ARC; Ltr. from James C. Magee, MG, TSG, to Hon. Norman H. Davis, Chrm. ARC, July 24, 1943, SGO 211 Nurses; Memo to TSG from Julia C. Flikke, Supt. ANC, July 2, 1940. File, AG 322.31 (7-2-40); Ltr. from Julia C. Stimson, Pres. ANA to Miss Mary Beard, Dir., Nursing Service, ARC, Sept. 3, 1940, File 052.3, Archives, ARC; Ltr. James C. Magee, Maj. Gen. TSG to Maj. Julia C. Stimson, Aug. 14, 1940, File 340.5-2 (Op.Sv.) Hist. Div., SGO; Ltr. from G.C. Marshall, C/S to Miss Julia C. Stimson, Aug. 14, 1940, File 322.21 (C/S) (7-3-40) War Dept., Record Room; Ltr. from G.C. Marshall, C/S to Miss Julia C. Stimson, Pres. ANA, Dec. 7, 1940, Photostat of original, File 052.3 Archives, ARC. Interview G.C. Marshall, S/S, Dec. 1, 1948.

5. Memo W 635-18-43.

6. Florence A. Blanchfield, *Organized Nursing...Three Wars*, on file Hist. Div., Office of the Surgeon General.

7. See Annual Rpts WRGH, for World War II period.

8. Annual Rpt., WRGH, 1943.

9. Unpublished manuscript, Hist. WRGH, (Used for World War I Hist. of Med. Dept.) on file library, WRAH.

10. Telephone conversation with Charles J. Considine, May 24, 1951; Guy W. Bennett, Jr., April 25, 1951.

11. Annual Rpt. MD PSS, 1940, on file Office of the Commandant.

12. Telephone conversation Miss Anne Grey, Personnel Division, SGO.

13. Conversation with Brig. General Royal Reynolds, M.C., Ret., at the Library, WRAH.

14. Annual Rpt., MD PSS, 1940, *op cit.*

15. Annual Rpt. of Technical Activities of the Army Medical School for FY Ending June 30, 1941, on file, Office of the Commandant.

16. *Ibid.*

17. Annual Rpt., AMS, 1942, *op cit.*

18. Annual Rpt., of Technical Activities of the AMS...1942, *op cit.*

19. *Ibid.*

20. Annual Rpt., of Technical Activities of the AMS...1943, *op cit.*

21. Annual Rpt., MD PSS, 1943, *op cit.*

22. Margaret Leech, *Reveille in Washington 1860–1865,* Harper & Brothers, New York and London, ca 1941, page 107.

Two Difficult Years

1944–1945

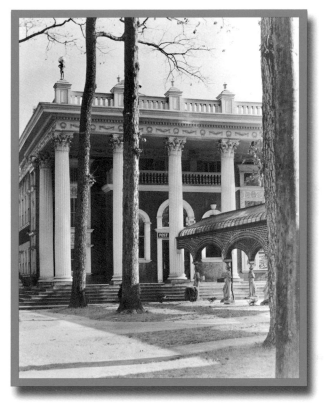

Post Theatre No. II, Forest Glen

"In attempting to arrive at an accurate diagnosis of any condition not plainly evident, one of the most essential steps is a complete history."[1]

Major General Shelley U. Marietta's five-year tenure as Post Commander at the Army Medical Center covered the most difficult administrative period in the entire life-cycle of the organization. This was especially true of the hospital, whose lineage encompassed the old station hospital at Washington Barracks, and which had survived the expansion program of three wars. The 18,000 new patients admitted in 1944, a 296 per cent increase over 1941, with only a fifty per cent increase in personnel,[2] required maintenance of institutional activities at the same high level of the year before.

The Convalescent Section, purchased from the National Park Seminary in 1942 and revamped for hospital use, included approximately 185 acres of beautiful and valuable land. Nevertheless, it was an additional administrative problem for the commanding general, as functionally it was a second institution, requiring all the installation support activities of the parent plant. Servicing the buildings was difficult because of their age and because they were not designed for patient care. Some ambulatory patients objected to being transferred to the suburban area because of the increased transportation difficulties to the city; others objected because of the generally semi-rural isolation and the necessity for commuting to Walter Reed by shuttle bus for clinics and consultations. None, so far as is known, objected because of actual domiciliary accommodations or the food service, which was generally conceded to be superior. As if one subinstallation activity was not enough to harass the management, the War Department's increasingly urgent pleas to conserve manpower necessitated by the military personnel shortages of 1944, resulted in increased emphasis on retraining of combat casualties and return to active duty. During 1944, therefore, the Army Medical Center acquired temporary possession of a former Civilian Conservation Corps camp at Beltsville, Maryland, about seven miles northeast of the main hospital and some four miles from the Forest Glen Section. Restoration and equipping the rough frame buildings, cleaning and servicing the grounds, establishment of a highly organized physical training program, installation of a small library and dispensary made Camp Ord, the Beltsville extension, an independent and self-sufficient station. Here the men wore fatigue clothes rather than Class A or convalescent clothing, and they were required to participate in organized athletics. It was a wholesome carefree type of existence, and to all outward appearances the men enjoyed their existence in a womanless world. The same system of shuttle buses, daily deliveries of newspapers, mail and supplies were used as for the Forest Glen Section. The rehabilitation program at Camp Ord applied to male patients only, not to WACs and nurses,[3] and continued until March 7, 1945.

Something New is Added

A war period presents unique problems for military commanders in general and hospital commanders in particular. The Army, which is seemingly forgotten or ignored in peacetime, unless requests for Congressional appropriations appear too high, suddenly becomes of prime interest to the nation. As Nicholas Senn, distinguished military surgeon of the Spanish-American War period said, "The military spirit is epidemic in our country; Kindle it and it spreads like a flash of lightening, from north to south and east to west."[4]

Thus, as the population was mobilized, scientists gave their best through Research and Development programs. Educators streamlined their academic courses in an effort to prepare additional manpower. Industrialists laid aside routine affairs and directed their

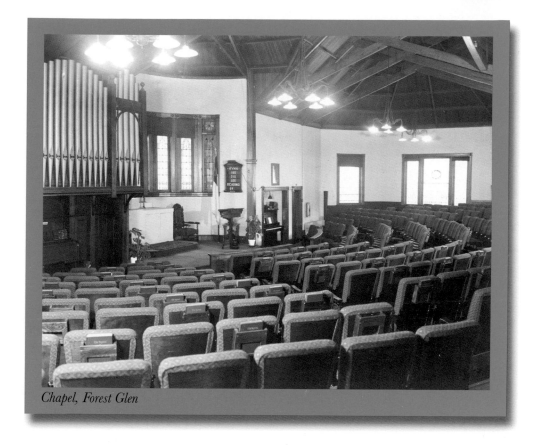

Chapel, Forest Glen

efforts toward winning the war. It is undoubtedly true that the young men of the country make the greatest sacrifice, for nothing can replace the loss of life or of human function or eradicate the horror of some war experience from the impressionable minds of the young.

The number of military rejections for psychiatric disability had, by 1944, become alarming, and the number of non-effective and/or discharges on this diagnosis was a cause for grave concern to military commanders faced with meeting manpower requirements for combat.[5] Encouraged by the public information provided by some medical writers, psychologists and lay writers in "slick" magazines, psychiatry had become an increasingly publicized branch of medicine during the fifteen years prior to the war. Many Americans discussed complexes, frustrations, inhibitions and defense mechanisms casually and with the complacency of the fully informed. In some quarters, conservative educators were reputedly beginning to evaluate and question the effects of the rather marked twenty-year trend toward progressive education and ponder the imponderable: the relationship between academic, religious and cultural discipline and the stable personality. On the whole, however, there then appeared to be no indisputable evidence as to the cause and effect of the many mental hygiene problems encountered by the Army.

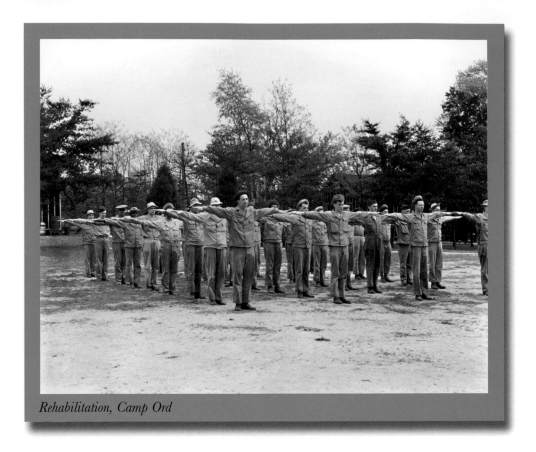

Rehabilitation, Camp Ord

At Walter Reed, accommodations on the Neuropsychiatric Section were expended rapidly. Medically, the professional functions of that section were primarily those of observation, classification and disposition of patients. Although the hospital was declared a specialized center for the care and treatment of neuropsychiatric disorders,[6] during the early part of the war the prevailing War Department regulations required that a medical diagnosis be entered on the *Certificate of Discharge with Disability* (CDD). By 1944, however, the regulation was changed, as veterans had complained vociferously that a diagnosis of psychiatric disorder affected employment opportunities. In a sincere attempt to ameliorate the situation, or preclude questionable entries by physicians not too familiar with psychiatric disorders, Medical Department policy was amended to provide a *Neuropsychiatric Board*, to act in the official capacity of a *Consultation Board, Disposition and Case Board*, but which was concerned only with cases having neuropsychiatric disorders without complicating organic diseases. Further, a clinical psychologist was assigned to the Neuropsychiatric Section at Walter Reed on June 30, 1945, to establish a suitable psychological testing program which included:

1. *Wechsler-Bellevue Intelligence Scale*
2. *Rorschach Psychodiagnostic Test*
3. *Murray Thematic Apperception Test*
4. *Shipley-Hartford Conceptual Quotient Test*
5. *Minnesota Multiphasic Personality Inventory*
6. *Bender-Gestalt Test*
7. *Sentence Completion Test*
8. *Stanford-Binet Intelligence Test*[7]

This section had always received an especially high type of auxiliary personnel services. The Occupational Therapy Shop, under the direction of Mrs. Emmy Sommers, was one of the finest in the Army. Mrs. Sommers had come to America in 1913, and to Walter Reed in 1918, where she and her husband both worked with the rehabilitation program of that period. A rare personality, generous, gentle and kind, she was an artist in tapestry weaving as well as other skills, and few if any other civilian employees at the Army Medical Center could claim such distinctive special preparation for their work.[8]

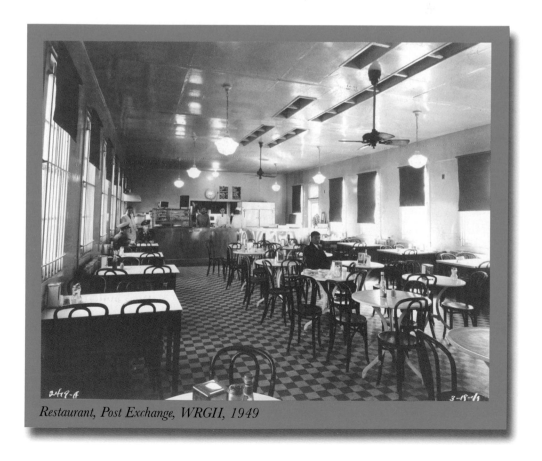

Restaurant, Post Exchange, WRGII, 1949

The special Occupational Therapy Shop, in the basement of the Neuropsychiatric Section, served the entire hospital for a number of years and until the World War II expansion program necessitated additional space, personnel, equipment and programs of especial benefit to the large number of patients with orthopedic and traumatic injuries. The Red Cross social workers, the Gray Ladies and the civilian hospital employees who worked with neuropsychiatric patients were usually selected and were trained for this type of work, either prior to receiving hospital assignment or through on-the-job-orientation courses.

It is a generally accepted fact that music produces varying reactions in people; some are stimulated; some are soothed. Thus it is wholly possible that temporary vasometer or emotional tones might follow a designated course in "applied" music, but these effects would tend to follow the personality pattern of the individual, including his preferences for certain types of music. Therapy, the specific treatment of disease, implied the application of some measurable agent, and to a physician as well versed in clinical medicine as General Marietta, the term musical "therapy" was a misnomer.

He was, however, at various times during late 1943 and the early part of 1944, encouraged, rather insistently perhaps, to endorse a program of musical therapy. When the program was finally begun, distinguished local artists willingly gave their time and talent. The patients selected for exposure to "applied" music were chosen by the ward doctor, and for a time the program appeared popular. During the first part of 1944 and prior to assignment of a special musical therapy building at the Forest Glen Section, the auditions were held in the basement recreation room of the Neuropsychiatric Section, redecorated in accord with the idea of the program director. There utter quiet prevailed during the musical seances.

Many of the patients receiving therapy were psychotic or psychoneurotic, and on August 24, 1944, General Marietta appointed a committee to report on the progress and success of music as a clinical treatment. The investigating committee decided that some of the patients with functional disturbances seemed to benefit, but objective analysis was lacking. As a result, therefore, a second committee presented extensive recommendations for the study of brain waves, pain sensitivity, gastro-intestinal tone and traumatic symptoms. By the end of the calendar year 1944, it was still impossible to advance definite claims for the benefits of the program, which was, however, continued during most of 1945.[9]

The Maxillo-facial sub-section of general surgery was discontinued in 1944; thereafter such causes were sent to other Army hospitals selected by the Surgeon General's Office as special plastic surgery centers. Nevertheless, there were 11, 110 surgical procedures performed at Walter Reed in 1944, and 1,592 blood transfusions. The latter figure represented a one hundred per cent increase over the number of transfusions given in 1943. Of the 8,289 anesthetics given during the year, 32.3 per cent were inhalation anesthesia and 28.1 per cent were spinal. No new anesthetic reagents were used during 1944. As the Anesthesia Department was responsible for instructing officers and nurses who would probably be assigned to theaters of war, wisdom decreed the use of standard items available within the theaters.[10]

It was understandable that the X-ray Department was performing an increasing number of examinations which required surgical techniques. These included bronchography, arteriography, renography, ventriculography, encephalography and myleography. The million-unit X-ray machine was used 3,584 times during the year, and 225 patients received radium treatment. Approximately one-third of all hospital deaths continued to result from cancer; about one-third of the surgical specimens were tumors, and one-ninth of the total surgical pathology specimens were malignant. This was essentially the same cancer-ratio as before the war, the reason being that although the average age of the patient had decreased, selective and referred cases maintained the former level. As in the case of practically all of the hospital services during this period, the X-ray and radium work was under the direction of distinguished civilians appointed to active duty as reserve officers.

The flow of patients to the hospital was curtailed in 1945, with the inpatient census of new cases dropping to 16,878 admissions. Fortunately, battle casualties requiring long-term hospitalization were less than forecast by some military agencies, and so the Zone of Interior hospital facilities consistently were not as hard pressed as was expected. As a consequence there was, late in the year, an adequate supply of certain selected categories of technical personnel such as nurses, WACs and medical and surgical technicians.[11] Regional Hospitals, staffed jointly by Air Medical Corps and Army Medical Corps personnel but caring only for Zone of Interior patients, were by then in operation, an arrangement which permitted many of the general hospitals to become specialty centers.

The Out-Patient Service, Walter Reed General Hospital, afforded medical service in all the usual specialties and sub-specialties. Some 108,850 treatments were given during 1944, of which 15,870 were rendered to military personnel. The principal administrative change in that service provided for the assignment of full-time visiting physicians rather than the former practice of having doctors spend part of the day in the clinic and part in home-service calls. Although cessation of war in the summer of 1945 reduced the work-level in this department to some extent, other problems developed as patients began making more demands for attention and were critical if their needs were not met.[12]

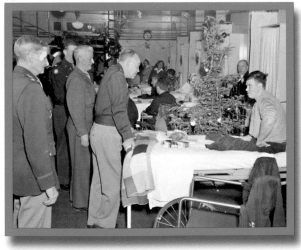

General Eisenhower and Patients

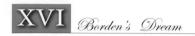

Reconditioning

A complete set of rehabilitation buildings was constructed at the Forest Glen Section during 1945, interconnected with covered walks. The occupational therapy work was of the usual type, including weaving, printing, leather work, carpentry, plastics, jewelry making, typing, business machine instruction, sign painting and drafting, automotive shop mechanics, electrical work, etc., a photographic shop and even a course in dancing for amputees. Two years later, during 1947, a course of instruction for amputees in drivers' training was given to 388 patients, with 110 men passing the approved AAA written and performance test; seventy-eight men were licensed to drive in the District of Columbia and Maryland. In 1946, the Capital Transit Company presented the Reconditioning Program with "Car 1100," a trolley for use in teaching men with artificial prostheses some of the new motions and adjustments to balance which they must encounter in their daily activities.[13] The reconditioning program had developed rapidly during the late war years, but to some of the older employees who had worked at the hospital in 1919 and 1920, conditions were reminiscent of that period. The same general type of patient was interested in the same general type of activities, often making flippant comments so characteristic of the American soldier whether he be called "doughboy," as in World War I, or "GI" as in World War II.

Once again the community responded wholeheartedly to the needs of "the boys" at Walter Reed. In addition to the government-sponsored reconditioning program, the Red Cross sponsored an *Arts and Skills* program, with the activities directed by volunteer workers. Many of Washington's best artists participated in the informal instruction of ward patients. Insofar as recreation was concerned, local volunteer artists, as well as the *Army Special Services* talent were used without stint, both on the wards and in performance at the Red Cross House. A long-standing Medical Department policy required that all recreation and entertainment programs be channeled through the Red Cross, which managed the many generous attempts to entertain the patients with card parties, teas, movies and guest boxes at the National Symphony Orchestra. During World War I the McLean family had loaned "Friendship House" as a rest home for officers, and during the second emergency Mrs. Evelyn Walsh McLean "adopted" entire fifty-bed wards at a time, her generosity including entertainment, refreshments and even custodial help to restore post-party order to the wards; on one occasion she even provided a galaxy of pastel-colored chenille Easter rabbits, much to the entertainment of the amused recipients.

The President occasionally visited the wounded veterans.[14] The Chesapeake and Potomac Telephone Company installed telephone booths in the Red Cross House, especially adapted to receive wheel chairs, authorized long distance calls for newly admitted patients from overseas, and provided writing paper for distribution on the wards. Even Samuel "Roxie" Rothsfel of World War I fame would have found an active competitor in Roy Rogers and his famous horse,[15] both of whom came in person. Neither, however, could compete with General Dwight D. "Ike" Eisenhower, who came on a special visit

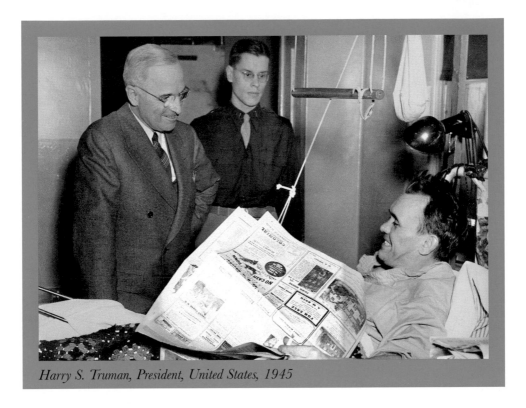

Harry S. Truman, President, United States, 1945

June 23, 1945, and found not only the patients and staff lined up to greet him but the surrounding neighborhood as well. The local Walter Reed radio broadcasting network mushroomed into a full-scale activity, with Mark Austed, later known on commercial radio programs as Mark Evans, as announcer. Patient-talent was encouraged to participate in broadcasts and skits presented on the station network.

The *Physical Reconditioning Program* was well-established, and all members of the staff, both officers and enlisted men, were graduates of the Army Service Forces special training schools. Class IV (bed patients) participated in approximately one-half hour of group (physical) exercises, conducted on daily schedules, and Class III (ambulatory) patients participated in approximately one hour of group activities in the gymnasium, swimming pool, etc. Popular sports such as archery, badminton and basketball were organized, with even wheelchair cases encouraged to participate in a form of handball. Outstanding authorities on sports were secured to address the patients and to demonstrate accepted techniques. Approximately sixty per cent of all military patients in the hospital participated in some form of physical reconditioning prior to cessation of hostilities.

The full impact of the evacuation from the European theater was felt in the spring of 1945, and from 514 amputees in January, the number increased to 1,051 by July. The Amputation Section was divided into sub-sections, according to the type of cases. In July 1945, a research laboratory on artificial limbs was established, and in Sep-

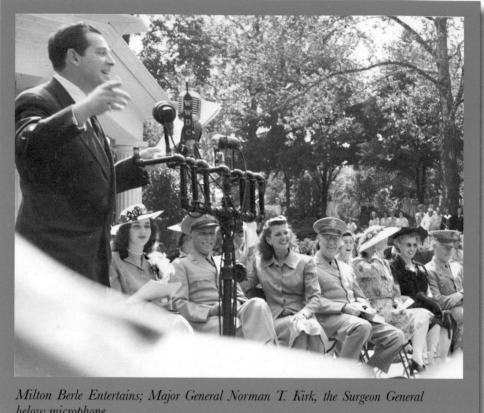

Milton Berle Entertains; Major General Norman T. Kirk, the Surgeon General below microphone

tember a directive from the Surgeon General's Office designated Walter Reed as a research and development center for the mechanical and cosmetic hand. One building was remodeled to house the offices, the mechanical laboratory and the plastic laboratory. In August 1945, Captain Monroe J. Romansky, who had worked for some months on penicillin experiments and therapy, reported that he had found a mixture of penicillin, beeswax and peanut oil whose effects lasted twelve hours after injection rather than the usual two and one-half to three and one-half hours.[16] The Walter Reed branch of the U.S. Post Office was distributing approximately 60,000 letters and packages each week, and so in spite of the still undeclared cessation of hostilities, the scientific and social life of the GI, medically the best serviced soldier in the world, gave little indication that it was time to turn swords into plowshares and begin life anew.

The *Educational Reconditioning Program*, a revived and certainly an expanded edition of the World War I reconstruction program, was likewise in full swing. By spring of 1945, all able-bodied patients were encouraged to take some accredited correspondence course, arranged by the *United States Armed Forces Institute* (USAFI) program,[17] and ward patients were provided with visiting instructors. Thirty-five volunteer civilian teachers were assigned to duty on the wards. In January 1945, only three officers and eight enlisted men were required for management of the organized program; by August, six officers and forty-four enlisted men, the latter group including WAC instructors, had regularly established ward schedules.

All classes of patients except short term and station hospital patients were interviewed and scheduled for some phase of educational reconditioning or diversional occupational therapy, with an estimated eighty per cent of the total number "exposed" to some aspect of the program. Attendance was sporadic and irregular for the large majority; at the Main Section, Walter Reed General Hospital, about thirty-five per cent of those who registered for courses attended regularly, and at Forest Glen, about forty per cent attended. Some patients failed to attend classes because of clinics and other legitimate excuses; but week end passes, furloughs and extended sick leave likewise took their toll. An estimated twenty per cent of the patients were uninterested and resisted participation in the educational program.[18]

Routine Affairs

In August 1945, a full-time dietician was assigned to the Out-Patient Service and Pre-Natal Clinic, in order to comply with the requirements for an approved student hospital training program. More attention was devoted to training for supervision and job relations. ASF Circular 50, February 10, 1945, prescribed a training program for Diet Kitchen Attendants, sixty-five of whom subsequently received such training at the hospital. In November 1945, construction of an addition to the Patients Mess (No. II) was completed. The improvements, or rather the extension, of the Mess Hall necessitated some renovation of the original structure, and in order to reconcile the old and the new, the fine old walnut-paneled walls of the older part of the structure were painted ivory. A new cafeteria service counter was put into operation, with a seating capacity of 216 and an overall serving capacity of 592. Semi-ambulant patients had table service.

The Dietetic Department was administration-conscious by this time. All accounting procedures were reviewed, and control on outside purchasing was tightened by employing competitive bidding for the purchase of items in short supply. New stock record cards were made with entries for all subsistence items, as a system of meal cost-analysis was installed. Food items were divided into classes similar to those used on the master menu. As a result of Change 4, AR 40-590, August 31, 1945, the *Post Hospital Fund* and the *Subsistence Accounts* were consolidated, effective November 1, 1945. Large quantities of cigarettes had been purchased by the Quartermaster General's Department, for overseas shipment, and early conclusion of the hostilities permitted the issue of such stocks to patients in Zone of Interior hospitals, some 40,000 being issued at Walter Reed in October.

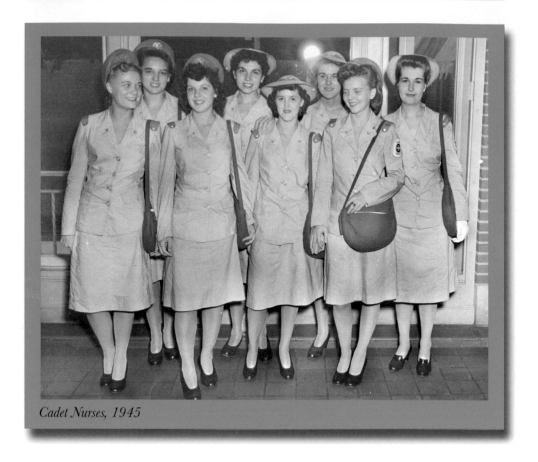

Cadet Nurses, 1945

There were 244 graduate nurses on duty at Walter Reed as of December 31, 1944, but no civilian nurses. Ten nurses completed the course in anesthesia. The Red Cross nurses' aide program, which brought strenuous objections from the national nursing organization in 1917 and 1918, and resulted in the establishment of the Army School of Nursing, became a Red Cross – Office of Civilian Defense program in 1941. It was designed primarily as a relief to hard-pressed civilian hospitals. By the time personnel shortages made this program appear interesting to the Medical Department,[19] the pattern of service to civilian hospitals only was so firmly established that OCD medical officials voiced some objection to the use of aides in military hospitals. Nevertheless, by March 1943, the first training courses for nurses' aides, for service in military hospitals, were authorized at Walter Reed General Hospital and Camp Gordon Johnson, Carabelle, Florida.[20] More than a year later, when the question of paid nurses' aides in military hospitals was a burning issue, some State Nurses' Associations protested to the Red Cross, the protest apparently arising from fear of competition with graduate nurses.[21]

The nurses' aide program, for both volunteer and paid aides, was popular and successful at Walter Reed and other Army hospitals, for the women rendered invaluable and irreplaceable auxiliary service in the care of the sick. Three training courses were

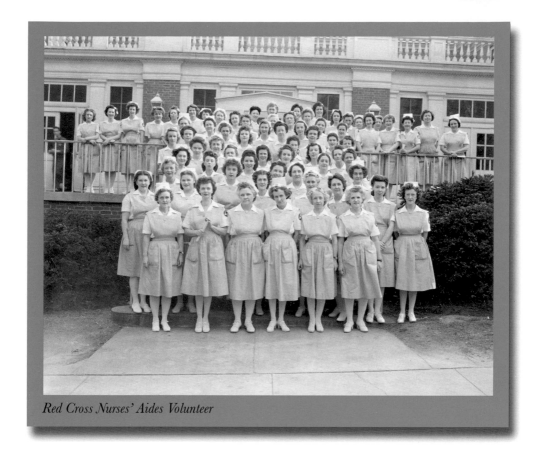

Red Cross Nurses' Aides Volunteer

given during 1945, and eighty-three women were graduated, thereafter rendering varying amounts of service to the trainer institution. The program was suspended at Walter Reed on December 8, 1945.

A percentage of U.S. Cadet Nurse Corps students, educated in civilian hospitals and at federal expense, could elect their last six months of senior cadet training in certain approved Army hospitals.[22] Selection and assignment of the students was made by the Civil Service Commission. All rules and regulations affecting the conduct and training of this group were endorsed by the national nursing organizations and the Nursing Division, Office of the Surgeon General. Local administration was the direct responsibility of an educational director, usually a reserve nurse on active duty with the Army Nurse Corps, assigned to the Chief Nurse's staff. The training program was carefully supervised in order to insure eligibility for examination by the various State Boards of Nurse Examiners, and licensing. When assigned to Walter Reed, the Senior Cadet nurses were housed in Delano Hall and accorded the privileges of Army Nurse Corps personnel. In the early winter and spring of 1945, a large part of the Women's Army Corps recruiting material was directed at providing medical and surgical technicians for Army hospitals, to obviate an anticipated shortage of nurses when the peak of the casualty load was evacuated from Europe. The women were recruited for and organized into hospital companies of one hundred women and one officer. Unlike the enlisted men, they were accorded specific ratings as a means of encouraging enlistments. The 92nd WAC Hospital Company was assigned to Walter Reed but inactivated December 26, 1945, with the personnel transferred to the 9901st Technical Service Unit (TSU), for men and women, in operation at the Post since June 29. Some of the residual morale problems which affected the early assignment of WAC to general duty had begun to subside, but the favoritism of special ratings for women who were performing the same functional duties as the corpsmen or male medical and surgical technicians, aggravated old grievances.

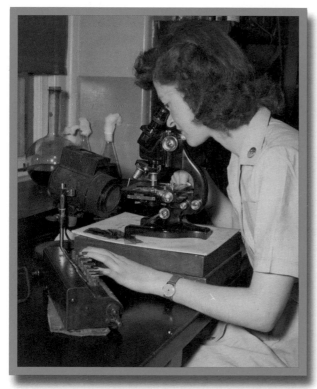

Further, during the spring of 1945 there was some competition for recognition between the female technicians and the volunteer nurses' aides,[23] as the latter were accorded some Post courtesies not available to the uniformed group, such as limited use of the Officers' Club, by then established in the building surrounding the Rea swimming pool. Thus whether in uniform or out, the individual's need for recognition affected the group attitude. If the Colonel's lady and Rosie O'Grady were, as Kipling said, "sisters under the skin," morale problems for men and women were also very much alike.

WAC Laboratory Technician

Technical Activities

During the fiscal year 1944, that is from June 1943 until July 1, 1944, the size of the classes admitted to the Army Medical School, Army Veterinary School and the Enlisted Technicians' School began to decrease, the first concrete evidence that the saturation point in technically trained medical personnel had been reached. A year later curtailed induction of new personnel had affected the training programs, but in contrast, the number of casualties had increased and the demands on the Army Medical School for diagnostic biologicals and plasma had increased markedly.

In addition to the work with plasma, the *Division of Surgical Physiology*, Army Medical School, was studying new mechanisms for furnishing whole blood, both for the various overseas theaters and the Zone of Interior hospitals. Virus and ricketsial diseases, improved immunogenic substances and bacterial dysentery were still under intensive study. This work was directed by Colonel Harry Plotz, M.C., a reserve officer on extended active duty, formerly with the Pasteur Institute of Paris. Three members of *The Typhus Commission* were assigned to this section and engaged in an intensive study of typhus. The 1943 nutrition experiment was concluded, reported and another experiment of this nature was begun. By 1945, however, the food and nutrition work of the Army Medical School was grouped with Quartermaster nutrition projects under study in Chicago, Illinois.

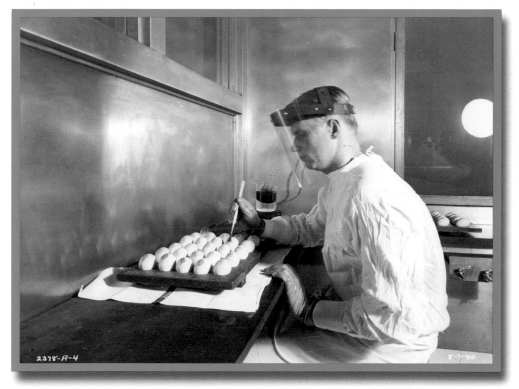

Production of Veterinary Biologicals

The organizational relationship of the various schools and departments remained the same. Housing these activities was no particular problem at this time, especially since the number of students had decreased. Personnel problems, the bane of the average production manager in any organization, continued to plague the directors of the various school programs, especially the Army Medical School. A similar complaint probably could have been advanced by many military commanders, but the director of the Army Medical School believed it most unfortunate that doctors of outstanding ability and special skills were, for promotion purposes, stymied by the T/O & E, which limited the job and grade. General Callender was especially sensitive to the fact that "men of outstanding ability, chiefs of sections and divisions, continue in company grades[24] (at) times instructing in the various classes their students of only a few years ago, now often at least two grades their senior in military rank."[25]

In the latter part of August 1943, the Civil Affairs Division (War Department administration) requested and was furnished 32,000,000 cc of typhoid vaccine of which only

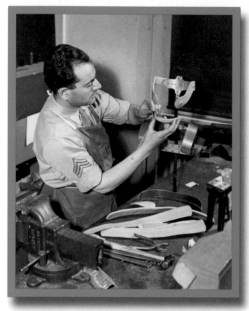

2,000,000 units was used by April 1944. In the meantime, UNRRA estimated a need for 100,000,000 cc of typhoid vaccine but actually made few requisitions. Thus a backlog or stockpile of vaccine was accumulated which provided some opportunity for temporary limited production of these items.

The *Tropical and Military Medicine* course had been especially popular with students from other governments, such as Canada, and staff members of both CAD and UNRRA, but by 1945, with the end of the war in sight, there was a marked decrease in such attendance. Such was not the case with seventy-five year old Dr. Mary F. Cushman, formerly a medical missionary in Angola, Portuguese West Africa, who was anxious to return to her former station despite the limitation of age.[26]

Skilled Worker in the Orthopedic Brace Shop, WRAH

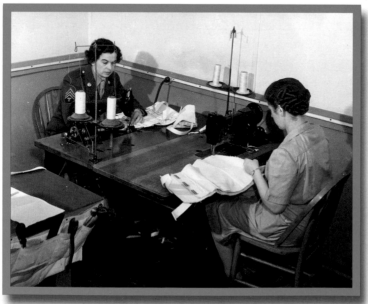

In addition to teaching functions, officers of the *Division of Parasitology* furnished large amounts of teaching material to practically all the medical schools in the United States and Canada and to public health and diagnostic laboratories throughout the United States. The routine work of the *Central Medical*

Skilled Workers in the Orthopedic Brace Shop, WRAH

Department Board and the examination of a large number of candidates for the United States military academy was, in part, accomplished by the staff of the Army Medical School and in addition to routine activities. As noted, refresher courses, terminated at the end of the fiscal year, were reestablished on a smaller scale as applicatory courses at Walter Reed General Hospital and administered from that institution.

The *Division of Pharmacy*, MD PSS, operated the pharmacy in addition to routine activities. The training course for pharmacy technicians, temporarily suspended in the fiscal year 1944, was reactivated on September 8, 1944 and continued until December 2.

In March 1944, the work in Plastic and Maxillo-facial surgery was transferred from Walter Reed Hospital to other Army installations, while the specialized experimental work at the MD PSS was terminated on March 31.

During 1944, the Army Veterinary School, under the direction of Colonel Raymond Randall, V.C., isolated for the first time in this area (eastern United States) the Venezuelan strain of equine encephalomyelitis virus, thus proving that the "disease occurs in man, producing a fatal infection." The production of Veterinary biologicals, research, food bacteriology and the examination of meat and food products continued to place a heavy load on the Army Veterinary School. The Army Dental School and Central Dental Laboratory continued their usual joint activities during this period but on an enlarged scale.

The *Medical Department Enlisted Technicians' School* continued until March 31, 1945.[27] The quota in medical, surgical, laboratory and dental technicians increased in July 1944, but the allotments of students to the various courses varied from month to month. As might have been expected, many of the more able young men of the country responded to early recruiting pleas; thus during the latter part of the intensified training program, School authorities noticed a drop in quality of student material from the standpoint of scholarship, interest and personalities. With the exception of trainees as orthopedic mechanics and electro-encephalographic technicians, the classes for Veterinary, Medical, Dental, Medical Laboratory, and Surgical technicians ceased after November 1944.[28] "Reduction of personnel incident to closing of the School began in November 1944 and was completed by the end of March 1945."[29] Thus it was obvious to military strategists and planners that the war was nearly over.

The Crest of the Wave

The largest number of patients admitted to Walter Reed during World War I occurred in 1918, when 13,752 men were treated. The largest number during the entire history of the hospital, 18,046 patients, was admitted in 1943, the third year of the Marietta administration. All administrative and professional problems were, therefore, magnified, and staffing the hospital became extremely difficult. One of the important but little discussed functions of the military hospital commander concerns public relations. Inasmuch as the hospital is a public service, the spread of interest manifest in such activities extends from the patient and his family to Congressional levels. Interested Congressmen, high ranking government officials, distinguished foreigners, newspaper

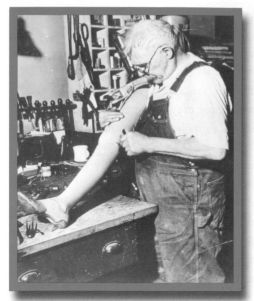

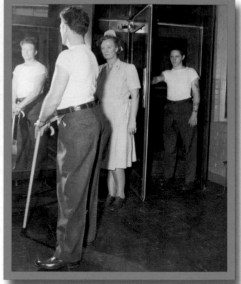

The Wounded Walk

Under His Own Power Again

columnists, periodical writers and nationally known entertainers visit the institution and must be accorded courtesy and provided with information. While such duties are an occasional responsibility in peacetime, they occurred with more frequency during the period of mobilization.

In addition to such "extra-curricular" affairs, administration and personnel management are time-consuming. Many of the patients were careless in their use of hospital facilities, creating manifold management problems. Further, the magnitude of government operations, and of the military hospitalization program, defied the understanding of many of the reserve officers or newly commissioned doctors, and many were impatient with what they believed to be unnecessary military "red tape," restrictions of their personal and professional liberties and independence of action. Some doctors found it difficult to accept and work with unfamiliar but standard items of medical supply rather than items of their own choosing. Personnel, both patients and staff, were made lonely and unhappy by involuntary separation from their families because of the acute housing problem in Washington.

As an attempt to prepare partially for the time when the Army of the United States would shrink in size and the splendid service of many distinguished civilian doctors would be lost to public service, in January 1945, a program of *Professional Refresher Training* for Regular Army doctors was established. The training was designed to restore professional confidence and familiarize medical officers serving in command or administrative positions for twelve months or longer with recent advances in medicine. By the end of 1945, eighteen officers had been assigned for refresher training in the usual specialties. Such preparation was a forerunner of an intensive professional training program, as for the fourth time in less than a hundred years some concepts of military medicine requirements for military surgeons would change.

The first change had occurred after the Civil War, when a more complete form of organization was of interest to medical planners, and as the rudiments of a public health and preventative medicine program followed the scientific awakening of the eighties. The second change occurred after the Spanish-American War, the end of an era of frontier doctors and saddle-bag medicine. An improved field medical service and the more complete militarization of the Army doctor characterized the twenty-year period following the investigation by the Dodge Commission. The Army Reorganization Bill of 1908, which provided an increase in pay and grades for medical officers, was hailed as a sure answer to the personnel procurement problems of the period. The third period, following World War I, was characterized by phenomenal growth in the general hospital program. The Medical Department was by then so large that the training program was divided into three distinct parts: the field medical training, given at Medical Field Service School, Carlisle, Pennsylvania; the laboratory training given at the Army Medical School; and the residency and specialized training for practitioners, given at the general hospitals.

As Medical Department programs broadened, in proportion to size and requirements of the Army, the three elements developed distinctive ideologies. As the philosophy of the medical profession began to change in favor of specialization, in the late thirties, so the philosophy of the Army Medical Department began to change, but less noticeably until encouraged by the complex social, political and economic changes of the World War II period and the closer contact with civilian medicine. Great emphasis was placed on the term "professional," used loosely to identify those doctors engaged only in the clinical care of the sick. The editor of *The Military Surgeon* had noted an impending change in 1910 and forewarned that "the man who thinks his whole duty is done when he treats the sick is mistaken."[30]

References

1. Capt. A.G. Wilde, Army Medical Records, *The Military Surgeon*, Vol. XXXIX, 1916, pg 591.

2. Annual Rpt., WRGH, 1944.

3. *Ibid.*

4. Lt. Colonel Nicholes Senn, *Medico-Surgical Aspects of the Spanish-American War*, Chicago, American Medical Association, 1900, pg 81.

5. Brigadier General Elliot Duncan Cooke, *All But Me and Thee*, Psychiatry at the Foxhole Level, Washington, Infantry Journal Press, ca 1946.

6. Annual Rpt., WRGH, 1944.

7. *Ibid*, 1945, pg 16.

8. Service Stripe, June 14, 1947; widowed during the thirties, on her retirement in June 1947, Mrs. Sommers returned to her home in Copenhagen, Denmark, where she ultimately married a childhood sweetheart, by then Denmark's leading tenor. Her life for the next ten years and until his death in 1949, was like the story of a modern Cinderella, for she moved in "high places" and attended festivals where her husband sang for the King. Ltr. from Mrs. Emmy Sommers to Miss Mary E. Schick, Nov. 21, 1950. On file, Library, WRAH.

9. Annual Rpt, WRGH, 1944; Interview, Major General Shelley U. Marietta, M.C., Ret., May 16, 1951.

10. *Ibid*.

11. Florence A. Blanchfield, *Organized Nursing and the Army in Three Wars*, on file Historical Division, SGO.

12. Annual Rpt. WRGH, 1945.

13. *Service Stripe*, July 6, 1946.

14. *Service Stripe*, April 28, 1945 (President Truman Visits Patients).

15. *Ibid*, April 21, 1945.

16. *Ibid*, August 11, 1945.

17. Known as Armed Forces Institute in 1943 and was very small; renamed in April 1945 and expanded.

18. Annual Rpt., WRGH, 1945.

19. Memo to CG, SOS, from John A. Rogers, Col., M.C., Exec. Officer, (for TSG) Subject: Nurses' Aides. Dec. 8, 1942, File 321 (Nurses Aides) SGO Record Room (O); 1st Ind. to above, Dec. 12, 1942.

20. Ltr. from Mrs. Walter Lippman, (Nat'l Dir. RCNA) to ARC representatives. Subject: Training Nurses Aides in Army Hospitals, March 29, 1943. File *Nurses Aides*, ANC, SGO.

21. See Nurses Aide files, Archives, ANRC.

22. PL 74, 78th Congress, June 15, 1943.

23. Blanchfield, *op cit*.

24. Captain or below.

25. Rpt. of Technical Activities MD FBS, AMC, FY 1944, Sect. I, on file, Office of the Commandant.

26. *Service Stripe*, June 16, 1945.

27.	Annual Rpt. MD PSS, FY ending June 30, 1945, Sect. V, on file, Office of the Commandant.

28.	Directed by the Training Division, SGO.

29.	*Ibid*, pg 2.

30.	*Military Surgeon*, Feb. 1910, pg 375.

Fragmentary Discussions

1946–1951

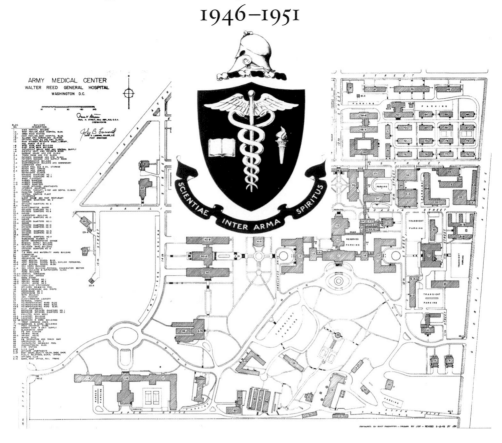

"The secret of success and the course of failure lie in the mental attitude which medical officers assume as individuals; that is, whether they elect to be in the Army or attached to it."[1]

Brigadier General George C. Beach[2] succeeded General Marietta as Post Commander on February 16, 1945, although the latter continued to make regular professional visits to the hospital to attend his old patient, George Pershing. Commissioned in the Medical Reserve Corps on September 15, 1911, and as a First Lieutenant on February 7, 1917, the greater part of General Beach's military service had been on Army posts[3] but the assignment to Washington was a return to the city where he had been attending surgeon and essentially the family doctor to a large contingent of Army personnel from 1926 to 1930. It was during these years that he became acquainted with many of the line and staff officers who later assumed positions of leadership and influence during and after World War II.

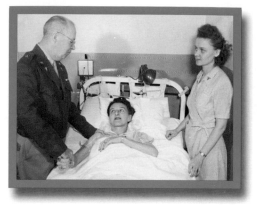

Brig. Gen. George C. Beach

His previous experience as commanding officer at the Brooke General Hospital, Fort Sam Houston, Texas, had provided him with a thorough knowledge of hospital administration, but General Beach was not of the militant executive type who attempts personally to regulate the infinite details required in directing so large an institution. Unlike "Noisy Jim" Glennan, who wandered restlessly about the building and grounds, or General De Witt, who prowled ceaselessly, his inquisitive fingers ever searching for a stray bit of dust and who, in spite of frequent attacks of gout, climbed nimbly on chairs or stooped to look under beds for the persistent invader, General Beach held his staff strictly accountable for the managerial housekeeping duties. It was therefore at the morning coffee hour that his carefully selected and highly competent assistants briefed him on daily problems, receiving, in turn, his wise counsel and guidance, his official sanction or disapproval of proposed actions or current problems. He was a gentle, lovable and understanding man, and his staff became a closely integrated "team", one that worked for him personally as much as for the professional management problems which were, in the final sense, his special responsibility.

He was pleasantly gregarious without being effusive, liked dogs, horse racing and hot spicy foods.[4] At some undated period in his career, friends of the Beach family substituted the names "Sandy" and "Coral" for the more orthodox names of George and Jessie, and as such General and Mrs. Beach were affectionately and better known to their many Army friends. Time and frequent usage converted "Sandy" to Sam, the name by which the quiet, kindly physician was usually addressed. Ward visiting and hospital inspection trips were customary routines for Army hospital commanders, but "Sam" Beach added a personal touch to such visits which did a great deal to overcome some patients' opinions that the visits were a routine and official inquiry. Daily he visited the seriously ill, and he never forsook the comforting habit of approaching the patient's bedside counting the pulse or otherwise bringing to the ill a recognition of his personal interest and professional competence.

The Army Medical Center and its best-known activity, Walter Reed General Hospital in particular, has passed through the busiest period of its history. The Obstetrical Service delivered almost one hundred infants monthly in 1945,[5] and the Quartermaster Laundry serviced enough separate items to serve a city of 7,000.[6] The Out-Patient Service maintained its reputation for being a hectically busy place in 1945; in 1946, 99,473 treatments were given, of which 13,915 were on military personnel. The service was still handicapped by the lack of continuity in personnel.

It was, therefore, principally through the effects of key civilians that established policies were maintained.[7]

All of the hospital and school buildings showed considerably more than the normal wear and tear of daily use, and they were, like some of the patients, in rather obvious need of repair and rehabilitation. Although apparently prescribed by enthusiastic and influential lay friends of the hospital familiar with the modern trends in institutional deco-

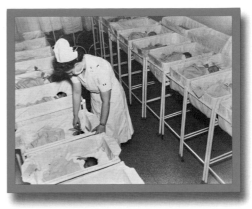

Nursery, 1950

rating, the two-toned paint scheme used in the halls and bedrooms of the hospital[8] was attributed to the wartime matériel shortage. The contrasting sections were separated by dado, object of some local criticism, but the results were profoundly satisfactory to the planners, who defended the pastels as more serviceable than the previously traditionally-used Army creme or tan color used throughout the hospital.

Washington, DC, was, during the war, ripe with fantastic and sometimes amusing tales of the misuse of public buildings by newly imported personnel unaccustomed to modern conveniences. Such rumors were not solely applicable to civilian buildings, for Walter Reed showed many evidences that the restless youths of World War II had less awareness of the costs of maintaining federal property than was desirable. Therefore, in spite of a seventy-five per cent turnover in employees, it was well that the decrease from some 16,000 patients in 1945 to slightly more than 12,000 in 1946 gave the command some opportunity to begin restorations.

At the beginning of the year 1946, the Detachment of Patients was responsible for the discipline as well as the personnel administration of all enlisted patients, and its activities were soon extended to include officers as well.[9] War Department Circular 215, 1946, authorized a one-grade promotion for all patients hospitalized for eighteen months as a result of combat wounds and who had received no promotion since being wounded. This policy increased the recordkeeping for the Detachment office, whose functional departments included payroll and allotments, records, assignment, classification, discharge, relief from active duty, retirement, courts-martial, disposition, decorations and awards, patients' funds, supplies, and the patient's baggage room.

As noted, Class III, ambulatory patients, attended the various occupational therapy activities, but Class IV, ward patients, had a special training program. All patients were interviewed, counseled and introduced to the Educational Reconditioning Program. Some took the USAFI courses and a few initiated college extension courses, but in all cases their records must be kept up to date.

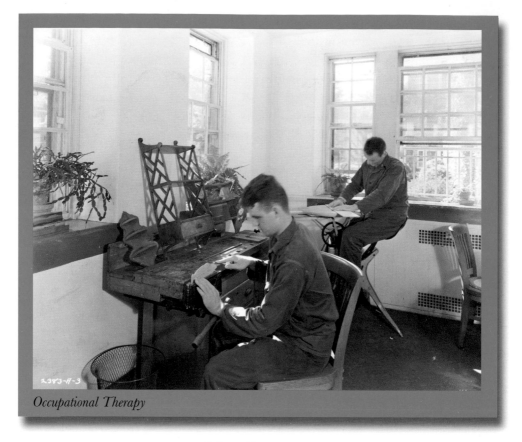

Occupational Therapy

New Patterns

The accelerated occupational therapy training course, which started in November, 1944, was terminated in April 1946.[10] In addition to this program, ninety-three volunteer workers in the Red Cross Arts and Skills Section worked with an average of 306 patients each month and gave a total of 7,649 hours in volunteer service during the year. A year later, from May 8 to 14, 1947, one hundred twenty-three volunteer workers in the *Arts and Skills Section* gave approximately 10,627 hours of time to hospital patients. This was a remarkable record, for many patients were restless and uninterested in crafts after V-J Day, wanting only to be on their way while the civilian employment situation was favorable.

In August, Walter Reed General Hospital became a center for Aural Rehabilitation,[11] with all the hearing cases from the temporary war service Borden, DeShon and Hoff General Hospitals concentrated at the Forest Glen Section. Construction delays necessitated an improvised program until October, at which time sections in lipreading instruction, speech correction and conservation, counseling, an ear mold laboratory, a hearing-aid laboratory, audiometry and otology laboratories were established.

A *Hospital Inspector's Office* was re-established as a separate and integral part of the hospital organization, utilizing the services of one officer, two Warrant Officers, one non-commissioned officer and a civilian secretary. The Hospital Inspector had varied duties and responsibilities, then including those of Training Officer. Over 300 inspections were made during the year, and all sections of the hospital were inspected at least once daily. This constant sanitary vigilance, combined with the reduced patient load, improved the cleanliness and general appearance of the hospital. Further, routine interviews were conducted with ward patients, and clinical records were checked with a view to determining the best physical, mental and moral well-being of the patients. Routine checks were made of the narcotics register, and precious and semi-precious metals were checked for their issue in the medical supply depot, through the Pharmacy and to the wards. Thus monthly auditing of these records and the Patients' Fund made the position of *Hospital Inspector* one of responsibility as well as one of infinite assistance to the Post Commander. Conscientious attempts were made to speed the discharge and disposition of all patients. This was an intricate and time-consuming process even in peacetime, but it was psychologically as well as administratively involved under the Army point system, for many patients with an insufficient number of points still believed themselves entitled to special consideration.

Insofar as permanent buildings were concerned, there was no new construction undertaken at Walter Reed during the year. There was, however, extensive renovation and modernizing of interiors, and a great deal of refurbishing. Ward 11B, on the third floor of the Main Building and proximal to the operating room, was completed as a new *Recovery Room* in February 1947. The arrangement provided three main sections, each with a nurse's station and two, three, four and five-bed units. In June 1947, Ward 8, the *Officers' Surgical Ward* on the third floor of the east wing, was converted into a luxurious *Presidential Suite*, the administration of which was placed under the direction of the Chief of the Medical Service. In the Army Medical School building the Central Dental Laboratory was reworked and improved equipment was added.

On November 15, 1947, the position of Deputy Post Commander was authorized as a result of provisions of the Officer Personnel Act of that year, (Sec.522, PL 381, 80th Congress, Officer Personnel Act of 1947, app. Aug. 7, 1947) and the position was filled by Colonel Clifford V. Morgan, Medical Corps, then Executive Officer of the Army Medical Center. It had long been the custom to have the second ranking medical officer assume command of the organization in the absence of the Post Commander. This arrangement was considered by many to be the administrative anomaly, inasmuch as the incumbent might have been continuously engaged in professional activities and thereby unfamiliar with the administrative activities of such a complicated command. Under the new arrangement the Commanding General was able to devote the greater part of his time to hospital activities and professional training programs which were Class II medical activities supervised by the Surgeon General's Office. In contrast the Center activities were Class I,

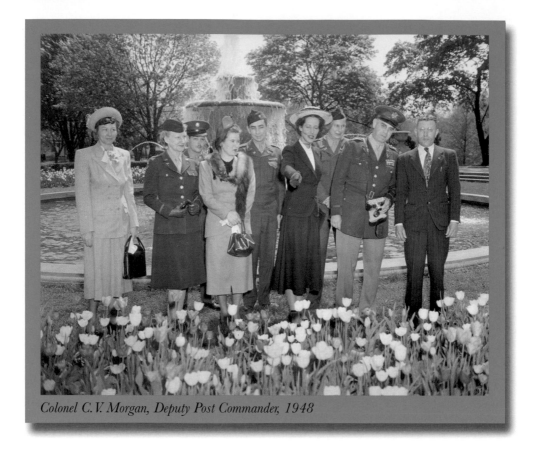

Colonel C. V. Morgan, Deputy Post Commander, 1948

or so-called housekeeping activities, with close administrative ties to the Military District of Washington. By the summer of 1948 Colonel Morgan was so thoroughly familiar with the current as well as the past needs of the Post that he offered the use of official records, historical photographs and old building plans further to facilitate completion of the slowly developing history "Borden's Dream," so long advocated by the Post librarian and already under way as a private project.

Likewise in November 1947, Lieutenant Colonel Ida W. Danielson, Army Nurse Corps, formerly Chief Nurse of the European Theater of Operations, succeeded Lieutenant Colonel Gertrude Thompson as Chief Nurse. Colonel Danielson came to the new assignment from a tour of duty in the Personnel Division of the Office of the Surgeon General. Insofar as administrative preparation for this assignment was concerned, she had a more varied background of administrative experience than any other Chief Nurse previously assigned to the staff of Walter Reed General Hospital. Tactful, gracious, blessed with a sense of finesse and the ability to persuade others to her way of thinking, she was an immediate success with the hospital staff. In a thoroughly generous spirit of appreciation, she credited much of her success as nurse-administrator to earlier training by Miss Dora N. Thompson,

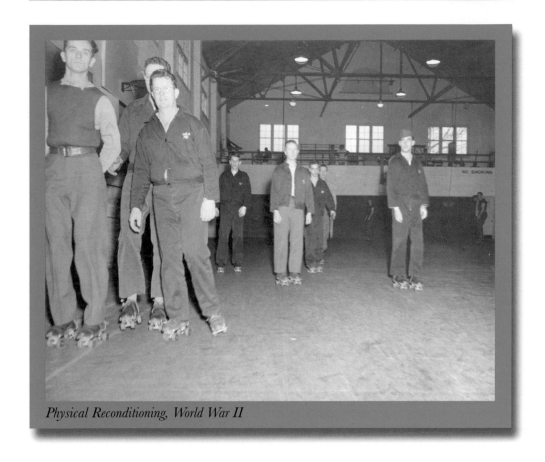

Physical Reconditioning, World War II

Superintendent of the Army Nurse Corps during World War I, and to Miss Jane Molloy, Walter Reed's first Chief Nurse.[12]

Outside Influences

Only 12,336 new patients were admitted to Walter Reed in 1947, this number being 659 less than admitted during the previous year when there were no civilian nurses on duty. At the close of the calendar year, however, there were fifty-one civilian nurses on duty in addition to the 206 Army Nurses. The point-release program for Army of the United States personnel affected nurses as well as doctors, and the Nursing Division, Office of the Surgeon General, believed a too-rapid demobilization was responsible for some of the personnel problems which developed a year later.[13] Certainly, the rapid turn-over in personnel was difficult for all concerned. National nursing policy groups strongly supported the principle that nurses should not engage in non-professional duties, and although the general ratio of employees to patients was high, some aspects of the local nurse shortage could be attributed to the change to the eight-hour schedule. Further, an increased amount of nursing time was required in the supervision of cooperative ward procedures, ward rounds and the orientation instruction of doctors on duty with the residency training program.

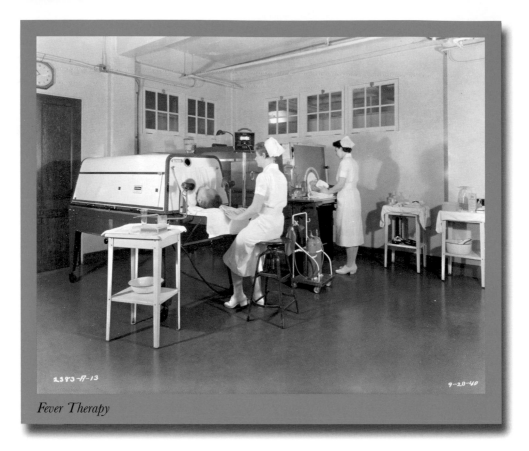

2383-A-13   9-20-48

Fever Therapy

Some minor intra-service reorganizations were accomplished during 1948, but none which affected the primary function, patient care. The personnel situation was more unstable than desirable, for the staff was preponderantly residents and internes, with only a few duty-officers for key assignments. This was undoubtedly a necessary arrangement, in order to conform to the ultimate objective of the Medical Department professional training program. Nevertheless, many patients both in the Out-Patient Service and in the wards found the interruption to the traditional doctor-patient relationship more exasperating than otherwise.[14]

It would have been extremely difficult, prior to World War II, to find many medical officers critical of their Corps, its objectives or the quality of professional care provided for the Army as a whole. Some medical officers, particularly the specialists, took periodic refresher courses at the Mayo Clinic, the Johns Hopkins Hospital and other great civilian training institutions, either at their own or at Government expense. The three principal branches of military medicine – professional field and supply – provided definite training programs, and the average medical officer had more than an even chance of selecting and remaining in his preferred specialty. On the whole the morale was good, and if the system of promotion by seniority penalized an impatient few, it nevertheless provided a sound and equable base for the many who contributed the usual thirty "best

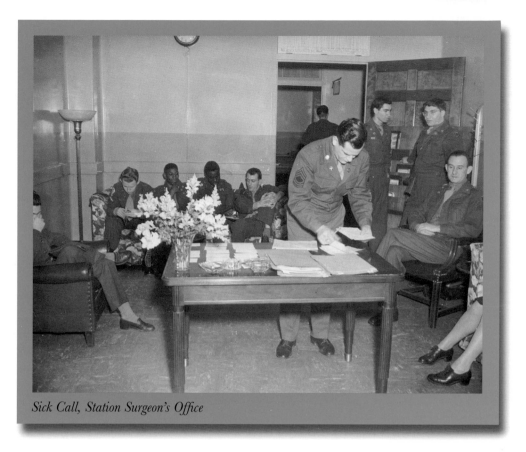

Sick Call, Station Surgeon's Office

years of their lives" to public service. In general special ability was recognized, and if there were an insufficient number of spectacular rewards for all, the respect of brother officers was pleasant balm.

The Army, at least, recognized that a special type of personality was required for military duty – men and women willing to uproot their homes without protest, willing to school their children in Alabama or New York, Virginia or Wyoming, Alaska or the Philippines, sometimes in four or five states in the course of a few years. The "Service" made many demands and offered few visible rewards except superior hospitalization and, on retirement, a modest income. On the whole, however, Regular Army personnel liked their way of life, and the majority were loyal, adaptable and satisfied.[15] Many, like Surgeon General Patterson,[16] preferred to specialize, but when they found the exigencies of the Service required a change to administration, the functional transition was usually accepted with good grace.[17] Thus as one Surgeon General noted in an Annual Report, "we should have (in the service) only such men as are adapted to its peculiar requirements."

It is surprising, therefore, that when Secretary of War Robert Patterson delivered a prepared address to the American Medical Association in June 1947, there was included for his pronouncement a statement that "Ever since the medical profession became officially associated with the Army more than 170 years ago...it has been evident that something was wrong, something was irritating the medical officer." As noted, the Medical Department of the World War II period was essentially a civilian organization, and the Medical Department officers were civilian physicians temporarily uprooted from the private practice of medicine. They were, by and large, men unaccustomed to group activity, to regimentation and to the necessity of conforming to the management policies of a large organization charged with the responsibility of meeting the needs of thousands rather than a few. It must be assumed, therefore, that the maladjustments of some World War II personnel had colored the publicly expressed opinion that complaints were due to uncertainty and dissatisfaction over an inability to practice the profession in a manner professionally satisfying,[18] i.e., clinical care of the inpatient. Such a viewpoint, doubtless would have surprised such loyal old soldiers as Hoff, McCaw, Straub, Birmingham, Arthur and Kean, who devoted their lives to the Medical Department and believed that on the whole, "across the board," in peace or in war, it gave the best medical service in the United States, perhaps in the world, as the American standard of living was notably high.

Not all local management problems were confined to the uniformed group, and the various Post Commanders would have been at a loss without the continuing and loyal

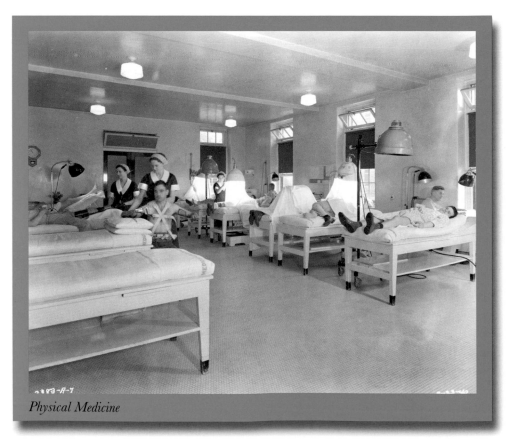

Physical Medicine

support of key civilian employees. By 1948, fifty-seven civilian employees had twelve or more years of continuous service and of this number twelve were employed before 1925. Concurrently, the *Civilian Personnel Section* of the Army Medical Center headquarters contended that more than 3,100 military and civilian persons were needed to carry out the functions of the installation,[19] which, with the addition of the usual 1600 patients, made the military reservation essentially a little city.

Many devotees of so-called scientific personnel management had appeared during the previous ten years, and such terms as "human relations", "human understanding" and the "human equation" were discussed as training agencies attempted to bring management and the worker closer together. The Adjutant General's Department had, during the war, sponsored special courses, including instruction for supervisors, and the stupendously large employment program of that period left an imprint on all government personnel agencies.

The "human relations" aspect of personnel management was, of course, essentially the consideration of the individual as a case, with his adjustment problems highlighted by a study of the social background. It was an old and simple game to the family physician, priest or lawyer, who had long employed the technique but failed to underwrite a specific nomenclature. As there was a very real need for this type of program in any

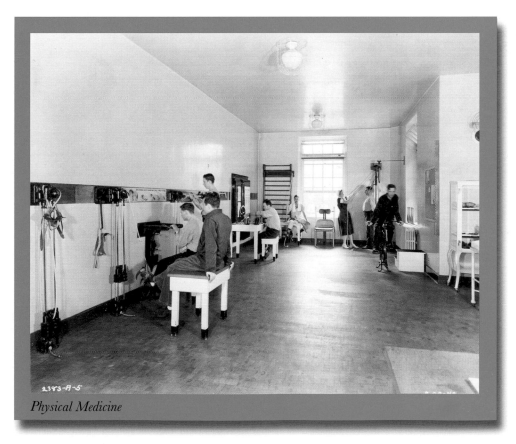

Physical Medicine

large and impersonal organization where some unnoticed "square pegs" could rattle unhappily in the "round holes", the *Personnel Section* at the Army Medical Center was divided into two principal departments. The *Military Section* was redivided into officer and enlisted, and the *Civilian Personnel Section* was divided into four principal sub-sections, which then required a staff of only thirty-nine persons to serve the 1,251 civilian employees of the Army Medical Center.

Fundamental Reorganization

General hospitals were transferred from the jurisdiction of the Service Command back to the Surgeon General in April 1946. On 11 June the War Department was reorganized; the nine Army Service Commands were abolished and six Army areas were created.[20]

In June 1946, the Surgeon General, Major General Norman T. Kirk, proposed establishing a 1,000-bed pathological hospital and a 250,000 volume library at the Forest Glen Section, Army Medical Center, to be operated in connection with the Army Medical Museum, renamed Army Institute of Pathology and still later the Armed Forces Institute of Pathology. Further, the Surgeon General proposed that an Institute of Research Medicine, Dentistry, Surgery, Radiation Therapy and a school of global medicine be incorporated as part of the new plan.[21]

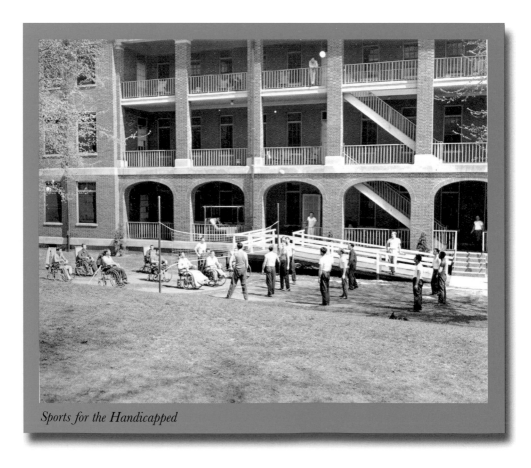

Sports for the Handicapped

Many of the doctors who served in the Army during World War II were extremely interested, for various public-spirited reasons, in the post-war Medical Department. The shortage of health workers, including doctors and nurses, had harassed the constantly expanding community medical services all during the war, and many national program planners had come to believe that an equable division of such personnel was not only practical but imperative in the event of another war. The training of doctors and nurses was a slow and costly business, and the nation could ill afford to waste their services. Some doctors, nationally known as specialists and board members, were interested in increasing the academic training and board membership of Army doctors to meet the more competitive requirements of civilian communities; some had a special interest in excluding doctors from administrative positions; some were interested in closer identification of the military and naval services in order to provide more economical use of professional skills, standardization of material and to provide a roster of inter-changeable personnel, the joint use of hospital facilities, etc. Some of these proposals grew out of dissatisfaction expressed by the Directing Board of the Procurement and Assignment Service for Doctors, Dentists, Veterinarians and Nurses, operative during World War II.[22]

With no immediate signs of hostilities in sight, the professional training and proper utilization of doctors were probably of more general interest to the average civilian than procurement of personnel. Consequently, one of the most overt signs of plans for a constructive program was the early post-war formation of *The Society of United States Medical Consultants of World War II*, which met at the Army Medical Center on October 18, 1946.[23] The consultants were former medical officers, by then returned to civilian life, and the group included many of the leading doctors in specialized fields.

Various plans were considered by both military and civilian groups which it was believed would please all concerned, and on April 18, 1947, General Kirk proposed a merger of the Army and Navy Medical Departments,[24] with a director chosen from the senior officers of the regular Medical Corps. He believed such an organization could be charged with operation of a common hospitalization program for the Armed Forces, preventative medicine services, vital statistics, etc. Further, he believed a common research program was feasible, with joint clinical and research laboratories, joint utilization of *The Army Medical Library* and *The Army Institute of Pathology*.

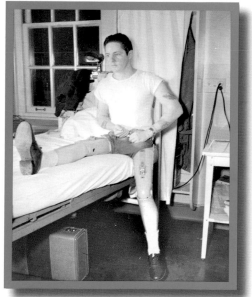

The Dignity of Man

The Training Program

Colonel Rufus Holt, Medical Corps, succeeded General Callender as Commandant of the School in 1946, thereby inheriting a difficult assignment at one of the most critical periods in the professional history of the Medical Department. A reorganization of the School program was then under study which would materially strengthen the technical training of all personnel categories, including a return to the twelve-month training for enlisted technicians, and the often-repeated recommendation that the enlisted men should be accorded technical grades on completion of the course.[25]

At the hospital, the *Peripheral Vascular Section* became a separate section on July 1, 1946, and *Radiology* and the *Radiation Therapy Section* were combined to form an independent *Radiological Service*. On May 1, the *Practice of Hospital Pediatricians* was established by Walter Reed (local administration) orders, with the annual report of the Medical Service for that year carrying its first full report of *Pediatrics* as a separate section, and a fifteen per cent increase in patients was noted.[26] Specialty sections in *Dermatology, Childrens' Orthopedics, Anesthesiology* and *Psychology* likewise appeared.

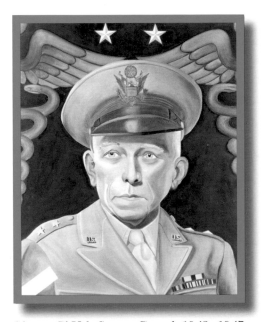

Norman T. Kirk, Surgeon General, 1943–1947. Photograph of watercolor painting made by patient in the Neuropsychiatric Section.

Practical training for civilian mess attendants was begun at the hospital in July 1946, under the direction of the Chief of the Dietetic Service. Further, technical training for enlisted men, previously conducted for eight weeks at Camp Atterbury, Indiana, or Ft. Sam Houston, Texas, was undertaken at Walter Reed. The men were supervised by the ward master, a sergeant or other non-commissioned officers, and the ward nurse. The ward doctor of the particular ward was named as the *Training Officer* for that specialty. In February 1947 the Surgeon General's Office authorized an anesthesia course for Regular Army nurses, and two special thirteen-month courses in anesthesia were offered in addition to a course in ward administration for which thirty nurses registered.

The early post-war refresher courses, such as the twenty-six-week course in tropical and global medicine, clinical pathology, and advanced Veterinary and Dental courses had proven insufficient to prepare Medical Corps officers to meet the professional requirements for civilian academic honors and board certification in some specialties. Insofar as man-hours could be evaluated, the staff of the various Schools were, in 1946, spending approximately five per cent of the time in administration; thirty-five per cent in diagnostic and routine laboratory procedures; twenty-five per cent on research and development; twenty-five per cent in production (biological, etc.) and ten per cent in instruction.[27] Additional instruction was contributed by civilian consultants and by military personnel of the Military District of Washington.

After one full year of experimentation with the refresher training program, General Beach noted some inherent difficulties such as haphazard presentation of teaching material and the tendency of the hospital staff to view consultants as "problem solvers" rather than as visiting teachers. The shortcomings, he believed, were not due to the system but rather to the individuals. He therefore favored affiliation with the medical schools of George Washington and Georgetown Universities as a smooth and easy way of weeding out some undesirable consultants as well as to secure better supervision and broader clinical facilities for the students, internes and selected residents.

Early in the twentieth century Jefferson Randolph Kean had noted the growing tendency of Medical Department critics, usually line and staff officers, to devalue the activities of Army doctors dissociated from the direct care of the sick, confiding to his diary that "at the time the prejudice was very strong against doctors holding any administrative position."[28] If reversed his observations could have been as timely in

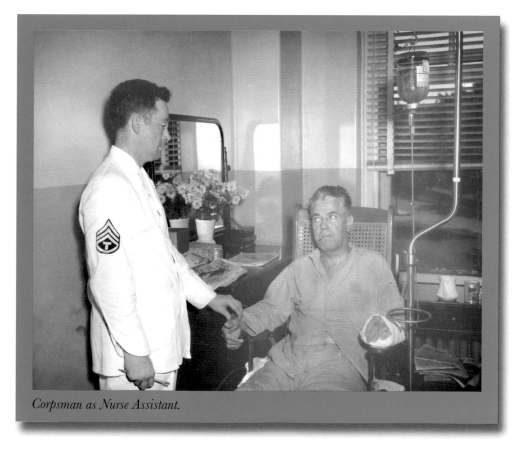

Corpsman as Nurse Assistant.

the post-World War II period as in the post-Spanish-American War period. In fact the degree of prejudice had increased markedly in the interviewing fifty years, although the criticisms now originated primarily from American physicians and from some of the smaller groups of allied health workers anxious to broaden their own fields of managerial responsibility. Thus as a result of the much touted prestige incidental to certification as a "Board Member," the post-World War II demands of Army doctors for advanced clinical training was reminiscent of the professional stampede of a half-century before, when doctors began abandoning their professional for military titles, unmindful, perhaps, of the maxim of Theodore Roosevelt that as military men they must "supplement in (their) calling the work of the surgeon with the work of the administrator."

The proposed teaching program was, therefore, of more-than-to-be expected significance, for it was destined to reshape some classic concepts of military medical preparedness. There was considerable talk of paying recognized specialists an emolument in addition to their Regular Army pay, and the possibility of such an inequity made many of the doctors anxious and uncertain regarding their future careers. A large number of the World War II Army Specialized Training Program (ASTP) graduates in medicine, with little or no practical clinical training, then were replacing experienced Army of the United States personnel eligible for separation, but few of these young men showed interest in Regular Army commissions and by and large they could think of no special changes in the Medical Department which would influence them to apply.[29] Many, reflecting both the dissatisfactions of some World War II personnel as well as the new philosophy of specialization and seemed to believe that the Army emphasized the vocation of soldier to the detriment of the profession of medicine.[30] Medical Department planners looked forward with dread to the depleted personnel situation when the ASTP doctors automatically would be released from service in spite of the fact that their generally critical attitude, fundamental dislike of military duties and insistence on performance of strictly clinical duties presented real problems in meeting and staffing problems in the small station hospitals and field installations. The military medical trend, therefore, was to place administrative officers in many positions formerly occupied by doctors in order to safeguard the latter category.

Circular No. 87, Office of the Surgeon General, November 21, 1946, authorized a *Basic Science* course in anatomy, physiology, bacteriology, biochemistry and pharmacology as part of the residency training program for Regular Army officers then being implemented for the Army Medical Department by hospital staffs. At the Army Medical Center, the

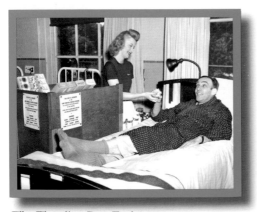

The Traveling Post Exchange

School faculty was charged with the responsibility of organizing the course. Because of the shortage of trained military instructors, the work was to be presented by civilians, selected for their wide experience in teaching, research and interest in postgraduate medical education. In order to correlate the academic and the clinical, the Director of the Basic Science course was designated *Professional Training Officer* at Walter Reed General Hospital. An active education committee was also established which consisted of the Commanding General, the Executive Officer, the Training Officer, the Chiefs of the Medical, Surgical and Neuropsychiatric Service, and a permanent secretary. This was, it will be recalled, exactly the same principle and general format of the old faculty board, so long operative in the history of the Army Medical School.

In the various specialties, *Internal Medicine*, *Surgery, Radiology*, *Urology* and *Obstetrics and Gynecology* led in popularity. An attempt was made to indoctrinate the students with the functional approaches to clinical medicine rather than to provide a mere accumulation of facts. Instructors were requested to emphasize this viewpoint. In an effort to eliminate unnecessary and unproductive duplication and to insure a continuation-type of instructional thought, assistant instructors were sent to the civilian laboratories and hospitals of the various senior instructors to secure notes and outlines. The course was, therefore, basically didactic. The limited amount of time precluded the teaching of laboratory methods and all laboratory demonstrations were prepared in advance.[31] The number of civilian employees at the School increased during this period, both because of the requirements of the Basic Science Course and the increased production of Japanese encephalitis vaccine. As a result, physical facilities of the plant were strained to the utmost.[32]

A *Residency Training Program* was begun in January 1947, primarily as an improved refresher course and as a stop-gap until a more formal training program could be established on a firm basis. Some forty civilian consultants were appointed by the Secretary of War, to participate in the clinical and pathological training of first year or *assistant residents*; second year, *residents*; and third year, *senior residents*.

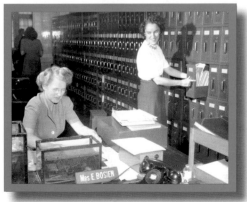

File Room, Out-Patient Service; Custodian of some 30,000 case histories

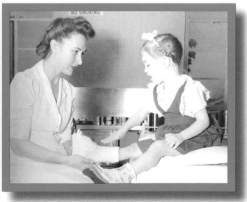

Geneva Aswell, expert orthopedic technician, 1949

The Army Medical School, Dental School and Veterinary School, regrouped as the *Medical Department Professional Service Schools* in 1934, became the *Army Medical Department Research and Graduate School* on January 10, 1947.[33] The new organization included the commandant and his assistants, directors of the three major professional divisions and, until transferred to the jurisdiction of the Army Medical Center Headquarters, on May 25, 1947, the *Photographic and Arts Unit*. Effective June 30, 1947, the Central Dental Laboratory was removed from the Dental Division of the School and placed with the Headquarters organization.[34] In 1927, Major Oscar F. Snyder, D.C., had taught operative dentistry at the Army Dental School and served as executive officer. In the summer of 1947, he returned, first as a Colonel and later as a Brigadier General, to direct all the dental activities of the Army Medical Department Research and Graduate School and the Central Dental Laboratory.[35]

In May 1947, Physiotherapy and its allied functions, at the hospital, were regrouped as *Physical Medicine*. A special training program was instituted in the early part of November 1947, in order to train ASTP officers in the fundamentals of physical therapy, occupational therapy and physical reconditioning. Military Occupational Specialty numbers (MOS numbers) had long been in effect as a means of classifying medical officers, and the Surgeon General's Office now added MOS-D-3180 to cover this new

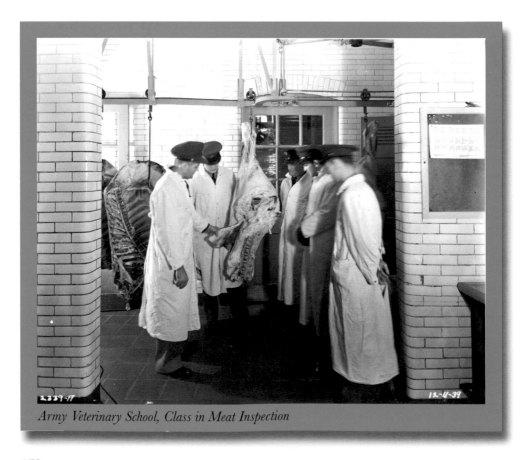

Army Veterinary School, Class in Meat Inspection

class. Dental internships began at Walter Reed July 1, 1947. Like other services, the Dental Service continued to have difficulty meeting personnel requirements, for dental technicians rarely reenlisted and dependents made a great inroad on the service.

In the last half of the calendar year 1947, eleven officers completed laboratory refresher courses varying from one to twelve weeks, and a few others had some refresher-type training before assignment to specific duties. Four enlisted men completed a twelve-week course as Veterinary Laboratory Technicians, and 352 persons, military and civilian, completed the five-day course in *The Medical Aspects of Atomic Explosion*, which was under the jurisdiction of The Army Medical Center for administration only.[36]

The Training Division and Research and Development Division of the Surgeon General's Office had not produced a reorganized school program at this time and so there were no changes in the organization of the various schools at the Center during the calendar year 1948. The atomic course was run primarily by the Surgeon General's Office; the Commandant of the Dental School was a Brigadier General and therefore senior in grade to his own superior officer, the School Commandant. Both circumstances tended to encourage a system that did not insure detailed and constant supervision of departments and sections by the commandant or his immediate assistants. As each department was under the direct supervision of at least one highly trained individual,

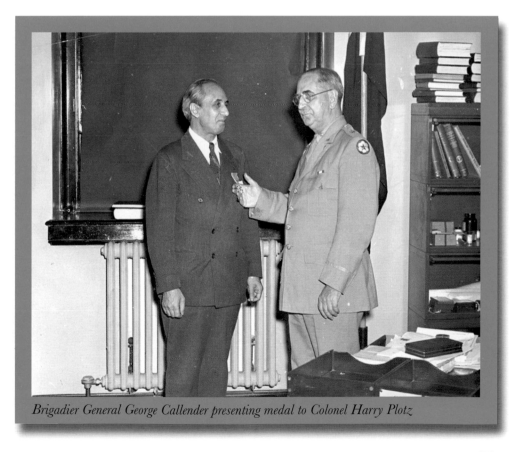

Brigadier General George Callender presenting medal to Colonel Harry Plotz

the director believed more detailed supervision would possibly be resented.[37] This was not a failure on the part of the command but rather that funds, personnel, matériel and housing were at that time insufficient for the program as envisioned.

The production of prophylactic and diagnostic biologicals varied in proportion to the size of the Army and the public health problems encountered by the Medical Department in domestic and overseas stations. It was not possible to secure all of the required biological products from civilian sources, since in many instances the commercial products failed to meet Army standards. Moreover, the *Army Medical Department Research and Graduate School* could provide some products more cheaply. The director believed, therefore, that the laboratories should serve as a pilot plant for working out commercially reproducible methods for the manufacture of new vaccines needed by the Army.[38]

An active recruiting program was under way during 1947 to provide competent civilian personnel as replacements for military personnel needed in other activities and thus insure continuing programs. As "ceilings" for civilian and military personnel are established in overhead military agencies, they are arbitrarily affected by budgetary limitations, manpower availability and/or fixed rations of personnel allowed for certain

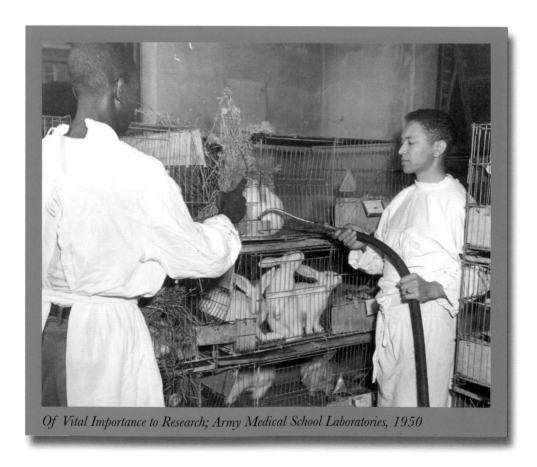

Of Vital Importance to Research; Army Medical School Laboratories, 1950

types of installations. Shortly after the recruiting program was implemented at the Army Medical Center, "the organization was again upset by the necessity of releasing about sixty civilians and immediately re-recruiting them as a result of restoration of the original ceiling on civilian employees. In spite of the inevitable frustration and confusion attendant upon such a fluctuating program,"[39] the functions of these important components of the Army Medical Center were discharged. It was, therefore, obvious to the Command that a long-range expansion plan should be developed, a plan that would provide the Medical Department in general and the Army Medical Center in particular, with a constant flow of adequately trained personnel.

Colonel Harry Plotz, Medical Corps Reserve, director of the Virus and Rickettsial work, died suddenly on February 7, 1947. His position was filled in July 1948, by Dr. Joseph Edwin Smadel, likewise a well-known civilian authority in this field.[40]

They Call It Unification

In June 1947, Surgeon General Kirk, one-time orthopedic surgeon at Walter Reed, was succeeded by Brigadier General Raymond W. Bliss, then Assistant Surgeon General but a one-time Chief of the *Obstetrical and Gynecological Section* at Walter Reed and well-known in Army groups as an able specialist in this field. Likewise in June 1947, the Office of the Secretary of Defense was created as a military structure in consonance with the provisions of the National Security Act of 1947. The War Department was replaced in name by the "Department of the Army," by General Order No. I, 1947. General Bliss therefore became Surgeon General during one of the most controversial periods in Medical Department history, for as a result of the war experiences, the encouragement of his predecessor, and the insistence of influential civilians interested in conservative and distributed use of medical personnel, there was a marked trend toward closer identification and unification of the three major services of Army, Navy and Air. As in the case of the War Department reorganization of 1942, which resulted among other changes in the formation of the Services of Supply (later known as the Army Services Forces), this was an exacting task.

As a result of acute interest in government studies, among many others, there were several actions taken in the early part of 1948 designed to facilitate unification of the medical services of the Federal Government. The first of these was the establishment by the Secretary of Defense on January 1, 1948, of an ad hoc committee known as the Committee on Medical and Hospital Services of the Armed Forces, more commonly referred to as the "Hawley" Committee (named for Maj. Gen. Paul H. Hawley, MC, ret., formerly an executive officer, AMC). This committee consisted of a civilian doctor as chairman and the Surgeons General of the Army and Navy, and the Air Surgeon, as members.

In February 1948, a committee to study Federal Medical Services was appointed and was commonly known as the "Voorhees" Committee. It was a task force of the Hoover Commission, which then was making searching studies of government functions. On

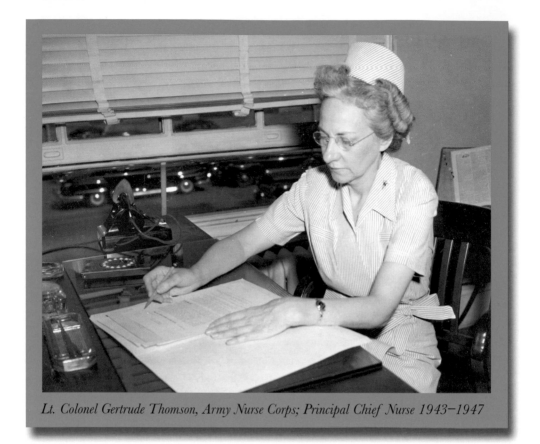

Lt. Colonel Gertrude Thomson, Army Nurse Corps; Principal Chief Nurse 1943–1947

May 21, 1948 a committee of the National Security Organization was appointed and was commonly known as the "Eberstadt" Committee. All of these committees made significant recommendations for economic reforms and reorganizations among the Federal Medical Services and especially pertaining to the military group.

In the summer of 1948 an Office of Medical Services, directed by a civilian doctor of medicine, was formed in the Office of the Secretary of Defense. In spite of the fact that such an office was first proposed by the Army Medical Department, the authority of this coordinating and policy office immediately became a controversial subject. As progress is ever painful, it is inappropriate to attempt an evaluation of its activities or its accomplishments at the operating level until sufficient time has elapsed to permit objective appraisal of its problems. The Medical Department became the *Army Medical Service* by General Order No. 23, 1950. Likewise in 1950, the Army dropped the nomenclature of general hospital, and the name *Walter Reed Army Hospital* made its appearance in the official records.

The Last Year of Reign

In September 1948, ground was broken for a Post theater, to be located near the thirty wards, on Dogwood Street. The Post Exchange, once the officers' Pavilion No. 1, during World War I, was destroyed by fire in April 1948. As a result, the

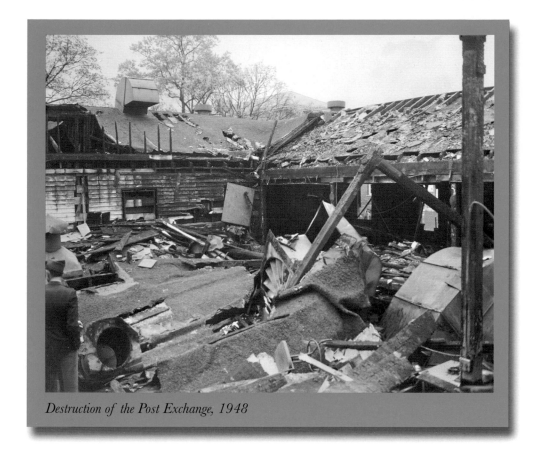

Destruction of the Post Exchange, 1948

enlisted men's game room, then occupying unsatisfactory quarters in part of the "Greenhouse Theater", on the Georgia Avenue side of the reservation, was moved to more desirable housing elsewhere. As it was necessary to provide commercial eating facilities for civilian and military employees, a snack-bar was established in the former recreation room.[41] Plans were well under way for a splendid Rehabilitation building, including gymnasium and swimming pool, and the modernization of the Officers' Club to include an air conditioned dining room. Athletic grounds for enlisted men were planned for the Forest Glen and the Main Sections, including two ball diamonds with backstops and bleachers, tennis courts and volley ball courts. In the latter case the courts erected across from the new Post Theater were constructed primarily through the kindness of a voluntary Engineer group from Fort Belvoir. The Post dial system for telephone was planned, budgeted and started during the year.

General of the Armies John J. Pershing, a domiciliary patient at Walter Reed after May 6, 1941, and for whom a special suite called "The Pent House" was eventually built on the third floor near the Officers' Surgical Ward, died on July 15, 1948. He had been both visitor and patient since the long-ago days of World War I, and as such he was almost an institutional "fixture."

On November 18, the Post Commander, Major General George C. Beach, died of a long-standing chronic complaint. This was the first time that a Post Commander of the Army Medical Center had died while on active duty, the only other death being that of a hospital commander, Colonel John J. Phillips, in September 1915. The funeral service for General Beach was conducted in the Memorial Chapel; the Troop Command, including the WAC detachment, and the Army Medical Center band formed a guard of honor. General Beach was a kindly and well-loved commanding officer, and patients and personnel alike grieved at the loss of so understanding and warm-hearted a man.

Quietly and without fanfare he had kept informed of personnel problems affecting key employees and with complete anonymity he reconciled situations which could have become morale problems. He was not the sort of man who enjoyed directing or commanding personnel to perform their job, for he was reasonable, quiet, judicial and persuasive, with the result that his staff worked for him personally as well as because of economic necessity.

General Beach's wide acquaintance among top-ranking military men such as General Dwight D. Eisenhower had apparently left him unspoiled. In 1947, as the time approached for Norman T. Kirk's retirement as Surgeon General,[42] it was common service gossip that "Sam" Beach could have the position for the asking, but he stated repeat-

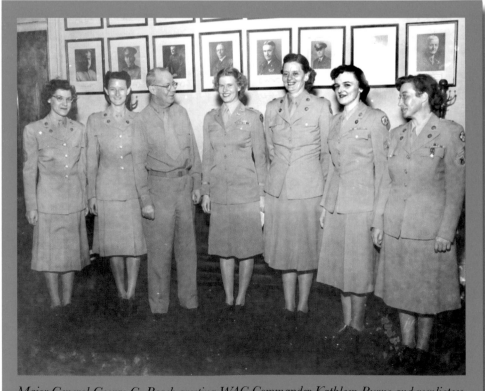

Major General George C. Beach greeting WAC Commander Kathleen Burns and reenlistees

edly in public and in private that he preferred to remain in the Army Medical Center where he could maintain close contacts with patients. When he died, and the employees contributed for a floral offering, a charwoman on duty in the School building hesitantly offered a twenty-five cent donation, as much as she could afford, because he had always said "Good Morning" to her as he passed on his way to his office at the Army Medical Center headquarters. Although an able hospital commander, it was as a humanist that General Beach was revered and remembered. It was especially fitting that he died in service, that within those walls where he greeted the great and spoke to the humble, where pain was the daily measure for many and birth the privilege of some, "Death silenced the soft footsteps of a man who loved his fellow man completely."[43]

Of Local Interest

On January 17, 1949, the nineteenth Post Commander, Brigadier General (later Major General) Paul H. Streit, reviewed the troops and accepted the command from the interim commander, Colonel Joseph U. Weaver. Like General Beach, he came to the Army Medical Center from the Brooke General Hospital, Fort Sam Houston, Texas. Surgeon General Bliss was open in his praise of the new Post Commander's managerial ability, under whose direction affairs at the Army Medical Center, as already planned, progressed with clock-like regulation and without interruption of the former program. The change-over in the Post telephone system was completed in the spring of 1949.[44] The new *Pediatric Section* was opened March 9,[45] and renovations were begun which would create a separate surgical section for children.[46] The Out-Patient Clinic by then employed a (civilian) female pediatrician. In 1950, a day nursery was established on the Post.

As a part of the expanded Medical Service training program, there was a fifty per cent increase in internships, beginning in July 1949. In October 1949, an experimental forty-eight-week course of instruction in practical nurs-

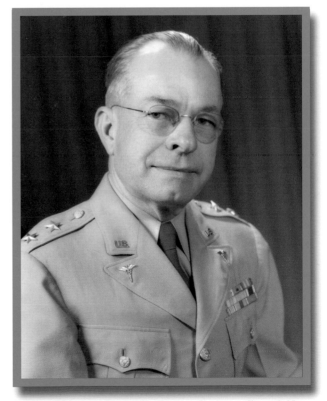

Major General Paul H. Streit, Commanding Officer January 1949–.

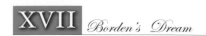

ing was opened at the Forest Glen Section to fifty enlisted members of the WAC; a year later the course was opened to both men and women. The faculty was composed of personnel from Army Nurse Corps and the Women's Medical Specialists Corps. General supervision of the course was conducted by the *Education Committee* of the hospital.[47]

Many of the buildings were repainted, and the post-war repairs were continued. On March 17, 1949, ground was broken for a splendidly equipped moving picture theater. And during the year plans were developed for converting the WAC Barracks, one-time home of the "Company of Instruction," into a luxurious Out-Patient Service, the finest of its kind in the Army. Trees and shrubs were re-marked, as in General Glennan's day, and an impressive marker calling attention to the *Army Medical Center* was installed at the 16th Street gate.

In October 1949, when General Streit had been Post Commander less than a year, the consultants to the Army Medical Library met for the first time at the Army Medical Center. The Army Medical Library had been unsuitably housed for years, and its plight was a cause for grave concern. Various efforts to relocate it near or subjoin it to the Library of Congress had failed, and both the internal management problems and lack of building funds had brought criticism on the Surgeon General's Office from librarians, scholars and distinguished doctors reluctant to see so fine an institution abused.

General Streit was somewhat familiar with Dr. Borden's plan for ultimate completion of the Army Medical Center, and during his first year as commandant he openly endorsed the four-way development of hospital, school, library and museum. Therefore in 1949 he made a quietly effective plea for giving the Library a permanent home.[48] Indefinite association of the Library and Museum was accepted by the majority of the Medical Corps of the Army as a fixed policy, and those officers interested in the completion of the Center considered any other disposition of the institutions sheer heresy. Any one of the Surgeons General after 1902 would have completed the Army Medical Center had the funds been available, and as late as 1947 the General Staff would have budgeted for the Library had the Surgeon General of that period given it a priority over other projects. In view of the changing "times" of the mid-century it is, therefore, interesting to note that in 1919 General Ireland proposed a comprehensive plan for completing the Center; Generals Patterson and Reynolds actively prosecuted this plan and struggled for funds against the insurmountable odds of an economic depression and the open hostility of some members of the civilian medical profession.

For many years fiscal officers in the Surgeon General's office had objected to charging the operating costs of the Library to the Medical Department (hospital) budget, but none considered giving the institution away.[49] At the time Surgeon General Magee was in office (1939–1943) the Librarian of that period was struggling desperately to secure a new building on Capitol Hill, and his program was completely agreeable to the Surgeon General. This was during the period when outside influences were openly stressing the civilian services provided by the Army Medical Library and emphasizing the national rather than the military value of the collection. General Kirk was, there-

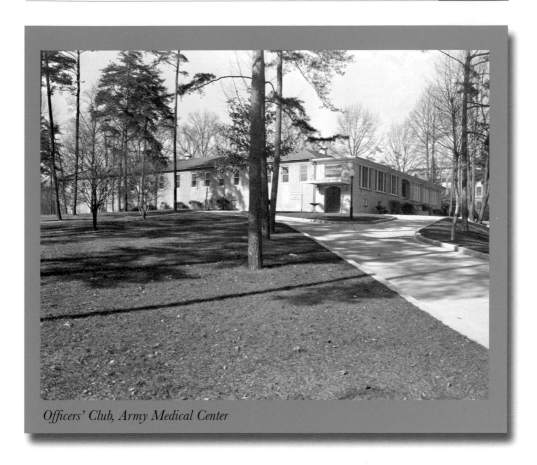

Officers' Club, Army Medical Center

fore, often told that because the volume of inter-library loans routed to civilian doctors presumably exceeded the service then required by the Medical Corps, the Library was improperly assigned to the Army. Frustrating budget experience of his predecessors had convinced him that the General Staff would not support the cost of a new building and so he proposed that the fine old institution become a semi-military project such as the Rivers and Harbors and flood control projects directed by the Engineer Corps.[50]

Unfortunately, from late 1946 until his term ended in 1947, the movement to reassign the Army Medical Library as a National Medical Library gained unusually active support from some of General Kirk's advisors, and the possibility of creating a National Medical Library in fact was discussed. Although it was the Army's greatest source of professional material in the fields of preventative medicine and medical intelligence, there was little defense of the institution as a military asset[51] or, in fact, little defense of continued military supervision. Meanwhile, the Museum, by then renamed in turn the Army Institute of Pathology and the Armed Forces Institute of Pathology, had active support from interested civilian and military pathologists. After formation of the "Hawley" committee for the study of Joint, Army, Navy and Air Force medical activities, the Surgeon General voluntarily presented the Library-Museum problems for consideration. In 1949, when it was apparently a question of having the

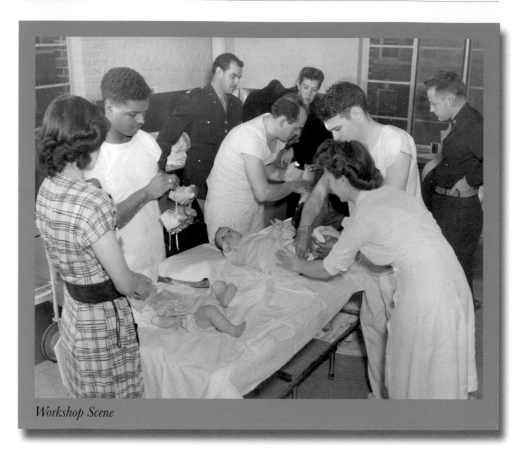

Workshop Scene

Army retain responsibility for one or the other of these great institutions, Surgeon General Bliss reversed the position adopted by his predecessors and stated that "the Army could not in good conscience ask that the Library be located at the Army Medical Center."[52] He chose maintenance of the Museum, or Army Institute of Pathology, and proposed consigning the "Army Medical Library" to the Naval Medical Center, thus separating it irrevocably from its parent organization and its primary function as a resource for the Army Medical Service Graduate Schools and the Institute of Pathology.

The matter was not immediately settled, and when the relative merits of various locations and stewardships later were re-studied by an objective committee selected by the National Research Council, the Committee proposed that the Library remain under military administration, preferably that of the Army. The Army Medical Center was proposed as a suitable location, with the Institute of Health, United States Public Health Service, as an alternate.[53] Further, an advisory board representing medical and academic groups was proposed.[54]

On July 10, 1951, an ordinary hot sultry summer day in Washington, a ground-breaking ceremony was held at the Army Medical Center for the new building of the Armed Forces Institute of Pathology, and the spectators who foregathered for the exercise heard the usual glowing words of praise that memorialize such ceremonies. High-ranking officials of the

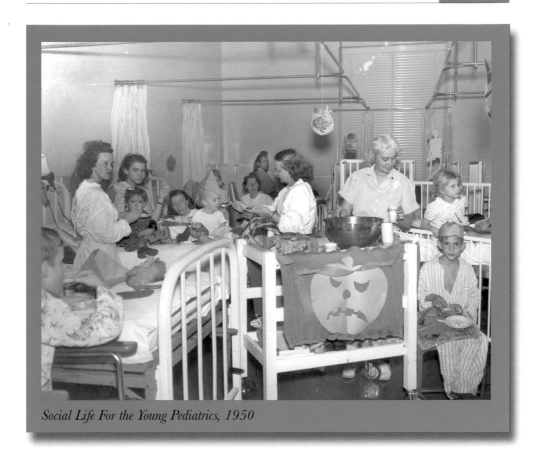

Social Life For the Young Pediatrics, 1950

three medical services, Army, Navy and Air, applauded the realization of the half-century old plan for locating the "Museum" at the Army Medical Center, but, strangely, only one, a Naval officer, Rear Admiral Joel T. Boone (Ret.), the new Chief Medical Director of the Veterans Administration, called attention to the decrepit and neglected condition of the Army Medical Library and its long-standing requirements for a new building.

The occasion marked one of the first public appearances of the Army's new Surgeon General, Major General E. Armstrong. In an appropriately eloquent speech he attempted to create for his listeners an imaginary scene at Seventh and B Streets, Southwest, location of the Museum-Library building since 1887. In so doing he advised that the spirit of Oliver Wendell Holmes was probably rejoicing that at last the Institute could be graciously as well as adequately housed. The ghost of the famous Major Walter Reed, he said, was undoubtedly viewing the scene from another world, proud of the scientific progress made in the fifty years since his death. One by one the shades of many of the great medical men of past generations were called on to witness this momentous occasion. All, said the Surgeon General, were rejoicing in the achievement in which they could take just pride – "But not Billings," murmured the editor of the recently terminated Index-Catalogue sadly, to himself, as he listened to the oratory – "But not Billings."

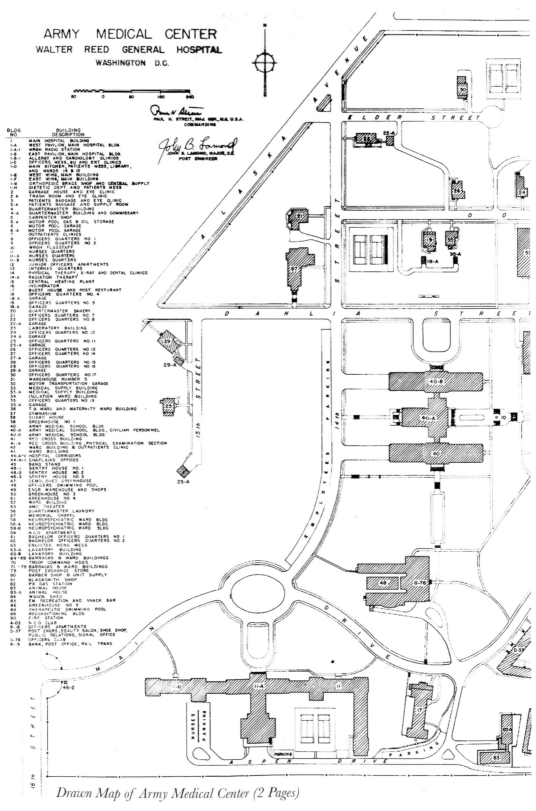

ARMY MEDICAL CENTER
WALTER REED GENERAL HOSPITAL
WASHINGTON D.C.

PAUL H. STREIT, MAJ. GEN., M.C. U.S.A.
COMMANDING

JOHN B. LAMOND, MAJOR, C.E.
POST ENGINEER

BLDG NO.	BUILDING DESCRIPTION
I	MAIN HOSPITAL BUILDING
I-A	WEST PAVILION, MAIN HOSPITAL BLDG.
I-A-I	WRGH RADIO STATION
I-B	EAST PAVILION, MAIN HOSPITAL BLDG.
I-B-I	ALLERGY AND CARDIOLOGY CLINICS
I-C	OFFICERS MESS, GU AND ENT CLINICS
I-D	MAIN KITCHEN, PATIENTS MESS, LIBRARY, AND WARDS 14 & 15
I-E	WEST WING, MAIN BUILDING
I-F	EAST WING, MAIN BUILDING
I-G	ORTHOPEDIC BRACE SHOP AND CENTRAL SUPPLY
I-K	DIETETIC DEPT. AND PATIENTS MESS
2	GARAGE HOUSE AND EYE CLINIC
2-A	TRASH ROOM AND EYE CLINIC
3	PATIENTS BAGGAGE AND EYE CLINIC
3-A	PATIENTS BAGGAGE AND SUPPLY ROOM
4	QUARTERMASTER BUILDING
4-A	QUARTERMASTER BUILDING AND COMMISSARY
5	CARPENTER SHOP
5-A	MOTOR POOL GAS & OIL STORAGE
6	MOTOR POOL GARAGE
6-A	MOTOR POOL GARAGE
7	OUTPATIENTS CLINICS
8	OFFICERS QUARTERS NO. I
9	OFFICERS QUARTERS NO. 2
10	WRGH FLAGSTAFF
11	NURSES QUARTERS
11-A	NURSES QUARTERS
11-B	NURSES QUARTERS
12	JUNIOR OFFICERS APARTMENTS
13	INTERNES QUARTERS
14	PHYSICAL THERAPY, X-RAY AND DENTAL CLINICS
14-A	RADIATION THERAPY
16	CENTRAL HEATING PLANT
16	INCINERATOR
17	GUEST HOUSE AND POST RESTURANT
18	OFFICERS QUARTERS NO. 4
18-A	GARAGE
19	OFFICERS QUARTERS NO. 5
19-A	GARAGE
20	QUARTERMASTER BAKERY
21	OFFICERS QUARTERS NO. 7
22	OFFICERS QUARTERS NO. 8
22-A	GARAGE
23	LABORATORY BUILDING
24	OFFICERS QUARTERS NO. 10
24-A	GARAGE
25	OFFICERS QUARTERS NO. 11
25-A	GARAGE
26	OFFICERS QUARTERS NO. 12
27	OFFICERS QUARTERS NO. 14
27-A	GARAGE
28	OFFICERS QUARTERS NO. 15
29	OFFICERS QUARTERS NO. 16
29-A	GARAGE
30	OFFICERS QUARTERS NO. 17
31	WAREHOUSE NUMBER 5
32	MOTOR TRANSPORTATION GARAGE
33	MEDICAL SUPPLY BUILDING
33-A	MEDICAL SUPPLY BUILDING
34	ISOLATION WARD BUILDING
35	OFFICERS QUARTERS NO 19
35-A	GARAGE
36	T.B. WARD AND MATERNITY WARD BUILDING
37	GYMNASIUM
38	GUARD HOUSE
39	GREENHOUSE NO I
40	ARMY MEDICAL SCHOOL BLDG.
40-A	ARMY MEDICAL SCHOOL BLDG., CIVILIAN PERSONNEL
40-B	ARMY MEDICAL SCHOOL BLDG.
41	RED CROSS BUILDING
41-A	RED CROSS BUILDING, PHYSICAL EXAMINATION SECTION
42	WARD BUILDING & OUTPATIENTS CLINIC
43	WARD BUILDING
44-A-V	HOSPITAL CORRIDORS
44-N-I	CHAPLAINS OFFICES
45	BAND STAND
46-I	SENTRY HOUSE NO I
46-2	SENTRY HOUSE NO 2
46-3	SENTRY HOUSE NO 3
47	DEMOLISHED GREENHOUSE
48	OFFICERS SWIMMING POOL
49	ENGR WAREHOUSE AND SHOPS
50	GREENHOUSE NO 3
51	GREENHOUSE NO 4
52	WARD BUILDING
53	AMC THEATER
56	QUARTERMASTER LAUNDRY
57	MEMORIAL CHAPEL
58	NEUROPSYCHIATRIC WARD BLDG
58-A	NEUROPSYCHIATRIC WARD BLDG
58-B	NEUROPSYCHIATRIC WARD BLDG
59	N.C.O. APARTMENTS
61	BACHELOR OFFICERS QUARTERS NO. I
62	BACHELOR OFFICERS QUARTERS NO.2
63	ENLISTED MENS MESS
63-A	LAVATORY BUILDING
63-B	LAVATORY BUILDING
64-69	BARRACKS B WARD BUILDINGS
70	TROOP COMMAND HDQS
71-78	BARRACKS B WARD BUILDINGS
79	POST EXCHANGE STORE
80	BARBER SHOP & UNIT SUPPLY
81	BLACKSMITH SHOP
82	PX GAS STATION
83	ANIMAL HOUSE
83-A	ANIMAL HOUSE
84	WAGON SHED
85	EM RECREATION AND SNACK BAR
86	GREENHOUSE NO 5
88	THERAPEUTIC SWIMMING POOL
89	RECONDITIONING BLDG
90	FIRE STATION
A-03	N.C.O. CLUB
B-18	OFFICERS APARTMENTS
D-37	POST ENGRS ,BEAUTY SALON, SHOE SHOP, PUBLIC RELATIONS, SIGNAL OFFICE
S-76	OFFICERS CLUB
B-5	BANK, POST OFFICE, RAIL TRANS

Drawn Map of Army Medical Center (2 Pages)

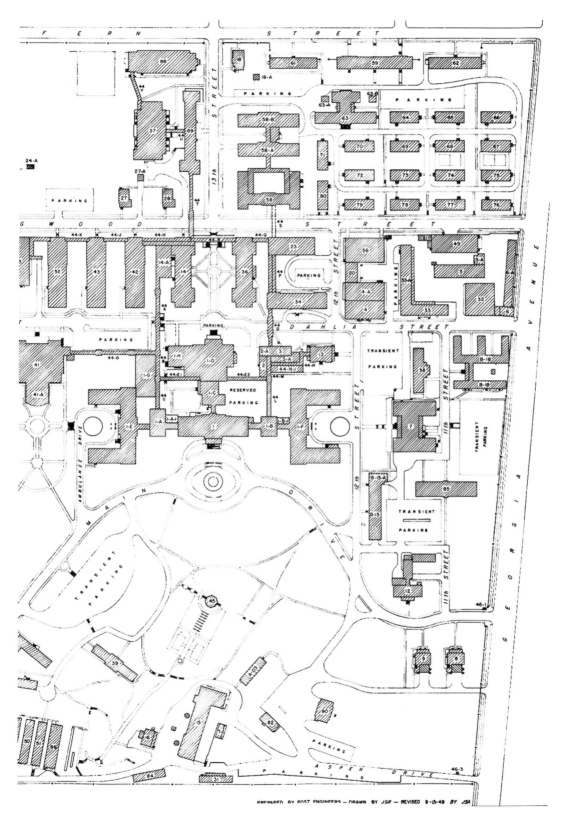

PREPARED BY POST ENGINEERS — DRAWN BY JSR — REVISED 9-15-49 BY JSA

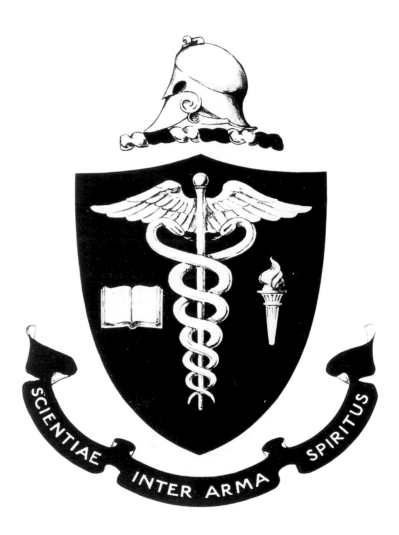

Shield, The Walter Reed Army Medical Center

And so it was that eighty-seven years and two days after the Battle of Fort Stevens Surgeon General Hammond's apparently far-fetched proposal for a military medical center in Washington City gave evidence of nearing completion. Lt. Colonel William Cline Borden was the human instrument in fact that brought about the building of the Walter Reed Army Hospital whose name so influenced public identification of the activity that on September 13, 1951, the Department of the Army finally made a colloquialism an official directive, and the *Walter Reed Army Medical Center*[55] became a matter of official record. *Borden's Dream* his critics called his plans for the colonial structure which, like the hero for whom it was named, was the Army's "First on the Scroll of Fame."[56]

References

1. Editorial, *Military Surgeon*, February 1910, pg 375.

2. Made temporary Brigadier General in 1943; a permanent Brigadier June 1, 1946; a Major General in January 1948, *Service Stripe*, (Jan. 31, 1948).

3. *Service Stripe*, July 27, 1946.

4. *Ibid*, March 24, 1945.

5. Annual Rpt., WRGH, 1945.

6. *Service Stripe*, April 21, 1945.

7. Annual Report, WRGH, 1946.

8. Interview with Maj. Gen. Shelley U. Marietta, M.C., Ret. May 16, 1951.

9. Annual Report, WRGH, 1946.

10. *Ibid*.

11. *Service Stripe*, January 25, 1947.

12. Retired in April 1951; her successor had not been named at the time the history was written.

13. Interviews with Colonel Florence A. Blanchfield, ANC, Ret., 1946–1950.

14. Based on general interviews over a four-year period.

15. Conversation with Major General Paul H. Streit, October 1950.

16. Interview with Maj. Gen. Robert U. Patterson, M.C., Ret., Aug. 29, 1950.

17. *Ibid*.

18. *Service Stripe*, June 21, 1947.

19. *Ibid*, July 31, 1948.

20. Sec. I, ASF Cir. 92, 11 April 1946 and Sec. III, ASF Circular 98, 19 April 1946; WD Circular No. 138, 14 May 1946; WD Circular No. 170, 11 June 1946.

21. *Service Stripe*, June 28, 1946.

22. Memo to TSW from Watson B. Miller, Adm. Sept. 5, 1946, with enclosure from Frank H. Lahey, M.D., Chm. Dir. Bd. P&AS. June 26, 1946. On file Office of the Adm. FSA.

23. *Service Stripe*, October 26, 1946.

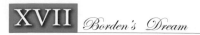

24. *Ibid*, May 3, 1947. Unification of the three combat services into a single National Security Organization was effected by Public Law 253, 80th Congress, approved 26 July 1947. The War Department was redesignated *The Department of the Army*.

25. Annual Report of Technical Activities of the Medical Department, 1946.

26. Annual Report, WRGH, 1946

27. Annual Report MD PSS 1946, Pt. I, pg 5.

28. Biography of Jefferson R. Kean, MSS on file, AML, Washington, DC pg 94.

29. A study on attitudes of ASTP medical officers toward service in the Regular Army, made at the request of the Office, Secretary of War, (by) WD Information and Education Division Troop Attitude Research Branch, Washington, 25, DC, 2 Nov. 1946 pg 1.

30. *Ibid*, pg 3.

31. Report of MD RGS, July 1, 1947 to December 31, 1947.

32. *Ibid*.

33. Section I, WD GO No. 5, 13 January 1947.

34. Annual Report of Technical Activities of the Medical Department, 1947.

35. *Service Stripe*, May 15, 1948.

36. Rpt...1 July 1947 – 31 December 1947.

37. Annual Rpt. of the Army Medical Dept., Research and Graduate School for the Calendar year 1948.

38. Annual Report...FY ending 30 June 1947.

39. Annual Rpt. AMDRGS...1947.

40. *Service Stripe*, July 10, 1948.

41. *Ibid*, October 29, 1948.

42. Brig. Gen. Raymond W. Bliss succeeded to this office on June 1, 1947. He had been at Walter Reed during the early twenties as the Chief of the Obstetrical and Gynecological Section of General Surgery.

43. *Service Stripe*, November 21, 1948.

44. *Ibid*, February 25, 1949.

45. *Ibid*, April 8, 1949.

46. *Ibid*, May 27, 1949.

47. *Ibid*, Sept. 2, 1949.

48. *Ibid*, October 28, 1949.

49. Conversation with Col. E.C. Jones, M.C., Ret., May 1938.

50. Conversation with Maj. Gen. Norman T. Kirk, M.C., Ret., June 23, 1951.

51. *Ibid*, May 1947.

52. Memorandum for Dr. Meiling from R.W. Bliss, Major General, TSG, USA, 22 November 1949. (MEDDA); Renamed "Armed Forces Institute of Pathology" on July 1, 1949.

53. Conversation, Major General Paul H. Streit, June 1951.

54. The large group of consultants to the Army Medical Library had proven unwieldy and impractical. From the functional standpoint, however, an advisory board, beyond the jurisdiction of military command channels appears impractical.

55. General Order #80, DA, 13 September 1951.

56. Eliza Cook, "The Englishman," Stanza I.

ADDENDA
Surgeons General of the Army Medical Department

1. Benjamine Church, Director General and Chief Physician of the Hospital of the Army, July 27, 1775–October 17, 1775.

2. John Morgan, Director General and Physician in Chief of the American Hospital, October 17, 1775–January 9, 1777.

3. William Shippon, Jr., Director General of the Military Hospitals of the Continental Army, April 11, 1777–January 3, 1781.

4. John Cochran, Director General of the Military Hospitals of the Continental Army, January 17, 1781–November 3, 1783.

5. James Craik, Physician and Surgeon of the United States Army, July 19, 1798–June 15, 1800.

6. James Tilton, Physician and Surgeon of the United States Army, June 11, 1813–June 15, 1815.

7. Joseph Lovell, Surgeon General, United States Army, April 18, 1818–October 17, 1836.

8. Brevet Brigadier General Thomas Lawson, Surgeon General, November 30, 1836–May 15, 1861.

9. Brevet Brigadier General Clement Alexander Finley, Surgeon General, May 15, 1861–April 14, 1862.

10. Brigadier General William Alexander Hammond, Surgeon General, April 25, 1862–August 18, 1864.

11. Brevet Major General Joseph E. Barnes, Surgeon General, August 22, 1864–June 30, 1882.

12. Brigadier General Charles Henry Crane, Surgeon General, July 3, 1882–October 10, 1883.

13. Brigadier General Robert Murray, Surgeon General, November 23, 1883–August 6, 1886.

14. Brigadier General John Moore, Surgeon General, November 18, 1886–August 16, 1890.

15. Brigadier General Jedediah Hyde Baxter, Surgeon General, August 16, 1890–December 4, 1890.

16. Brigadier General Charles Sutherland, Surgeon General, December 23, 1890–May 29, 1893.

17. Brigadier General George Miller Sternberg, Surgeon General, May 30, 1893–June 8, 1902.

18. Brigadier General William Henry Forwood, Surgeon General, June 8, 1902–September 7, 1902.

19. Brigadier General Robert Maitland O'Reilly, Surgeon General, September 7, 1902–January 14, 1909.

20. Brigadier General George Henry Torney, Surgeon General, January 14, 1909–December 27, 1913.

21. Major General William Crawford Gorgas, Surgeon General, January 16, 1914–October 3, 1918.

22. Major General Merritte Weber Ireland, The Surgeon General, October 4, 1918–May 31, 1931.

23. Major General Robert Urie Patterson, The Surgeon General, June 1, 1931–May 31, 1935.

24. Major General Charles Ransom Reynolds, The Surgeon General, June 1, 1935–May 31, 1939.

25. Major General James Carre Magee, The Surgeon General, June 1, 1939–May 31, 1943.

26. Major General Norman T. Kirk, The Surgeon General, June 1, 1943–May 31, 1947.

27. Major General Raymond W. Bliss, The Surgeon General, June 1, 1947–May 31, 1951.

28. Major General George E. Armstrong, The Surgeon General, June 1, 1951– .

POST COMMANDERS
Walter Reed Army Hospital

NAME	*RANK*	*CORPS*	*YRS OF COMMAND*
Borden, William Cline	Major	MC	Oct. 10, 1898 to June 15, 1907*
Arthur, William H.	Colonel	MC	1 June 1908 to 11 July 1911
Richard, Charles	Colonel	MC	Sept. 1911 to Sept. 1912
Birmingham, H.P.	Colonel	MC	Oct. 1912 to Aug. 1913
Fisher, Henry C.	Colonel	MC	1 Aug. 1913 to 11 May 1914
Phillips, John L.	Colonel	MC	May 12, 1914 to 18 Sept. 1915
Ashburn, Percy M.	Major	MC	19 Sept. 1915 to 5 Oct. 1916
Mason, Charles P.	Colonel	MC	6 Oct. 1916 to 27 Nov. 1917
Truby, Willard F.	Colonel	MC	28 Nov. 1917 to 27 Aug. 1918
Schreiner, Edward R.	Colonel	MC	27 Aug. 1918 to 15 Mar. 1919

Army Medical Center

Glennan, James D.	Brig. General	MC	Mar. 1919 to Mar. 1926
Kennedy, James M.	Brig. General	MC	Mar. 1926 to Dec. 1929
Darnall, Carl. R.	Brig. General	MC	12 Dec. 1929 to 31 Dec. 1931
Truby, Albert E.	Brig. General	MC	Jan. 1932 to 31 July 1935
DeWitt, Wallace C.	Brig. General	MC	Aug. 1935 to 25 Dec. 1939
Metcalfe, Raymond F.	Brig. General	MC	26 Dec. 1939 to 31 Jan. 1941
Marietta, Shelly U.	Major General	MC	1 Feb. 1941 to 9 Feb. 1946

| Beach, George C. | Major General | MC | Mar. 1946 to Nov. 1948 |
| Streit, Paul H | Major General | MC | 17 Jan. 1949 to |

* S.O. #239, Oct. 10, 1898; S.O #76, April 1, 1907

PRESIDENTS AND COMMANDANTS OF THE ARMY MEDICAL SCHOOL

1893 – 1898	Colonel Charles Henry Alden
1898 – 1901	[School closed during Spanish-American War]
1901 – 1902	Colonel William Henry Forwood
1902 – 1903	Brigadier-General Calvin DeWitt
1903 – 1906	Colonel Charles Lawrence Heizmann
1906 – 1909	Colonel Valery Havard
1909 – 1912	Colonel Louis Anatole LaGarde
1912 – 1915	Colonel Charles Richard
1915 – 1918	Brigadier General William Hempel Arthur
1918 – 1918	Colonel Weston Percival Chamberlain
1918 – 1919	Brigadier General Francis Anderson Winter
1919 – 1923	Brigadier General Walter Drew McCaw
1923 – 1924	Colonel Weston Percival Chamberlain
1924 – 1929	Brigadier General Henry Clay Fisher
1929 – 1930	Colonel Christopher Clark Collins
1930 – 1931	Colonel Charles Franklin Craig
1931 – 1931	Colonel Jay Ralph Shook
1931 – 1932	Colonel Edward Bright Vedder
1932 – 1935	Colonel Philip Weatherly Huntington
1935 – 1939	Colonel Joseph Franklin Siler
1940 – 1946	Brigadier General George Russel Callender
1946 – 1949	Colonel Rufus Holt
1949 – 1950	Colonel Elbert De Coursey
1950 –	Colonel William S. Stone

CHIEF NURSES
WALTER REED ARMY HOSPITAL[*]

Molloy, Jane G. (first C.N.)	21 June 1911 – July 1913
Burns, Sophy M.	July 1913 – April 1914
Hine, M. Estelle	May 1914 – October 1915
Bell, Bessie S.	October 1915 – October 1917
Sheehan, Mary E.	October 1917 – December 1917
Magrath, Katherine C.	December 1917 – August 1918
Stewart, Robina L.	August 1918 – January 1919
Clark, Margaret E. (Acting C.N.)	January 1919 – February 1919
Trench, Amy M.	February 1919 – June 1919
Williamson, Anne	July 1919 – April 1922
Reid, Elizabeth D.	April 1922 – February 1923
Flikke, Julia O.	February 1923 – May 1934
Keener, Lydia M.	May 1934 – January 1944
Thompson, L. Gertrude	February 1944 – October 1947
Danielson, Ida W.	November 1947 – 31 March 1951

[*]Information compiled from 201 files by Nursing Division, Office of The Surgeon General, 26 March 1951

CHIEF DIETICIANS
WALTER REED ARMY HOSPITAL

Mrs. Genevieve Field Long (civilian)	October 1922 – May 1925
Mrs. Grace Hunter (Young) (civilian)	May 1925 – May 1933
Helen C. Burns (Goarin), civilian-Major	May 1933 – August 1942
Helen A. Dautrich, Lieutenant-Major	August 1942 – July 1946
Nell Wickliffe, Captain-Major	July 1946 – September 1948
Hilda H. Lovett, Captain-Major	September 1948 – July 1952
Eleanor L. Mitchell, Major –	July 1952 –

Source of information: Lt. Col. Hilda M. Lovett, WMSC, Women's Medical Specialist Corps Division, SGO and Documentary Material in Historical Unit, SGO.

CHIEF OCCUPATIONAL THERAPISTS WALTER REED ARMY HOSPITAL

Alberta Montgomery (civilian)	1919 – 1933
Mrs. Emmy Sommers (civilian)	1933 – 1947
Roberta Aber (Lees), Captain	1947 – 1951
Mary Riley, Captain	1951 – September 1952
Katherine Maurice, Captain	September 1952 –

Source of information: Lt. Col. H. R. Sheehan, WMSC, Chief, Occupational Therapy Branch Physical Medicine Consultants Division, SGO

CHIEF PHYSIOTHERAPISTS, WALTER REED ARMY HOSPITAL

Emma E. Vogel (civilian but later a Colonel and Chief of Corps)	1919 – 1942
Evelyn MacDonald, civilian - 2nd Lt.- Captain	1942 – Aug. 1946
Elsie Kurener, Captain	1946 – Oct. 1947
Barbara Robertson, Captain	1947 – May 1950
Bruentta Kuehlthau, 1st Lt. - Major	May 1950 –

Source of information: Lt. Col. H. S. Lee, WMSC, Chief Physical Therapy Branch Physical Medicine Consultants Division, SGO

CHAPEL MEMORIALS*

GIFTS	*DONOR*	*MEMORIAL*
Field Stone	Ellen R. and Harriet C. Riley	Brevet Major Joseph Sim Smith, M.C., USA
Marble Altar, Reredos, Altar Rail	Mrs. Blair Spencer, George T. Summerlin, John V. Summerlin	Mrs. Henrietta Vandergrift Johnson
Altar Window	Katherine Weeks Davidge Sinclair Weeks	Martha Sinclair Weeks John Sinclair Weeks

Entrance Window	Mrs. Hugh Campbell Wallace	Ambassador Hugh Campbell Wallace
East Window (1)	Anna O. Connolly and Eleanor M. Connolly	Hon. Maurice Connolly
East Window (2)	Chaplain Edmund F. Estarbrook	Fanny Nescomb Estarbrook
East Window (3)	American Legion Auxiliary, Dept. of Pennsylvania	"Sons of Pennsylvania in the World War who gave their lives in the cause of liberty."
East Window (4)	Mary Willing Clymer Bayard	Mary Schubrick Clymer
West Window (1)	Army Nurses	Army Nurses who died in the World War
West Window (2)	Mrs. Edith Nourse Rogers	Hon. John Jacob Rogers
West Window (3)	Mrs. George Russell Cecil	Colonel George Russell Cecil
West Window (4)	Mrs. Elsie C. Crabbs	Colonel Joseph T. Crabbs
West Window (5)	American Women's Legion	"Those who carried the Flag Forward (1917–1919)"
Flagstone floor and foundation	Mrs. Edith Oliver Rea	Henry Robinson Rea
East buttress (1)		Medical Department, United States Army
East buttress (2)	Mabel T. Boardman Alice Clapp	District of Columbia Chapter American Red Cross
East buttress (3)	Daughters of the American Revolution	
East buttress (4)	Charter members of the Memorial Chapel Guild, AMC	
West buttress (1)	Disabled American Veterans of the World War	
West buttress (2)	Spanish War Veterans	
West buttress (3)	Knights of Columbus	World War Dead
West buttress (4)	American Legion	
Chapel Lights	Princess Margaret Boncompagni	Margaret Wicliff Brown
English-style lantern (Main entrance)	Medical Dept, personnel at Walter Reed General Hospital	Brig. Gen. James M. Kennedy

PEWS

East	(1)	Edith P. Chapman	2d. Lt. Charles Wesley Chapman
"	(2)	Harriet Granger Jackson	2d. Lt. Oliver Phelps Jackson
"	(3)	Geo. Andrews Benny, Jr.	Cpl. Philip Phillips Benny
"	(4)	Masonic Club, AMC	
"	(5)	Gray Ladies, Pittsburgh Chapter, ARC	War Service Memorial
"	(6)	Grace Occumpaugh	Sara Darrow Occumpaugh
"	(7)	Miriam B. Hilton	Walter Edward Hilton
"	(8)	Chaplain Alfred C. Oliver, Jr.	J.E. Lake Oliver
"	(9)	Mrs. Richard Fourchey Mrs. William E. Lewis	Maj. Gen. James M. McMillan (Civil War)
"	(10)	Mrs. Wallace Chiswell	Cornant C. Nelson William T. Chiswell
"	(11)	Cecilia B. Sniegoski "The Polish Gray Lady"	Count Casimer Pulaski Brig. Gen., Rev. War
"	(12)	The Department	Mrs. Frank B. Emery, Pres. of Dept. of Pa. American Legion Auxiliary
"	(13)	"Dugout Gang" Former World War I patients at Walter Reed Bertha York Webb sponsor.	
"	(14)	Gray Ladies, N.Y. chapter, ARC	Joint Disease built Hospital and Recreation Service NY Chpt., ARC
"	(15)	Gertrude Lustig	Emma Gene Reinhardt
"	(16)	Mrs. Alfred M. Craven	Augustine Saux
"	(17)	Alida Frances Pattee	Walter Scott Pattee
West	(1)	Alumnae	ASN graduates "who have given their lives in the service of humanity."
"	(2)	Graduate Nurses WRAH	

"	(3)	Graduate Nurses WRAH	
"	(4)	Student Nurses WRAH	
"	(5)	Constance B. Jordon	Eldridge Jordon Marcus A. Jordon
"	(6)	Lt. Col. Richard J. Donnelly	1st. Lt. Herbert J. McDermott
"	(7)	Mrs. Christy Dalrymple Brown	Sgt. Joseph Francis Brown
"	(8)	Mr. & Mrs. Samuel Baughman	Faber Dolle Baughman
"	(9)	Mrs. Marie Fagon Walter	Lt. George L. Walter, Jr.
"	(10)	Gift of his parents	Sgt. Francis J. Osterman
"	(11)	Polish people living in Washington	"To the Sons of Poland who served in the United States Army during World War I"
"	(12)	Kathleen Cecil Morgan	Col. George Russell Cecil
"	(13)	Sophie C. Stanton	Sgt. Edwin M. Stanton
"	(14)	Am. Leg. Auxiliary, Dept. of Virginia	"The Virginia Soldiers who lost their lives in the World War"
"	(15)	The Roy McKinley Basford Unit of the American Legion Auxiliary	Roy McKinley Basford
"	(16)	Flander's Field Unit, American Women's Legion	"The World War Dead"
"	(17)	American Women's Legion	" " " "
Baptismal Font		Occupational, Physio-Therapy and Dietetic Departments of Walter Reed General Hospital.	
Chapel Floor		Mrs. Herbert J. Slocum	Col. Herbert J. Slocum
Pulpit		Mrs. E. Hope G. Slater	Mary Gwynn
Lectern		Mrs. Lucy C. Willock Lillian Willock	Frank Scott Willock
Bible		Enlisted Men at Walter Reed Gen. Hosp., Then the Christian Endeavor Society	"To the Glory of God."

Brass Altar Cross	Mrs. Brady G. Ruttencutter	Margaret A.A. Baker
Brass Candle-sticks and Vases	John A. Liggett Mrs. Merritt W. Ireland	William Harvey and Rebecca Mills Liggett
Chancel Chairs (1)	Caroline B. Burrell	Rev. Jos. D. Burrell
" (2)	Chaumont Unit, American Women's Legion	Brig. Gen. Robert H. Dunlop, U.S.M.C.
" (3)	Mrs. Lillian Sanchez Latour	Francisco Sanchez Latour
Chair Stalls	Edith Anne Rea Benney	Mrs. Edith Ann Oliver
Prayer Desks (1)	Gray Ladies at Walter Reed General Hospital	Mary Norton Lower
" (2)	Jessie Kennedy Frost	Sgt. Kennedy Conklin
" (3)	American Red Cross Staff at Walter Reed General Hospital	
Skinner Organ (three-manual)	Princess Margaret Boncompagni	General William Franklin Draper
Missal Book " Stand	Thos. S. Blandford	Elizabeth Hill Blandford
Silver Cross Two Silver Vases Two Double Candlesticks	Mrs. Walter Reed	Major Walter Reed

McCOOK MORTUARY CHAPEL

Altar, Reredos	McCook Family	Daniel McCook (and 8 Sons); John McCook (and 5 Sons). "The Fighting McCooks"
Altar Rail	Mrs. Charles A. Craig-head, Mrs. Thomas Dunlop	Lucy McCook Baker
Flagstone Floor	Sen. and Mrs. David A. Reed	"In memory of those whose graves are unknown."

Cathedral Chairs	Henry Oliver Rea	Henry W. Oliver
Lectern	Med. Adm. Corp of Walter Reed Gen. Hosp.	Deceased Members of the Sanitary Corps and the Med. Adm. Corps.
Lights	Alice J. Clapp	Louis Ward Mercur
Windows (1)	McCook family	Martha Latimer and Catherine J. Sheldon McCook, wives of Daniel McCook and John McCook
" (2)	McCook family	Capt. Francis R. McCook
Gothic Tower	Mrs. Henry R. Rea	Brig. General James Denver Glennan
Chapel Bell	Gray Ladies Volunteer Service, ARC, Walter Reed Chapter	
Bell Rope	Eben L. Comins	
Communion Service	Gray Ladies	
Bedside Communion Service	Mary E., James F., and John L. Schick	Rev. John M. Schick, D.D.
Electric Clock (Chaplains Office)	Masonic Clubs of D.C.	
American Flag	Am. Gold Star Mothers	
Red Cross Flag	Miss Margaret Lower	
Hymn Boards	Am. War Mothers	
Limestone Plaque Main Chapel	"A few of the many who loved her - 1933"	Armide DeSalles McClintock
(R.C.) Vestment Case	Catholic Congregation	
(Vestments)	Reverend Mothers Rosalie and Theresa Hill	Nine Catholic Chaplains killed in WWI
Jewish Ark (Scroll of the Law, two silver horns with bells, a silver breastplate, a silver pointer and the Ark Headpiece)	Children of Harris and Fannie Schiff	Parents

Hand-illuminated record of memorials. (Prepared by Miss Juanita Gould, Ass't Lib.)	Gray Ladies
Altar hangings, linen and cushions	Chapel Guild Organization

*Felthman S. James, comp., "The Story of the Memorial Chapel", WRGH, AMC, Wash., D.C., published by Chapel Guild...pam., on file Lib., WRAH.

APPROXIMATE* ANNUAL ADMISSIONS, WRAH

1909 – 760	1931 – 6,871
1910 – 569	1932 – 8,064
1911 – 594	1933 – 7,796
1912 – 565	1934 – 8,366
1913 – 867	1935 – 7,981
1914 – 964	1936 – 7,505
1915 – 1,169	1937 – 7,600
1916 – 1,350	1938 – 7,503
1917 – 4,197	1939 – 8,079
1918 – 13,362	1940 – 8,467
1919 – 9,111	1941 – 8,025
1920 – 5,407	1942 – 10,818
1922 – 5,289	1943 – 18,046
1923 – 5,286	1944 – 18,009
1924 – 5,138	1945 – 16,878
1925 – 6,808	1946 – 12,955
1926 – 6,726	1947 – 12,336
1927 – 6,858	1948 – 11,053
1928 – 7,448	1949 – 12,412
1929 – 8,012	1950 – 14,702
1930 – 7,122	

*Compiled from WR and SGO Reports. Sometimes at variance because of difference in fiscal and calendar year.

MEDICAL OFFICERS ON DUTY
AT THE WALTER REED GENERAL HOSPITAL

Colonel John L. Phillips .... Medical Corps, U.S. Army
Major Paul S. Halloran .... Medical Corps, U.S. Army
Captain William H. Moncrief .... Medical Corps, U.S. Army
Captain John A. Clark .... Medical Corps, U.S. Army
Captain Percy L. Jones .... Medical Corps, U.S. Army
Captain Howard H. Johnson .... Medical Corps, U.S. Army
Captain Ralph H. Goldthwaite .... Medical Corps, U.S. Army
Lieutenant Thomas J. Leary .... Medical Corps, U.S. Army
Lieutenant Chester R. Haig .... Medical Corps, U.S. Army
Lieutenant George F. Lull .... Medical Corps, U.S. Army
Lieutenant Charles C. Hillman .... Medical Corps, U.S. Army

ARMY NURSE CORPS
Estelle M. Hine, Chief Nurse

Mary C. Barker	Jean G. Mackenzie
Jessie M. Braden	Margaret M. MacNeill
Ila Broadus	Evelyn E. Mericle
Ethyl L. Dumbrille	Pearl Murphy
Louise Fennelle	Madeleine M. Pampel
Gertrude A. Hines	Emma M. Rousseau
Ruth Holland	Mary E. Sheehan
Mary E. Jordan	Marie Speckert
Louise Knapp	Elizabeth Spencer
Gertrude H. Lustig	Frances M. Steele
Margaret J. MacDonald	Alice M. Tappan

Mary E. Welsh

ENLISTED MEN ON DUTY
AT THE WALTER REED GENERAL HOSPITAL

Sergeant 1st Class Fred S. Owen	Sergeant Cyrus G. Wood
Sergeant 1st Class Quentin J. Barker	Sergeant John J. Pempey
Sergeant 1st Class James E. Young	Sergeant George E. Lavalley
Sergeant Thomas B. Carpenter	Sergeant Gregory Cipriani
Sergeant Luther C. Copley	Sergeant Charles D. Mudd

Corporal George J. Levy

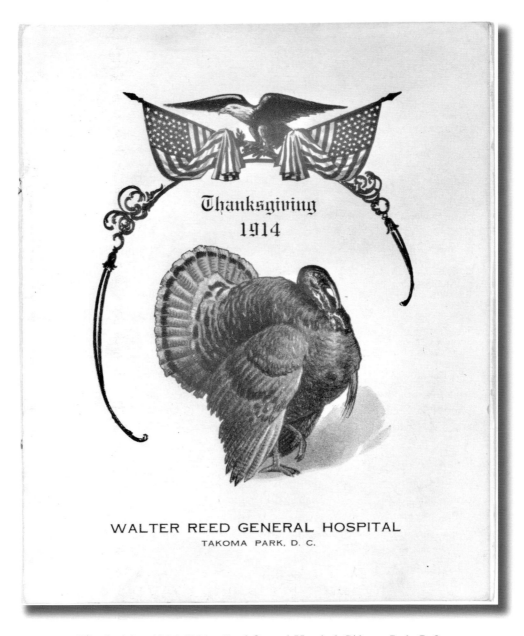

Thanksgiving 1914, Walter Reed General Hospital, Takoma Park, D.C.

ACTING COOKS

Thomas H. Cook

Noah Foster
Civilian Cook: William Jackson

James J. Logan, Jr.

PRIVATES FIRST CLASS

Archie S. Black
John E. Bohman
Albert Brenner
Edgar Dorsch
Hugh Drinkwater
Erastus E. Edwards
Nathan Gillman

Ivon B. Goldsworthy
Charles H. Jeffries
Wescott C. Joslin
James B. Judge
John Mullen
Max Riesenberg
George Roberts
Axel G. Worm

Stephen R. Royall
James A. Speer
John A. Spellbring
Enoch W. Stewart
Thomas Tuthill
Ennis C. Wallon
Joseph C. Willett

PRIVATES

Edward G. Baines
Francio St. Boulanger
James W. Brown
Edward R. Davidson
Tom L. Dorman
Martin L. Effross
John Engle
William S. Gideon
William P. Hart

Arthur R. Jernberg
Leo Lewis
Edward J. McCrea
John McKeller
Frank Maganno
James J. Magee
Sam Middleton
Aloyous Martin
William O'Hara

Harold S. Pickering
Frank Sandlin
Richard A. Scott
Albert P. Shannon
John H. Smith
William G. Strause
Charles Swoboda
Meltiades G. Tegopoulos
Francis M. Whitmore

QUARTERMASTER CORPS

Q.M. Sergeant Denis J. McSweeney
Sergeant John Polasko

Corporal Theodore M. Geupel
Corporal James F. Kight

PRIVATES FIRST CLASS

Curtis A. Jackson
Frederick C. Koschnitzke
Stephen J. Lonergan

John R. Lucas
Walter Powell
William D. Schuster

Louis A. Phelan

EXTRACT FROM LAST WILL AND TESTAMENT OF GENERAL FRED C. AINSWORTH[*]

"It is my desire that a permanent library be established at Walter Reed General Hospital, Washington, D.C., to be known as the Fred C. Ainsworth Endowment Library. If there shall be a permanent library at the said hospital at the time of my death or if no suitable space can be provided in the said hospital or in any building connected with for the purpose of establishing such a library and if such library already established or to be established shall therefore be known as the Fred C. Ainsworth Endowment Library but not otherwise, I give and bequeath to the sum of $10,000 to the person or persons, board, agencies, organizations, corporations or to the United States government who or which may be deemed by my executors hereinafter named to be best qualified to carry out my desires in this respect and who or which shall agree to the foregoing provision as a condition precedent to taking this bequest. I direct that the discretion of my own executor shall be final and conclusive in deciding as to whom if anyone the foregoing bequest shall be paid and also as to what if any agreement or undertaking to abide by the said provision shall be required of whomever shall receive the said bequest. I further direct my executor shall make its decision in regard to the foregoing matter within one year from date of my death and that receipt of whomsoever shall receive this bequest shall be a full discharge and acquittance of my said executor in respect thereof. I impose no duty or obligation on my said executor to see to the use of that application therefore."

[*]Read over the telephone by Mrs. Elizabeth Kerwin Dore to Mary W. Standlee and Anabel Bryant, October 18, 1951 at 12 noon.

LIST OF BUILDINGS AND DATE OF CONSTRUCTION

BUILDING NUMBERS	NAME	DATE BUILT
1	Main Building	December 1908
1A	Main Building Annex	May 1915
1B	Main Building Annex	May 1915
1C	Main Building Annex	December 1914
1D	Main Building Annex	January 1928
1E	West Wing, Main Building	April 1928

1F	East Wing, Main Building	April 1928
1G	Main Building, Annex	March 1944
1H	Main Building, Annex	April 1946
2	Trash Room - Eye Clinic	July 1930
2A	Trash Room - Eye Clinic	July 1930
3	Eye Clinic - Blood Bank	July 1930
3A	Eye Clinic - Blood Bank	December 1940
4	Quartermaster Building	January 1910
4A	Quartermaster Building and Commissary	July 1932
5	Carpenter Shop	January 1910
5A	Oil & Gas Storage	July 1939
6	Garage, Transportation	January 1910
6A	Garage, Transportation	January 1910
7	Out-Patient Clinic	March 1910
8	Officers Quarters	March 1910
9	Officers Quarters	March 1910
11	Nurses Quarters	November 1929
11A	Nurses Quarters	July 1931
11B	Nurses Quarters	December 1933
12	Officers Apartments	April 1911
13	Internes Quarters	November 1913
14	Dental & X-ray Clinic	July 1930
14A	X-ray Therapy	October 1943
15	Heating Plant	1919
16	Incinerator	June 1920
17	Guest House	December 1920
18	Officers Quarters	purchased June 1920
18A	Garage	purchased June 1920
19	Officers Quarters	purchased June 1920
19A	Officers Quarters	purchased June 1920
20	Bakery	July 1932

21	Officers Quarters	purchased October 1920
22	Officers Quarters	purchased October 1920
22A	Garage	purchased October 1920
23	Laboratory & Morgue	July 1930
24	Officers Quarters	purchased October 1920
24A	Garage	purchased October 1920
25	Officers Quarters	purchased October 1920
25A	Garage	purchased October 1920
26	Officers Quarters	purchased July 1920
27	Officers Quarters	purchased July 1921
27A	Garage	purchased July 1921
28	Officers Quarters	purchased July 1921
29	Officers Quarters	purchased October 1922
29A	Garage	purchased October 1922
30	Officers Quarters	purchased October 1922
31	Wagon Shed	August 1921
32	Motor Transportation Garage	October 1919
33	Medical Supply	April 1922
33A	Medical Supply Annex	December 1925
34	Isolation Ward	July 1930
35	Officers Quarters	purchased October 1922
35A	Garage	purchased October 1922
36	TB & Maternity Building	July 1930
37	Gymnasium	June 1945
38	Guardhouse	November 1922
39	Greenhouse #1	January 1923
40	School Building	June 1925
40A	School Building & Hdqs. WRAMC	September 1932

40B	School Building & Hdqs. WRAMC	September 1932
41	Red Cross	September 1927
42	Wards	January 1928
43	Wards	January 1928
44-N-1	Chaplain	September 1945
45	Band Stand	June 1941
46-1	Sentry House	December 1941
46-2	Sentry House	December 1941
46-3	Sentry House	December 1941
49	Eng. Warehouse & Shops	July 1941
50	Greenhouse #3	1926
51	Greenhouse #4	November 1928
52	Wards	July 1930
53	Post Theatre	February 1950
56	Laundry	July 1932
57	Chapel	May 1931
58	N.P. Wards	December 1930
58A	N.P. Wards	October 1941
58B	N.P. Wards	October 1941
59	NCO Apartments	December 1933
61	BOQ	June 1941
62	BOQ	June 1941
63	Mess Hall	June 1941
63A	Lavatory Bldg.	June 1941
63B	Lavatory Bldg.	June 1941
64-80	Troop Command	June 1941
81	Warehouse #5	June 1942
82	PX Gas Station	1940
83	Animal House	March 1942
83A	Animal House Annex	December 1943
84	Wagon Shed	June 1942
85	Cafeteria & Forms Control	January 1943
86	Greenhouse #5	1941
88	Swimming Pool	September 1945
89	Reconditioning Building	June 1945
90	Fire House	June 1946
B-15	Post Office	1917

B-15A	Bank and Transportation Office	July 1944
B-18	Officers Apartments	1917
D-37	Post Engineer, Post Signal Office Welfare Division, Nursery	1918
G-76	Officers Mess	1918
A-03	NCO Mess	1917

CORRIDORS	_DATE BUILT_
44A	January 1928
44B	January 1928
44C	April 1928
44D	January 1928
44E-1	January 1928
44E-2	January 1928
44H	January 1928
44J	January 1928
44K	July 1930
44L	April 1928
44M	July 1930
44N	July 1930
44O	July 1930
44P	July 1930
44Q	July 1930
44R	July 1930
44S	1940
44T	1940
44U	1940
44V	1940

Forest Glen purchased in 1942.
Glen Haven built in 1941 - transferred to Walter Reed September 1947.

The Book Lady

"Let all things be done decently and in order."[1]

Four things bounded her well-ordered life and each in its way contributed to that undefined but total composition, the personality: a definite philosophy of work; a determination to ask no favor of anyone; a deep and innate distrust of the constancy of human affections; and The Library, Walter Reed General Hospital, business address for thirty-one years. Of the four, the last loomed largest in her life.

The only daughter of a scholarly Dutch Reformed minister, she was born in Meyersdale, Pennsylvania, July 28, 1885[2] but moved to Washington at the age of fifteen. The father was a man of strong and magnetic personality, well-beloved by his congregation and his President, Theodore Roosevelt. The child was precocious, vigorous and quick-tempered. Together they read the classics, studied language and mathematics and took long walks, discussing, meanwhile, religion, philosophy and the sacredness of human confidence. It was, therefore, the kindly loving father whom she adored above all others and who encouraged the academic thirst of her already active mind while teaching her disciplined self-control. Her only playmate during the first decade was a slightly older brother, with whom she romped and competed on equal terms. A beautiful, gracious and efficient mother shaped other characteristics and traits which, tempered by the reticence required of a parsonage family, developed the enigmatic personality of Mary Elizabeth Schick, to whom the fulfillment of duty was an honor and public service was a pleasure.

In the early years of the twentieth century only a few professional fields were open to young women of refinement, and so after graduation from Washington's Central High School, she attended Hood College, in Frederick, Maryland, where she studied music. In 1906, when a few educated young ladies from good families were offered positions as library assistants in the Public Library, a friend persuaded her to apply.

She was immediately successful as a reference librarian, and though she facetiously professed a preference for scrubbing the Library's handsome marble steps rather than lead the academically isolated life of a cataloguer, by 1910 she had decided on librarianship as a career. She was already known for her tact, graciousness and dignity when at twenty-five, properly chaperoned, she went to Philadelphia to be examined for entrance to Drexel Institute. The absence from home was complicated by a promise to return to Washington for employment, and although a number of excellent positions were open to her on graduation, including an offer from Herbert Putnam, Librarian of Congress, on May 30, 1911 she accepted the position as librarian at the U.S. Soldier's Home, the first woman to be so appointed in that institution. She began immediately to have the antiquated library remodeled and redecorated, and she discovered that eliminating the treasured cuspidors, used carelessly by some of the ancient inmates, required masterly

---

[1] I Corinthians, XIII, 40.
[2] *Service Stripe*, June 29, 1951.

tact. During the afternoons she read aloud to blind domiciliary patients in the Home hospital, and it was here that she became acquainted with the hospital commander, the dignified, reserved and ascetic "Noisy Jim" Glennan. Mary Schick remained as librarian for the Soldiers' Home until 1917, when she resigned for war work with the Information Service of the National Defense Council. This assignment was followed by an entertaining and valuable period as a special assistant in the U.S. Bureau of Efficiency.[3]

Socially graceful, quick-witted and with a remarkable ability to manage people with or without their consent, she nevertheless made neither personal nor official demands on others. Colonel Glennan had recognized her talent for leadership, and when he was assigned as commanding officer of Walter Reed in March 1919, he began trying to entice Mary Schick to join his staff on the promise of a free hand in building the Medical Department's finest hospital library. Afternoon tea, a regular ceremony at the Soldiers' Home Library, became the custom at Walter Reed, and her warm friendliness encouraged the commanding officer and other staff members to attend. Thus from the beginning she was an intimate part of the Post life, and the births and deaths, the marriages and promotions of Army personnel became of deep personal interest. The great and the near-great who visited the hospital came to her Library on guided tours. She believed it an obligation to attend all official functions to which she was invited, and she seemed unaware that she was often asked as dinner guest because of her sparkling conversational adaptability and not, as she mistakenly believed, because of the prestige of "The Library." She came, therefore, to pity many of her professional contemporaries who moved from place to place in search of more highly-graded positions. Some made more money, but she believed none had such an interesting life.

Her philosophy of work was a philosophy of service. She believed, without equivocation, that the individual wishes of employees should be subjugated to the welfare of the institution. Regardless of the quantity of books circulated or shortages in personnel she kept "The Library" open on holidays until the problem was settled by hospital regulations. Rather than impose unwelcome restrictions on her staff she often worked the holiday hours. Many who came to that quiet refuge to borrow a book remained to lean on her desk as they committed their woes to her keeping, for she never betrayed a confidence.

She was a person of strong convictions, which she unhesitatingly expressed if pressed, and her repartee was quick and telling. Although an incomparable raconteur, she never mentioned herself, and her conversation represented the essence of brevity, pointed and pungent. Thus like G.K. Chesterton she believed that "merely having an open mind is nothing. The object of opening the mind, as of opening the mouth, is to shut it again on something solid." She admitted without apology that she found the conversation of men more stimulating than the usual "small talk" of women, although she listened to their troubled trivia with apparent attention. She cared little for children, nothing for animals

[3] Ibid.

and rarely touched a human being if contact could be avoided. As a rule people felt at ease with her, for she was an excellent listener, and her impersonal manner loosened the tongues of those who had an insatiable need of an understanding audience.

Her thrift in administering "The Library" was as well known as her impersonal manner. Her moods were changeable, and she was sometimes dogmatic, even inconsistent. She was always keen-minded, professionally well-informed, punctual, impatient of stupidity. Her neatness and personal fastidiousness was a subject for comment, and she somehow managed to appear cool and immaculate in the hot humid Washington summers which she despised. Her heavy reddish-gold hair had begun to gray in her late twenties and at forty its perfectly marcelled waves fitted her head like a spun silver cap. Her erect, almost military posture, which she credited to the many years of pew-sitting under the surveillance of her Presbyterian-born mother, was the envy of less formal friends and associates.

She longed to travel more frequently than permitted by the requirements of her full schedule of work, and so she read and bought guidebooks with enthusiasm. Above all other things she dreaded the age of enforced retirement from her beloved Library, or to become physically dependent on others for geriatric care.[4]

She had played the Chapel organ during the late thirties and until the longer work-week of the World War II period absorbed her free time, and she played for weddings and funerals, to full congregations and to empty pews. Best of all, however, she liked her practice hour at the Chapel, for then she could give the organ its full volume. One of her favorite melodies during this period was "Londonderry Air," which she thoroughly enjoyed before acquaintance with the sentimental words, "Would God I were a tender apple blossom." She annually denounced the Yule season as a celebration for children and servants but quietly gave presents, fed the hungry and visited the aged. It was Mary Schick who subsidized "The Library" janitor between paydays; who advanced funds to her soldier-helpers for rent, obstetrical service or a new suit of clothes, who quietly loaned money to friends who appeared more prosperous than she. She had a keen interest in and understanding of the financial page of the *New York Times*, and she managed her own stocks and bonds as successfully and thriftily as she managed "The Library." Cultured, cryptic and business-like, she gave a lifetime of service to the hospital, happy in her sphere and "queen" of all she surveyed.

She was knowledgeable of the theatre, the symphony and the opera, and her familiarity with books and authors was almost legendary. There were nearly forty thousand recreation books in her Library, and the monthly purchase exceeded the majority of the branch libraries of Washington's public system. By 1950, *The Medical Library* and *The Ainsworth Library* contained a combined eight thousand volumes. More than one hundred medical journals and periodicals were received each month and circulated to interested staff members prior to permanent filing. An extensive inter-library loan business was conducted with the Army Medical Library, which she had long wanted to

---

[4] Ltr from Lt. Helen A. Taggart, ANC, Ret., July 6, 1951.

see located at the Army Medical Center as planned. Thus under her expert guidance the hospital library at Walter Reed became one of the largest of its kind in the United States.[5] She could discuss surgical literature with her faithful friend, Colonel Keller; the stock market with General Metcalfe; deplore the high cost of living with a disconsolate "GI," quickly find the shortest historical novel in "The Library" for a desperate high school sophomore, or exchange clever stories with her best non-fiction reader, "Big Jim" Kimbrough.

Although she never sought the company of juveniles, many adored her. Army children, she said tartly, grew up under her desk. Some returned as staff physicians, or as proud young mothers with struggling gurgling youngsters to be duly admired; others merely returned to see her. Walter Reed was the Medical Department's Mother House for training, and its doctors and nurses were reassigned to small station hospitals throughout the United States. Some wrote to her for guidance in establishing libraries or to purchase books. Many who went overseas in World War II sent for books for

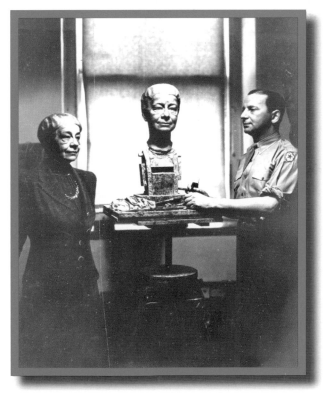

An Artist at Work; Lt. Niesen Tregor, MSC

[5] S. Kathleen Jones, *Hospital Libraries*, American Library Association, 1939, pgs 66, 80; *Service Stripe*, March 10, 1945.

their units, and in spite of the excellent facilities afforded by the Army Medical Library, Walter Reed-trained doctors often preferred having her undertake their medical reference work. For years she had procured special purchases of medical books for staff members, buying the volumes on her account and then waiting patiently until "next month" for payment, if the purchaser was hardpressed. It was not surprising, therefore, that the president of one of the large Medical Book Companies counted on her as one of his "best friends in the library business,"[6] for her orders were large, her records were exact and always in order and her own bills paid with clock-like regularity.

In the years from 1923 to 1941 only two librarians, the Misses Schick and Gould, and three soldier-helpers accomplished all the library work, including a readers' advisory service to bed patients. It was during this period that Miss Schick earned the title of "The Book Lady," as gray-haired, gray-uniformed and with a small four-wheeled book-laden cart she visited the wards. In late 1941, when Miss Gould transferred to a Navy library and before her replacement was secured, Miss Schick attempted to serve all the wards alone rather than request an authorization for additional personnel. The increased activities of the World War II period ultimately forced her to expand the staff and confine her own activities to administration. Such an arrangement did not restrict her personal contacts, however, for old-timers invariably sought her out with a glad cry - "Why Miss Schick, are you still here?" And they always reminisced, for she represented a continuity in the life of the hospital that was solid, respectable and gracious. Like Kean's description of the hospital's noble facade, she was authentic.

She had, through the years, carefully collected and hung portraits of the hospital's many commanding officers, and some of the Surgeons General, but close association with occasionally pompous members of the military population of the Post had convinced her, to her own satisfaction at least, that civilian employees were not included as intimates in the military group. As a consequence, she steadfastly refused to provide "The Library" with an acceptable photograph or portrait of herself. When her old friend of Soldiers' Home days, Norman T. Kirk, became Surgeon General in 1943, he ordered a terra cotta model made of her leonine head, for permanent assignment to "The Library." As the features lacked the "laughter lines" worn deep by her friendly smile, some of her associates thought it was an empty-eyed and cold-looking creation, and so for several years she kept it shrouded and in the Ainsworth Library, on top of Colonel Keller's old empyema files. Now and then a photographer from the *Medical Illustrations Section* of the Army Medical Center headquarters would try his luck at photographing "The Book Lady," but few achieved any real likeness, her friends complaining that her pictures lacked the warmth of her personality and seemed severe.[7]

[6] Ltr from Edward T. Speakman, Jr. (C.M.B.C.) to the writer, July 5, 1951
[7] Sculptured by Lt. Niesen Tregor, MSC.

Although long afflicted with hypertension, as well as a minor heart ailment which she carefully refrained from mentioning to her family, in 1946, for the first time since beginning her forty years of public service, Mary Schick was away from her work for a three-month surgical illness. Once recovered she returned to duty with the same zest and the same determination that characterized everything she did. By the early summer of 1951, however, her brisk step faltered occasionally, and once or twice she admitted, rather disdainfully, to having a headache.

On June 25, 1951, during the afternoon tea hour and while entertaining her staff with a clever story, she experienced a sudden and temporary loss of consciousness. She was hospitalized in spite of determined protests, but two hours later, while again playing the inimitable raconteur, she suffered a massive cerebral hemorrhage.

Few have been privileged to choose their exit from life, but hers was as she wished. At 9 PM, the closing hour for her beloved library, the Great Physician turned the key for Mary E. Schick, *The Book Lady* of Walter Reed who was always too busy with her daily duties to write the story of the hospital that she wanted for her own Library. She died as she had lived, quietly and without distress, with "all things...done decently and in order."[8] The news spread

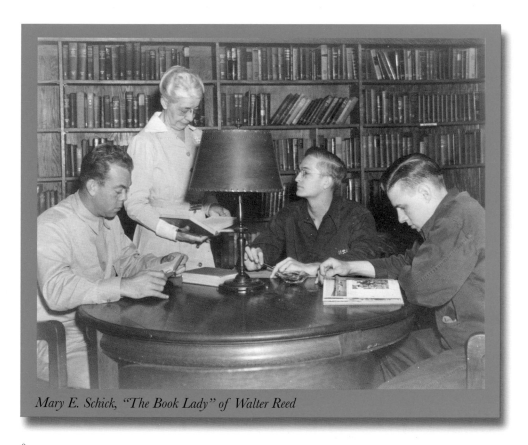

Mary E. Schick, "The Book Lady" of Walter Reed

[8] Ltr L.K. Multon to P.H. Schick, June 28, 1950.

quickly, and letters of condolence came from far and wide, for to her friends, to many of the sick and wounded soldiers whom she had befriended through the years, "The Library," quiet oasis in the busy life of the hospital, and the librarian were one and the same. The letters were always the same - that the hospital had lost an irreplaceable employee, the person writing had lost a best friend, and the world was richer because she had lived. Many came to pay their last respects and there were, of course, "the many, many thousands not there. Those would be the hospitalized soldiers over the years, and many others, for whose good (she) gave of her wisdom, of her strength, of her heart, and of her joy."[9] Doctors, nurses, patients and friends had often found comfort in her selfless service, and because of her versatility in friendship some had remarked that she was "made all things to all men."[10]

In the years following publication of "A Tree Grows in Brooklyn," librarians, like school teachers, became the object of gentle literary ridicule. There were an increasing number of stories, plays and cartoons which depicted a librarian as a mousey, bookish and detached creature, one who looked and acted frustrated and afraid of the world. As a rule some amused friend provided "The Book Lady" with the current samples of such wit or art, which usually found their way to the waste basket. Among the few personal items which she retained in her desk, however, was one of James J. Metcalf's poems called "The Librarian," for which she could have been the model.

> *The good librarian is one...Who knows not only books...*
> *But how to handle people and...To judge them by their*
> *looks...Who also knows a thousand facts...Or finds them*
> *in a hurry...To satisfy the doubtful minds...That cogitate*
> *and worry...From ancient words to current news...And*
> *how to spell a name...The wars that shaped geogra-*
> *phy...And who was most to blame...The best there is in*
> *juveniles... In poetry and fiction...The latest thing in*
> *science and...The key to better diction...The good librar-*
> *ian is kind...And yet politely stern...Whose knowledge is*
> *abounding but...Who does not cease to learn.*

In her fine almost Spencerian handwriting she had made notes on a small library card which indicated that she had consulted the hospital's cardiologist in 1939, and the Chief of the Medical Service in 1942. Their conclusions were apparently the same. There was no enlargement of the heart, although both physicians had detected a "slow, soft murmur;" both had informed her, as doctors often do, that she had an

[9] I Corinthians XIII, 40.
[10] I Corinthians IX, 22.

"interesting" condition. She had been told that she could take limited exercise on level ground, should avoid exhaustion and nervous tension. Adherence to such instructions, they had said, would give her "several years longer" to live.

Someone had apparently asked her to make a brief talk on her activities as a hospital librarian, for she had made other miscellaneous notes on a scratch pad, among which was the phrase "Have always worked hard." Her affairs were in order; her accounts were correct.

One small task, residue of her early days at Walter Reed, remained incomplete - the history of the installation which had received from her a lifetime of devotion. She had begun collecting newspaper clippings in the early twenties, for library visitors were always suggesting that she write an institutional history. The busy, happy years slipped away from her, however, and during the early forties she began urging a younger staff member to write the story, undertaken as a casual extra-curricular activity in the winter of 1943. It should, she said, record indelibly the personalities of the many hospital commanders, the intimate almost family loyalty of the staff, and it should tie firmly the past to the present. She had agreed to serve, with her old friend Jimmy Kimbrough, as an informal advisor during the preparation of the manuscript, and with her customary poignant intellectualism she had derided the censorial efforts of those desirous of degrading history to the level of public relations media.

It was the late Raymond Dodge who said "To indoctrinate his subordinates with his main principles of action is one of the tasks of a great leader." If, therefore, this small informal volume had been prepared for publication rather than as a local reference work, the dedicatory page should carry the sort of inscription that has so often appeared on book plates, "Mary E. Schick, Her Book," for in undertaking the task the pupil, who is neither librarian nor historian, has merely borrowed the mantle of the teacher.

Index

A

B

E

F

G

H

I

J

K

L

Mc

M

N

S

T

U

V

W

XYZ

M.I. Surg. 20, 1907

THE WALTER REED GENERAL HOSPITAL OF THE UNITED STATES ARMY.

By MAJOR WILLIAM C. BORDEN.

SURGEON IN THE UNITED STATES ARMY.

IT will be noted that the establishment which we are considering is designated The Walter Reed U.S. Army General Hospital. Of the reason for naming the hospital after Walter Reed there is hardly need to speak. It is the custom of the service to name army posts after those officers no longer living who have been distinguished in the service. In the Capitol city no more appropriate name could be given to a permanent army general hospital than that of the man much of whose life was spent there, and whose yellow fever work was of such inestimable value to mankind; while the connection of the hospital with the Army Medical School, in which Dr. Reed so long served as a teacher, makes the name doubly appropriate.

As to the term "general hospital," this has in the military service a special significance, and means, not necessarily a hospital to which all sorts of cases are admitted, but one which is quite directly under the control of the Surgeon General of the army. The Army Regulations, paragraph 1467, state that "General hospitals will be under the exclusive control of the Surgeon General and will be governed by such regulations as the Secretary of War may prescribe. The senior surgeon will command the same, and will not be subject to the orders of local commanders other than those of territorial divisions and departments to whom specific delegation of authority may have been made."

Aside from the special hospitals, such as the field hospital established in time of war, there are in the medical service two kinds of hospitals—the post and the general hospital. The post hospital is for the care of the sick of a military post or station, a

(20)

special building for this purpose being erected at each established military garrison. The post hospitals do not, except in unusual cases, receive any cases from outside nor care for any other than those immediately attached to the station at which the hospital is placed

The general hospitals on the other hand, are alike in taking cases from the army at large, the patients being sent to these hospitals under special regulations, and coming not only from stations throughout the United States but from its territorial possessions. There are in the United States at the present time four general hospitals. Of these, two are special hopsitals and

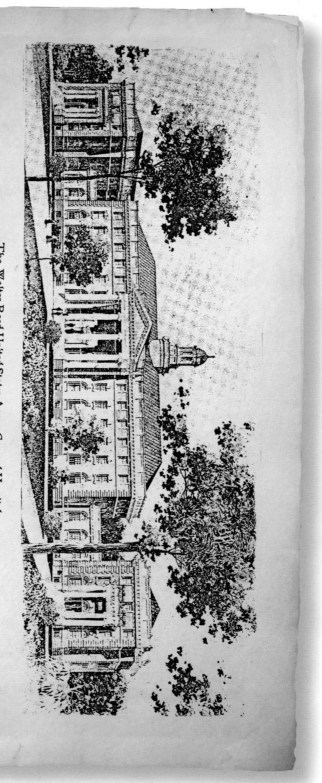

The Walter Reed United States Army General Hospital.

two are general hospitals, in the accepted medical significance of the term.

Of the special "General Hospitals," one is at Hot Springs, Arkansas, and is for the treatment of such diseases as rheumatism, neuralgia and like troubles, which the waters of the Hot Springs of Arkansas have an established reputation of benefiting, except that cases of venereal disease are not admitted. Admission is restricted to cases of the kind above mentioned, and the hospital is entirely a special one.

The other special hospital is located at Fort Bayard, New Mexico. At this hospital only cases of tuberculosis are admitted, the location, on occount of the elevation and dryness of the atmosphere, being particularly adapted to the treatment of pulmonary tuberculosis.

Of the army general hospitals which are general in the medical acceptance of the term and admit all classes of cases, one is located at the Presidio, San Francisco, California and the other, the immediate predecessor of the Walter Reed Army General Hospital, is located at Washington Barracks, D. C. Previous to the Spanish-American war there were no general hospitals of this character in the army. During the Spanish-American war, as is usual in time of war, a number of large general hospitals were established, and of these the two above mentioned have been continued since that time. Of the two, the General Hospital at San Francisco is the larger, for the reason that it acts as a receiving hospital for most cases of disease and injury sent from the Philippines. The work done at this hospital has been very great and most creditable.

The other army general hospital for all classes of cases is located at Washington Barracks, D. C. As before stated, this hospital is the immediate predecessor of the Walter Reed Hospital, and a brief account of it and the place it fills in the medical department of the army is, therefore, germane to our subject as showing the work which will be carried on in its successor. This hospital was established by General Orders, 140, dated September 8, 1898, which set aside the post hospital at Washington Barracks as a general hospital. This hospital has therefore been in a large way an extemporized one. The post hospital at the Barracks was built some fifteen years ago, and, while an excellent example of the post hospital as then built, was not intended for, and therefore could not entirely fill, the requirements of a general hospital. The writer was assigned to the command of this hospital by Special Orders No. 239, dated October 10, 1898. At that time there were over two hundred patients, some of whom occupied the hospital building and others were in tents on the ground near it. With the approach of winter it was necessary to provide better accommodations for those in tents, and two temporary wooden buildings with kitchens and accessory buildings were erected. The hospital also utilized an old hospital building which had not been torn down when the new hospital was erected, and some wooden buildings were put up for use as shops, stables, etc., the whole establishment being of a make-shift nature. The hospital building itself, however, was in good repair, and the operating and sterilizing rooms were put in excellent condition by equipping them with the most modern apparatus. The hospital worked along under these conditions for some time. Soon another feature was added to it. For several years a detachment of enlisted men of the Hospital Corps known as a "Company of Instruction" had been located at Washington Barracks. This company was used as a school for teaching recruits to the Hospital Corps the elements of anatomy, physiology, nursing, Hospital Corps drill and like subjects, in order to equip them for duty as nurses and for the field service required of the Hospital Corps. The Company had also been used in connection with the Army Medical School for instructing the junior medical officers attending the school in Hospital Corps drill, the establishment of field hospitals, and like work connected with the Hospital Corps. It was evident that if the Company of Instruction could be attached to the hospital instead of the post of Washington Barracks, thus making it a part of the hospital organization and so directly under the commanding officer of the hospital, it could then be used for work connected with the Army Medical School without any clash of authority and with the fullest efficiency so far as assignment

24 *MAJOR WILLIAM C. BORDEN.*

to duty and instruction were concerned. Therefore, by General Orders No. 3, dated January 8, 1900, the Company of Instruction was transferred from the control of the commanding officer of the Barracks to the General Hospital.

With the reopening of the Army Medical School in October, 1901, the writer was made Professor of Military Surgery in that institution, thereby putting the hospital in direct connection with the school, so that it could work with it and be utilized for the clinical instruction of the students, particularly in military surgical methods, and for teaching them hospital administration and the general details of hospital management as they pertain to the military service.

The general hospital now assumed the position of a military station, under the command of the commanding officer of the hospital, and consisted of two units, the hospital proper and the company. It will be noted, therefore, that the hospital was not now a hospital in the common acceptance of the term, but a military post, having the functions not only of a hospital but of an educational institution for enlisted men and for students at the Army Medical School.

The desirability of maintaining such an institution both for the treatment of the sick and for work in instructing Hospital Corps men and for teaching in connection with the Army Medical School was at once evident. Equally it was evident that such work could not be properly carried on in a group of extemporized buildings, many of which were poorly constructed for temporary use only. It was the necessity for the continuance of this establishment which gave rise to the appeal to Congress, through the Secretary of War, for funds for the purchase of a suitable site, and the erection of a proper hospital thereon, and which has eventuated in the Walter Reed U.S. Army General Hospital soon to be erected.

The work done in the present hospital, and which is to be continued and amplified upon the completion of the new one, shows the general character and purposes of the hospital. Serially stated, the hospital will be used for the following named purposes:

(*a*) For treatment of special cases.

(*b*) For training enlisted men of the Hospital Corps for nursing and other duties.

(*c*) For instruction in connection with the Army Medical School.

(*d*) In case of war, to be expanded and used as a base hospital. Cases of illness and injury are constantly arising in the military service which require special skill and special appliances for their treatment in order to save the men to the service, to reduce the pension list, and to give men disabled in the service of their country the benefit of the most advanced medical and surgical knowledge. The post hospitals at military stations are equipped for the ordinary run of cases, but it is too expensive to equip all the hospitals in the army, irrespective of their size, with the special and often costly apparatus required for the treatment of difficult cases. Equally it is impossible to have all the surgeons skilled in all the specialties of medicine and surgery. The advance of medicine and surgery has produced a large number of complicated and costly appliances, and has necessitated the training of medical men for their use and in the observation and treatment of special diseases. The proper treatment of cases requiring special skill and special apparatus can only be given at hospitals especially equipped for the purpose. The conditions relative to the treatment of special cases are similar in the army to the conditions in civil life. In civil life difficult and obscure cases occurring in the country and in towns and small cities are sent to medical centers where there are large hospitals fully equipped and with specially trained medical men in attendance. It is evident that under the conditions which obtain in military surgery similar methods must be pursued. The post hospitals must be supplemented by larger institutions, fully equipped with special apparatus and appliances, and officered by men who pay special attention to surgery, clinical diagnosis, diseases of the eye, ear, nose, throat, etc. On account of the small size of the main building at Washington Barracks all these requirements could not be carried out, but it is hoped that in the Walter Reed Hospital all these necessities will be met. In spite of the disadvant-

26   *MAJOR WILLIAM C. BORDEN.*

ages which obtain at the present hospital, quite a large number of patients have been treated, and this may be taken as an indication of the usefulness of a general hospital in the treatment of special cases which are sent to it. From the establishment of the hospital up to September 8th, 1906, 6,674 cases have been treated. Of these 4,922 were medical cases and 1,752 were surgical, nearly all of the latter being operative.

As to the character of the disabilities treated at the General Hospital (and a like kind will be treated at the Walter Reed Hospital), it may be said that most of them are of a sub-acute or chronic nature. The preponderance of this class of cases over the acute kind is due to the fact that the majority are not of local occurrence, but are sent from all parts of the United States, and some from the Philippines. They are usually cases of an obscure nature, or those which, after prolonged ordinary treatment, require more special or operative measures. At the same time a fair percentage of acute cases is received, these being mostly from the posts in the immediate vicinity of the hospital, or cases arising in the Company of Instruction, the detachment on duty in the hospital, and soldiers and officers on furlough or leave in the city or passing through. The number of acute cases, in connection with the chronic ones, is sufficient to make the clinic at the hospital an entirely general one, and therefore useful for clinical instruction in connection with the Army Medical School. With the increased size and facilities of the Walter Reed Hospital the clinical advantages will be correspondingly increased. Also, owing to the peculiar function which a general hospital has of treating those cases which have been found to require special appliances or special skill, the proportion of obscure and difficult cases is great. From a medical standpoint this makes service at the hospital particularly interesting, as difficult problems in diagnosis, prognosis and treatment are constantly arising.

A further function which the hospital will have is the treatment of officers who would otherwise be on sick leave. With no facilities for treatment other than those available at military posts, it has been customary in the past to give officers requiring special treatment, sick leaves of absence. In such cases the officers are removed from supervision of superior officers and medical officers. In consequence the treatment adopted is not always to the benefit of the officer, and the service suffers through long delay in restoring the officer to duty or by producing conditions which may lead to permanent disability. The interests of the service and of sick officers are better subserved if, instead of sick leave, a fully equipped hospital is available to which officers may be ordered and there treated by competent medical men who are fully alive to safeguarding the interests both of the officer and of the United States.

Another important function of a general hospital is the observation of officers presumably incapacitated for service. The conditions of the military service are such that officers frequently have but desultory medical attendance. Their medical history is, therefore, imperfect, and their real physical condition when claim of permanent disability is made is often a matter of conjecture. It is important, if disability is not permanent, that this fact be ascertained and the officer saved to the service. Equally, to safeguard the interests both of the Government and the officer, it is necessary when disability exists that an accurate opinion be arrived at, both as to the nature of the disability and its cause. Observation at a hospital equipped with modern diagnostic apparatus is frequently the only way in which these questions can be authoritatively settled. The General Hospital at Washington is being constantly put to this use to the fullest satisfaction of all, and the value of the Walter Reed Hospital to the Government in this way will be constant in the future.

In connection with the preceding remarks relative to the treatment of officers and enlisted men, it may interest the members of the profession who are in civil life to know that the professional work of a medical officer of the Army has a definite economic value, a value which can be accurately measured in dollars and cents. This arises from the fact that soldiers incapacitated for service on account of diseases or injuries acquired in line of duty receive pensions, and officers retired for similar cause are entitled to retired pay throughout the remainder of their lives. Conse-

28   *MAJOR WILLIAM C. BORDEN.*

quently if a medical officer removes any evident disability from an enlisted man of the army and returns him to duty, he saves the Government the amount of the man's pension which he would have received in case of discharge for disability, and, in the case of an officer, saves the Government an annual outlay to the amount of the officer's retired pay. The value of the work done at an army hospital in saving money to the Government can therefore be, in certain cases, estimated, and when the writer appeared before the Appropriations Committee of Congress asking for an appropriation for a new general hospital, he presented to that body an argument for the appropriation based in part upon the work done in the General Hospital, at the Barracks and its value in saving money to the Government. This argument was presented in September, 1898, and it showed that up to that time forty-three officers had been operated upon for disability, who, had the trouble not been removed, would have been retired from the service. The monthly retired pay of these officers ranged from $93.65 to $281.25, and had these officers been retired their retired pay would have been, per year, $79,253.40. Also it was shown that 480 enlisted men had been saved to the service, whose pension rate would have been from $6.00 to $65.00 per month, making a saving per year for pensions of $53,812.08—a total yearly saving to the Government of $133,065.48—the equivalent of three per cent interest on an investment of $4,435,516.00. This estimate of saving was from surgical cases alone, no estimate being made on the 4,201 medical cases which had been treated up to that time, for the reason that while it is possible to accurately determine the result of an operable surgical disability, the same cannot be said in regard to a medical case; but that the saving from medical cases is large cannot be disputed. These figures will serve to show what can be expected from the work at the Walter Reed Hospital, and the economic value to the Government of providing a hospital equipped with all modern appliances at which difficult cases can be properly treated.

As before stated, the hospital has a further function, that of training enlisted men of the Hospital Corps in nursing and other duties. Recruits for the Hospital Corps come from all vocations in civil life and most of them are entirely unfamiliar with nursing, Hospital Corps drill and military duties. In fact it may be said that a large number of the recruits have never seen the interior of a hospital, and the great majority of them have not the faintest idea of how to care for the sick. These recruits have been laborers, school teachers, pharmacists, stenographers, physicians, in fact represent almost every vocation. It is from this material that nurses have to be made and non-commissioned officers educated, so that the Hospital Corps can do its multitudinous duties of caring for the sick, both in peace and war. The Company of Instruction now attached to the General Hospital at Washington consists of about 150 men. In this company a systematic course of instruction in nursing, first aid and Hospital Corps drill is given by means of recitations, lectures, drills and practical work in the wards of the general hospital. As soon as instruction is completed the men are sent for duty to various military hospitals in the United States and the insular possessions. Since the establishment of the General Hospital at Washington, in 1898, over 2,300 men have passed through the company. With the establishment of the Walter Reed Army General Hospital much greater facilities will be afforded for the theoretical and practical training of the company.

A further use to which the general hospital will be put, and has been put, is for instruction in connection with the Army Medical School. The Army Medical School was established in 1893, and yearly sessions have been held at the School with the exception of an interval during the war with Spain. This school is one of the military service schools authorized by the Secretary of War and placed under the general supervision of the War College by General Orders 155, November 27, 1901. In this school, medical graduates who are candidates for appointment to the Medical Department from civil life and selected officers from the National Guard of the different states are trained in the duties of medical officers; the school is carried on in the Army Medical Museum, on the corner of Seventh and B Streets, Southwest. It is essential to the success of training in this school that the students be instructed in hospital administration as applied to military

30   *MAJOR WILLIAM C. BORDEN.*

hospitals, military surgery, Hospital Corps drill, establishment of field hospitals, and like subjects which pertain particularly to military medical methods. As the curriculum of the school is now arranged, student officers attend clinics at the general hospital, where they are instructed in military surgery and in the use of instruments and appliances furnished for the use of medical officers. The use of the hospital for clinical instruction in connection with the Army Medical School (as stated by the Surgeon General in his report for 1903, page 126) "has a value as an essential part of the instruction of young medical officers and enlisted men of the Hospital Corps which cannot be estimated." In this connection the Surgeon General (in his report for 1903 page 18) states, "The distinctive features of the course at the school are, first, the large measure of personal attention paid to the student's individual work by instructors in the laboratories and surgical demonstrators, which it is believed is not exceeded, if equalled, in any post graduate school." The combination of the general hospital and school, as was the case with the English army hospital and school, established at Netley after the Crimean war, and the celebrated French hospital and school at Val-de-Grâce at Paris, offers advantages which are great and evident.

In laying out the general plan of the grounds on which the Walter Reed Army General Hospital is to be built, provision has been made for a site for an academic building for the Army Medical School, and it is hoped that in time a building entirely adequate to the purpose may be erected, thus giving a military medical institution with all necessary working units.

The Walter Reed Army General Hospital will also subserve the purposes of a base hospital capable of almost indefinite expansion in time of war. In all previous wars in which the United States has engaged, troops in considerable number have been assembled in Washington and its vicinity. The number of the sick from the troops, assembled in and near Washington and sick from other commands who while being shipped to different parts of the United States in passing through Washington are retained in this city, has in the past always necessitated the establishment of one or more large general hospitals here. The establishment *de novo* of large general hospitals is always accompanied with considerable delay, expense, some confusion and unavoidable discomfort to the sick. With the nucleus of a general hospital already established and in running order the expansion of the hospital to any desired size can be done practically, without delay, and at a minimum expense—the nucleus being provided with all necessary apparatus, both medical and surgical, with operating rooms, and with the administration in working order, nothing is required but the addition of temporary wards to care for the sick in the very best manner. The establishment of a general hospital in the District of Columbia, not only for the use of the army in time of peace, but for its expansion in time of war, is one which immediately appeals to the military expert as thereby a contingency is prepared for in advance, fully in accord with the time honored maxim, "in time of peace prepare for war." When, therefore, such an establishment meets so many requirements, namely, special advantages for the care of the sick in time of peace, the training of Hospital Corps men for their duties in nursing, the training of medical officers fresh from civil life in administrative and other duties which pertain particularly to the military service, and expansion in time of war, the great use of such an institution in the military service is evident.

The location of a new general hospital to be built in the District to replace the old one at Washington Barracks required careful selection. A board was appointed by the Secretary of War of which the writer was a member, and notice was sent to all the prominent real estate men in the city to submit plots of ground. Some forty different offers were made, and the board in its work canvassed the entire District. In locating the site the board was governed by the considerations that although the hospital was not a city hospital it should be located within convenient reach of the main railroad depot, on a good road, and should have street-car facilities, adjacent water main and sewer, also the site should be well elevated, well drained, and have sufficient size to give good air space about the hospital and to allow the erection of other buildings which would eventually be required. Equally, the site should be sufficiently large to allow

32   *MAJOR WILLIAM C. BORDEN.*

the erection of numerous temporary pavilion wards for use in time of war. With these various considerations in view the board finally recommended the purchase of 43½ acres of ground, fronting on Brightwood Avenue, and extending through west nearly to Fourteenth Street.

This site is therefore in the most northerly portion of the District, and is almost exactly five miles distant from the Treasury, the Capitol and the new Union Depot. Street-car facilities are now furnished by the Brightwood Avenue line, and when the Fourteenth Street line is extended, as it will be, to the District boundary, the site will be most convenient to this car line as well. In time of peace the Brightwood Avenue road, which is finely macadamized, affords an excellent way in which to bring patients from the railroad terminal. In time of war, if necessary, direct railroad communication can be made with the Metropolitan branch of the B. & O., as this passes within about a quarter of a mile to the east, and a branch road could be run into the grounds without difficulty; or Silver Spring station, which is less than half a mile away, can be utilized. From Fourteenth to Sixteenth Street in this part of the District is but one block, and on the west of Sixteenth Street is Rock Creek Park with its high ridges, where temporary camps can be placed if such are required.

The terrain of the site is itself most excellent, for while the site is not level, it consists practically of five main elevations upon which the different groups of buildings can be advantageously placed, and the slopes from these are such that perfect surface drainage is assured. Probably in no other part of the District could so many advantageous conditions be found, and when Fourteenth and Sixteenth Streets are extended these fine approaches will be available on the west, putting the hospital in most perfect communication, so far as fine roads are concerned, with the central portions of the city.

The hospital itself is designed to be built on the pavilion system, with a central administration building and wings placed laterally, all facing the south. With the present appropriation of $200,000 only the central building will be erected, this being planned to include for the present the administrative offices, the wards, kitchens, operating room, etc., for a total of seventy-five patients. The hospital is designed on the colonial type of architecture, and all the adjacent buildings erected in the future will conform to it. It is to be built of red brick with white stone facings, and will have all modern improvements. The ventilation of the hospital will be by the plenum-vacuum system, the air being filtered on entry and carried over coils of hot-water pipe before being distributed to the different rooms. The air ducts have been so constructed as to change the air in the offices and halls three times and in the wards four times per hour. The heating will be by hot water, mechanically circulated, and the radiators will be only of such size as to supplement the warmed incoming air and to make up for radiation. Lighting will be mainly by electricity, only a sufficient number of gas lights being installed to furnish light should the electric current fail. The plumbing will be most modern in character. No plumbing will be installed in the operating room, this room being kept entirely free, the necessary wash stands, sinks, etc., being placed in adjacent rooms. The floors of the wards and offices will be of wood—as it is believed that experience has demonstrated that a wooden floor can be kept sufficiently clean and gives the pleasantest surface upon which to walk—except in those situations where much wear will be had, such as the main hall of the lower floor, which will be laid in Terazzi and marble.

Finally, some statement may be made relative to the expansion of the hospital and its combination with other units as a part of a medical military educational institution. The Medical Department stands greatly in need of a fully equipped army medical school, and the site of the Walter Reed Army General Hospital offers excellent facilities for uniting such a school with the hospital and with companies of instruction of the Hospital Corps, so making a complete educational unit. Equally, in time the library and medical museum of the Surgeon General's office, now at the corner of Seventh and B Streets, Southwest, will have to be provided for elsewhere. The city improvement plan, which will undoubtedly be quite closely adhered to in the future, disposes of this brick building. For this reason, Congress

34   *MAJOR WILLIAM C. BORDEN.*

has not favored further appropriations of money for extensive repairs or extension. The Army Medical School is now carried on in the building, but the quarters are cramped and not suitable; nevertheless, Congress will not enlarge the building to accommodate the school, as the building is not in accord with the city improvement scheme. With the elaboration of the improvement scheme it will be necessary to do away with this building, and then a new and suitable one should be erected. The library is such an important institution that it should be continued in its individual existence rather than be absorbed into the Library of Congress. It is hoped that with a suitable place for locating the library, and with the members of the medical profession advocating it, a proper building may be erected on the site of the Walter Reed Hospital when the necessity for such a building occurs. The total expansion upon the site, therefore, covers a medical military institution having for units the academic building of the Army Medical School, and its adjuncts; the Walter Reed U.S. Army General Hospital; barracks for two companies of the Hospital Corps—one a company of instruction and the other a reserve ambulance company; and, finally, the library and museum of the Surgeon General's office. This scheme, properly carried out on an adequate scale, will give an educational institution for the use of the army in accord with its needs and somewhat on the lines of the large army medical schools and hospitals in Europe. It is now an accepted fact that the practitioner of medicine and surgery graduated in the civil schools must have a supplementary education in the special work of the Medical Department in order to fit him for the duties of a medical officer. The special requirements of the practice of medicine and surgery as adapted to the army in peace and in war must be taught, and thorough instruction must be given in theoretical and practical hygiene as it relates to the military forces. Also, with the extension of our possessions to the tropics, the subject of tropical medicine, which is not extensively taught in the civil schools, must be given due attention in the Army Medical School. With an academic building of suitable size and properly equipped with laboratories, lecture rooms, etc., supplemented by a general hospital having facilities for clinical and administrative teaching, combined with companies of the Hospital Corps being instructed in their duties and used for instruction of student officers, and with the library and museum of the Surgeon General's office upon the same site, a complete medical military educational institution of great value would be had. It is hoped that in time such an institution may be obtained in its entirety, and that it can be built upon a scale worthy of the object for which it is intended and of the Capitol city in which it is placed.

ABILITY FOR SERVICE AFTER WOUNDS FROM MODERN WEAPONS.

AS recipient of the Langenbeck fund, Schaefer (Berlin) made extensive studies in the field of the Russo-Japanese war. After the battle of Mukden he was enabled to examine over 7,000 wounded who again recovered sufficiently to return to their commands. The losses were undoubtedly great, but the percentage of loss not so unprecedented as the early reports showed. The percentage of wounded compares with that averaged in the Franco-Prussian war. The officers suffered more than the privates. The chances of the individual are shown in a table giving an average of forty-four dead and wounded in every one hundred men of the First Siberian corps. The relation of dead to wounded was 1–5.5. He reports upon the progress of the wounded. The percentage of deaths after wounds was remarkably small. Though many dead on the field were not reported, the prognosis for the wounded who were carried alive from the field, seems more favorable than in former wars. Surprisingly large was the number of wounded who were again able to report for service. Schaefer found about one-half of the wounded, after the battle of Mukden, able to serve after a period of three months. The report contains a classification of the wounds, as to the parts wounded and the nature of the missiles and weapons. Fifteen per cent of all wounds were caused by artillery fire.—*Annals of Surgery.*

ORIGINAL EDITS

Page(s)	Remarks

11.   Clearer syntax on Seventh Street Road.

11.   The issue is the early history of the geographical location of WRGH. Something like the suggested change is more specific and guides the reader's thinking.

15.   Inserted sentence. It is helpful to the reader to know why this skirmish is described; it is interesting and important to present, but the reader can use a reminder.

15 - 16   This paragraph interrupts the logical flow; it logically falls at the top of page 13.

18 - 21   Recommend newer (or British) format for repetitive citations:

1. First citation of reference is given in full, followed by (hereafter, author, short title - e.g., Ashburn, Medical Department).

2. Repeated citations use author, short title and page.

Pictures   Recommend retaining

1. Sharpshooter's Tree
2. Lay Mansion.

3. Has been used in other MS - then the years, but modern readers need the ambulance picture to contribute to the sense of crudity in medical transportation. 'Tis true about this means being subverted to other uses.

2

CHAPTER II

my copy says proportious fe — size

Remarks

Page(s)	

proportions

22.
I'm not sure what a ~~propositions~~ of the Surgeon General's Library means. The change is a small boast for our side.

small posts few medical officers

22.
The Army was the reverse of concentrated - there were over 250 posts.

22.
Nursing education comment is true, but not germane here to the flow of logic. Lister lectured in U.S. in 1867 and convinced most of the East Coast surgeons by 1868-69. Lister did not invent the germ theory of disease - this was Pasteur and Koch.

23.
No so. "Listerism" was enthusiastically adopted in Europe and America by 1870-75. The only "holdout" - for nearly 20 years - was London. After all, what could a Scotsman know? Actually - I recommend deletion of all of last paragraph page 23 and top of page 24. The Sternberg facts are true, but can be better used later on. — *are used later on*

24.
I agree with Phalen quotation - but it really refers to Lovell's views in 1818. Its a little unfair to use here without explication as added.

25.
Department of Columbia was the Northwest Pacific.

25.
Since Sternberg was TSG, he clearly believed in the germ theory. Malaria vector discovery was of course still 4 years away.

26.
Military manners was what Hoff added to the Corps.

33.
Delete - with change in Chapter 1, this no longer follows.

33-35.
The last half of p. 33, all of p. 34 and 35, seem disjointed and unconnected. A smooth paragraph or so on the Red Cross Nurse and and Clara Barton would be appropriate, but these pages interrupt the flow of narrative about the AMEDD and AMS. A major revision is indicated here. I think pages 1-3 plus these need recombination into a section on the Army Nurse.

36.
Carrier state in typhoid was outlined in 1880's; Typhoid Board also showed its existence.

36.
The Typhoid Board documented the previously suggested food, fly, finger transmission; suggested the carrier state on epidemiological (not laboratory) evidence, and pinned responsibility for sanitation on the line commander. Perhaps its greatest result was forcing the introduction in 1901 of a course

CHAPTER 3

Page
Remarks

40

Sternberg is quoted out of context and erroneously. He is being conceptual; he knew very well the etiology, ecology and solution to typhoid. This introductory paragraph is in error.

40

Since there was no available technology, it is not fair to criticize early theorists for not doing laboratory work. The revision makes the sentence non-perjorative.

40

Ross published in 1898 - this sentence belongs on page 42 to maintain chronological order.

41

What is the evidence for the perjorative cast to these sentences?

42

The deaths in the camps were typhoid, measles and pneumonia. The Dodge Commission reference isn't particularly relevant here. The lead sentence flows neatly into the next paragraph.

44

When did Sternberg ever train under Welch? They were age contemporaries.

44

Kean sentence?

45

Reference for direct quotation?

46

Carter did not provide the "modus operandi" - e.g., The research protocol. Carter showed with epidemiological studies of single family outbreaks that there was an incubation period in the mosquito before it became infective.

53-54

Delete as not relevant; no one <u>would</u> have asked their advice. This part was also deleted from the published article.

54

Reference 82. Has enough time passed to attribute these remarks?

55.

The allusion to Ross is unclear. Ross always acknowledged his debt to Manson who proved in 1877 that mosquitoes transmitted filariasis. Theobold Smith documented vector transmission of Texas cattle fever in 1893. Recommend deletion - its not really an issue.

Pictures

Recommend retaining:

CHAPTER 3

1. The Young Doctor (Reed)
2. Letter, Reed to Borden
3. Post Hospital, Washington Barracks
4. Reed, 1902

CHAPTER 4

Remarks

Page	
64	Is there a reference to this delightfully wrong MCP remark of (which?) TSG? Sternberg?
65	What behavior problem?
66 & 69	I think this is Company 1, not I (Eye)? Or is it shorthand for Company of Instructions?
68	What do you think about inserting the story (from D.L. Borden) of Borden's "who owns the jail" argument with the Post Commander at Washington Barracks? It is a good anecdote to make this point.
70	The sudden intrusion of the AWC doesn't track here.
71	The Ainsworth story is fun (have you see Mabel Deutrich's The Struggle for Supremacy, 1962?) However, it simply doesn't seem to fit in here. We have been following the Hospital Corps, and then we go to O'Reilly. Recommend this be deleted here and saved for potential insertion elsewhere.
71	Was this as Exectuive Officer of OTSG?
72	Lynch arises - and then?
72	Maybe they had, but the issue was closed since Lawson's time. Who wanted to keep MC's as First Lieutenants now?
73	Reference for 80% figure? I have been looking into Board exams and results with the view of writing a paper. About half to two-thirds of applicants failed and about half of those flunked the physical exam. What are your thoughts?
75	Reference for Arthur as MCP?
75	Do you know if Arthur's sketch of the Examining Board was of actual examiners? And if so - who?
76	What is a "colonial" hospital?

CHAPTER 4

Remarks

76   Deletion: See previous note.

77   Pure speculation. Recommend deletion.

78   I assume this means the Army Medical Library, but there is no prior reference. Recommend deletion here and save quote for future use.

78   Worth quoting the bill?

79   Whoops! Where did this come from? I think the thrust is to lay the groundwork for the naming of the new hospital, but is this the right set of words? Looking ahead to Chapter 5, I can't make a transition. Which leads me to an overall observation on this chapter; it is choppy (as in oceans). Consider the topic:

1. Medical Department reorganization.

2. Enlisted training.

3. Nurses.

4. Borden, Washington Barracks.

5. Borden, new General Hospital.

6. Army Medical School.

Consider that Chapter 3 covers yellow fever and then Reed and the yellow fever work, and then Reed's death and the "claims to fame" issues. A flowing, smooth story. It seems to me that Chapter 4 should continue the story of:

1. Medical Department reassembly after Reed's death.

2. Borden, the man (Washington Barracks) and Borden and the new hospital.

The remainder of the material should be put into separate chapters, later, because it is important to get down the Army Nurse story,

CHAPTER 4

Page

Remarks

the Hospital Corpsman story, and the Army Medical School story. I am afraid that too strict an attention to chronology leaves the rope of events rather unraveled for the reader. Let me know what you think. *Personally, as a non-historian, I believe in chronology.*

Pictures   Recommend retaining:

1. Surgical demonstration by Borden.

2. Examining Board.

3. Borden's Dream.

References   #12 - What is an "equivalent"?

#34 - Has enough time passed so sources can be cited?

CHAPTER 5

Page	Remarks
83	Nomenclature change from Company 1?
83	I can't figure out what a "Cuban Expeditionary Brigade" would have been formed for in <u>1906</u>. Can you help me? Reference?
87	"In May 1909 - the month his brain-child, the Walter Reed U. S. Army Hospital opened to patients - he became Dean of the George Washington (Columbian College) Medical School."
88	This paragraph interrupts the flow of description of construction. Let's save it and insert it later when discussing the School. Perhaps page 102?
89	"Colonial" as in architectural style? I would have thought it was more Federal in style?
92	Tetchy! As compared to what?
94	Let us consider if this is the right place to go back to the deleted pages (1-3, etc. seq.) and tell the ANC story from the beginning. To me, there is a logic, because in introducing nurses to WRAMC, let us introduce the Corps and its history to the reader.
95	What could be ironical?
96	Insert is for temporal accuracy; "outright defiance" is becoming more common.
98	"Unimpressive" to whom? Would "colorless" convey the message?
98	I don't follow "accident or design." Assume they were all appointed on orders, so "accident" seems unlikely?
99	What "manual"?
100	"little was said "--by whom?
100	Why is Birmingham stuck in here?
101	What is the Nelson (#88) reference? May wish to cite Deutrich's book which has the full story on Ainsworth.

But I have not read Deutrich's Book — nor was it in existence when this MS was prepared. You will have to bridge that gap if you can't accept this.

CHAPTER 5

Remarks

102   Reference 91; may want to use Siler's book - it has the whole story, circa 1930's.

102   Reference 94; I will check this in Siler - I remember a different date.

103   Reference 96. I will run this down, but I think it is like the Girard story - more myth than fact.

103   Basically, this page covers work at the AMS, but it is not clearly apparent to the uninformed reader. May need to re-cast and expand somewhat for emphasis.

Pictures   Recommend retaining:

1.   Old Main (is that LTC Arthur's car?)

2.   Colonel Arthur

3.   Anderson boys.

4.   Russell vaccine

5.   AMS - 1910

6.   BG Richard

CHAPTER 6

Page

Remarks

References   #12 - is there a more complete citation?

#84 - what does the "as proposed" by Rogers mean?

Pictures   Recommend retaining:

1.   COL Birmingham
2.   BG Fisher
3.   COL Phillips *and daughter (later an editor for some big publishing house - Ref to her app. is in notes - in references.*
4.   COL Ashburn
5.   AMS - 604 Louisiana Avenue

CHAPTER 6

Remarks

Page	
113	These paragraphs on the AMS, VD, etc, interrupt the flow here; they fit neatly around page 126. Needs a sentence or so to make clear that "venereal disease" (Largely gonorrhea) was not treated ~~only~~ with salversan which was used to treat syphilis. *even I Knew that—*
116	"dominie"? Why this word? How can we know this? It is an assumption - are there data? The next few sentences contradict this statement.
121	One can't fall from an elevator shaft. Did he fall down the elevator shaft?
123	Can't read insert. Did Reid precede or succeed Hine?
123a	Please sort LTC Maxwell's insert into text and reference. Do you want this included? If so - where?
124	"reprisals" for what? Is this confused with appropriate "punishments" by an acknowledged strict disciplinarian?
124	Chronology is confusing. Kean gets ARC job in 1916, Delano leaves Army in 1912 to go to ARC - this, I assume is what re-unites them. What does reference to her superintendent's job mean?
125	Who was this female artist?
125	Reynolds footnote needs to be made a reference.
127	What does a "technical" ally mean?
128	deletion; this is personal opinion; may be true, but is not an historical statement.
130	I'm confused. Who was insurgent? Whose side was the AMA on?
129 - 131	All this material on the AML is dropped in here essentially out of context and it interrupts the flow of the narrative which is directed at the DC and then back to WRAMC. This material should be saved and inserted elsewhere.

119? Note?

see back

CHAPTER 7

Remarks

Page

137   ✓   What research?

137   Given the facts of Gorgas' tour, the "him" refers to Gorgas, not
           Birmingham?

138   I think an explanation of these "National Army" promotions should be
           added to enlighten the modern reader.

138   Where did Mason go? *Check the military record!*

139   Reference #17. I assume that Bastion said Truby was a good internist
           and that Truby said he preferred clinical medicine to administration.
           However, the citation makes it come out vice-versa. Recommend 2
           references and split #17 in half.

139   Was Willard Truby related to Albert Truby? *Cousin (first)*

140   What has fatigue got to do with average patient stay? In fact, in all
           mobilization planning and operations, patient stay decreases - in part
           because of the more transient nature of recruit illnesses and in part due
           to pressure to keep beds empty to meet evacuation surges. *Call it*
           apprehension — war neuroses — fear — Just be happy! →

140   Sentence not clear to me. Who was responsible for medical supplies -
           QM or WRGH Property Division? *Im not sure — but even to*
           1934 — +2 — there was a question about who ran things — MDS — or g.m.?

141   Sterile water? Why?

141   But "insane" was no longe the classification?

142   I bet its not "strange." The FY 1917 report ended on 30 June and
           probably was prepared in March or April 1917. The WRGH reports
           addressed calender years. As the text says, 1917 <u>was</u> the year of all
           the construction.

142   "ground soil" is interesting. Do you mean raw sewage or just plain
           dirt? *Just plain dirt — (I hadn't lived in Japan then) — "*
           and a nurse used that term in describing their "progress

144   Isn't this more of an architect's sketch than a painting? At least, that is
           what the legend says. *yes totally*

144   Quota of what?

see back

CHAPTER 7

Page	Remarks
162	Please tell me what these insignia were.
162	Do you mean prerequisites for command? Does "compensation" mean the pay of increased grade?
163	"thirty-sixth, etc." I assume you mean Arthur, not Welch? Antecedent to "he" is unclear.
163	This could be interpreted to mean that Ireland was the first commander of the Company of Instruction. I thought Hoff and then Deshon preceded Ireland?
163- 164	On page 163, Arthur has ambitions to be TSG; then "the Ireland gang" get it for Ireland, then Arthur blasts Noble. Temporal sequencing is not clear. Was Arthur a member of the "Ireland gang"? Arthur surely knew that Ireland had sent Noble to "Limoges" - why did he invite Noble at that late date? I do not understand Arthur's rôle and behavior - it needs explanation.

But the ~~Ireland gang~~ an intrusive ~~...~~) over

References

#1 - What is the Nelson reference?
#38 - delete
#40 - is this meant to be Ashburn? or the WW I history, which the use
    of a volume number would suggest?
#48 - delete.
#64 - delete - not needed to make the point in the text.
#71 a - insertion of reference.

Pictures.

Recommend retaining:

1. COL Mason (with sword)
            or
   COL Mason in office (I prefer the latter).
2. Medical Library.
3. COL W. F. Truby.
4. Hospital 1917.
5. Aerial view, 1918.
6. Mrs. Sommers.
7. War Service Library - old Red Cross hut.

*You know the modern Army. I know
the old Army - let's not "nit pick".
In general, I think your suggestions are
excellent, and, if you note, I don't quarrel.
Mind, I dissected frogs legs and tamped
boots, but I have no claim to editorial
fame — even punctuation*

181-182	"Special Note." These 3 paragraphs on Glennan belong on page 174, added to the end of the other comments on him. It gives us Glennan all of a piece.
187	$500.00 or $50,000? The latter figure seems more correct.
188	Recommend deletion. Historical fact, but it interrupts the Sawyer story and by now, Wood was no longer of interest to the medical profession in any "medical" way. See VOL II of the Hagedorn biography.
188	Recommend omission. All true, but of no bearing on the WRAMC story.
193	Omit - it dangles.
References	33, 50, 53, 54, 55 would have to be dropped if recommended omissions occur. 37, 38, & 39 would have to be moved to match up with move of Glennan paragraphs.
Pictures	Recommend retaining:

1. Nurses residence - Butternut Street

2. Old Lay House - 1919

3. Prince of Wales - 1920

4. Service Club

5. Dean and Lumsden

6. Officers Quarters, Butternut Street - 1919

7. Keller at work

2

CHAPTER 8

THE GARDENER

Page	Comment

170   150 letters would suggest that he <u>did</u> interest them.

172   Is the first quotation from the <u>Star</u> as well?   *apparently*

174   The implication escapes me. Was Keller going to flunk his

        entry exam?

175   Can one be quiet and reserved and also be a blusterer?

176   I added the phrase, since I assume that is what happened and

        it completes the story for the reader.

179   Recommend omit - the point is made.

179-180 Do you mean the Chief (Keller) saw all patients once a week?

        I can't believe that patients were visited only weekly by any

        attending surgeon.   Further, Keller <u>had</u> to be making rounds

        from the beginning of his practice, and <u>teaching</u> rounds from

        the day he began as Chief. The rest of the paragraph is melo-

        drama. Recommend deletion.

180-181 Recommend deletion from "Further to method." Detailed re-

        counting of this kind of statistical data, unless to make a point

        about workload in certain areas, or the increase of a special-

        ized operation, is an obstacle to the narrative.

181   Miss Lower sentence is out of context. Remove here, insert

        as appropriate.

CHAPTER 9

THE ARMY MEDICAL CENTER

Page	Comment

Do you really believe that statement? a descent yourself in what's been happening to the esprit of...

198   I put these ARC functions in past tense, because they no longer
        do most of them; it would be misleading to today's reader.

199   Hard to support. Author's opinion, but there have been 3
        wars since then and esprit-de-corps is in the eye of the be-
        holder. Recommend deletion of bracketed words.

Miss Dchick's opinion!

200   Hokum!   *Miss Dchick again — She was there, I wasn't!*

202   This is probably where the earlier deletions on the ANC from
        earlier chapters should be inserted.

OK

209   If the internes came as First Lieutenants, how could they re-
        fuse commissions? Or could they resign their commissions
        right away? *etc.* *To the est of my recollection, they were uniform Army but had to "make" the regular army*

213   Alas - 9A is now gone.

218   The concepts are true, but blurred and the point was made in
        the earlier chapters on the school. Recommend deletion.

References   Need complete citation for reference 1. Reference 49 can be
              dropped.

Pictures   Recommend retaining:

1. First Easter Egg Roll

2. AMS - 1923

3   ANC - 1922

4. Rehabilitation

5. Dental Clinic - 1922

6. Mrs. Walter Reed and Glennan - 1924 - bottom picture

7. Formal garden

8. Cornerstone, AMS

9. AMS

10. AVS - 1923

11. Training Corpsmen - 1924

CHAPTER 10

THE PRIDE OF THE MEDICAL DEPARTMENT

Page

Comment

226

Makes the staff look like ghouls. Omit; "an bloc" statistics

are blocks (pun intended). What do you think of an Appendix with

all such data as these, chronologically arranged, and reserving

text space for discussion of trends?

Don't think much of it! W credit show steady growth at a glance.

228

Wasn't it $13/month?

230

What does "pseudo-scientific" mean? *have to verify —*

234

118 student nurses? That many?

239

Why quotations without a reference? *See page for revision*

240

Kelser's work was done at the Tropical Medicine Board in the

Philippines, with no command relationship to the School (al-

though the staff rotated assignments). Why include it here?

Certainly - but it was program for the Department. I knew him, also - Reynolds and St. John, as I recall, also served at the School -

240

Pictures

Minor work on dengue vectors - recommend omission. *Does it hurt to give them a little boost?*

Recommend retaining

1. 1929 - ARC Building and West Wing

2. 1929 - Isolation ward

3. 1930 - Medical ward

4. 1931 - Delano Hall

5. 1929 - Faculty

6. Russell in Lab

You should have from Ernest gentry. He was a professional writer when around!

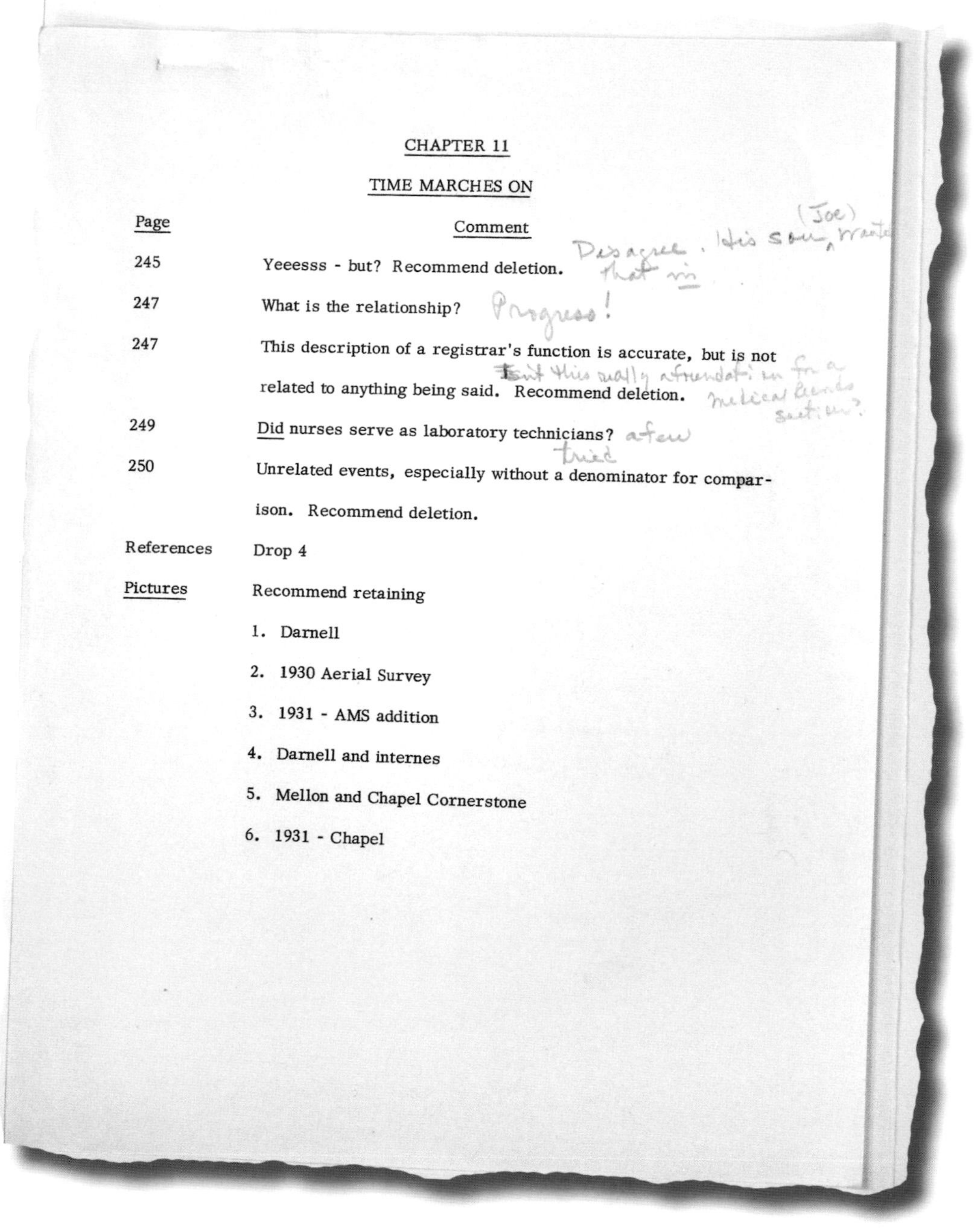

CHAPTER 11

TIME MARCHES ON

Page	Comment
245	Yeeesss - but? Recommend deletion. Disagree. His son (Joe) wanted that in
247	What is the relationship? Progress!
247	This description of a registrar's function is accurate, but is not related to anything being said. Recommend deletion. Isn't this really a foundation for a medical events section?
249	Did nurses serve as laboratory technicians? a few tried
250	Unrelated events, especially without a denominator for comparison. Recommend deletion.
References	Drop 4
Pictures	Recommend retaining

1. Darnell
2. 1930 Aerial Survey
3. 1931 - AMS addition
4. Darnell and internes
5. Mellon and Chapel Cornerstone
6. 1931 - Chapel

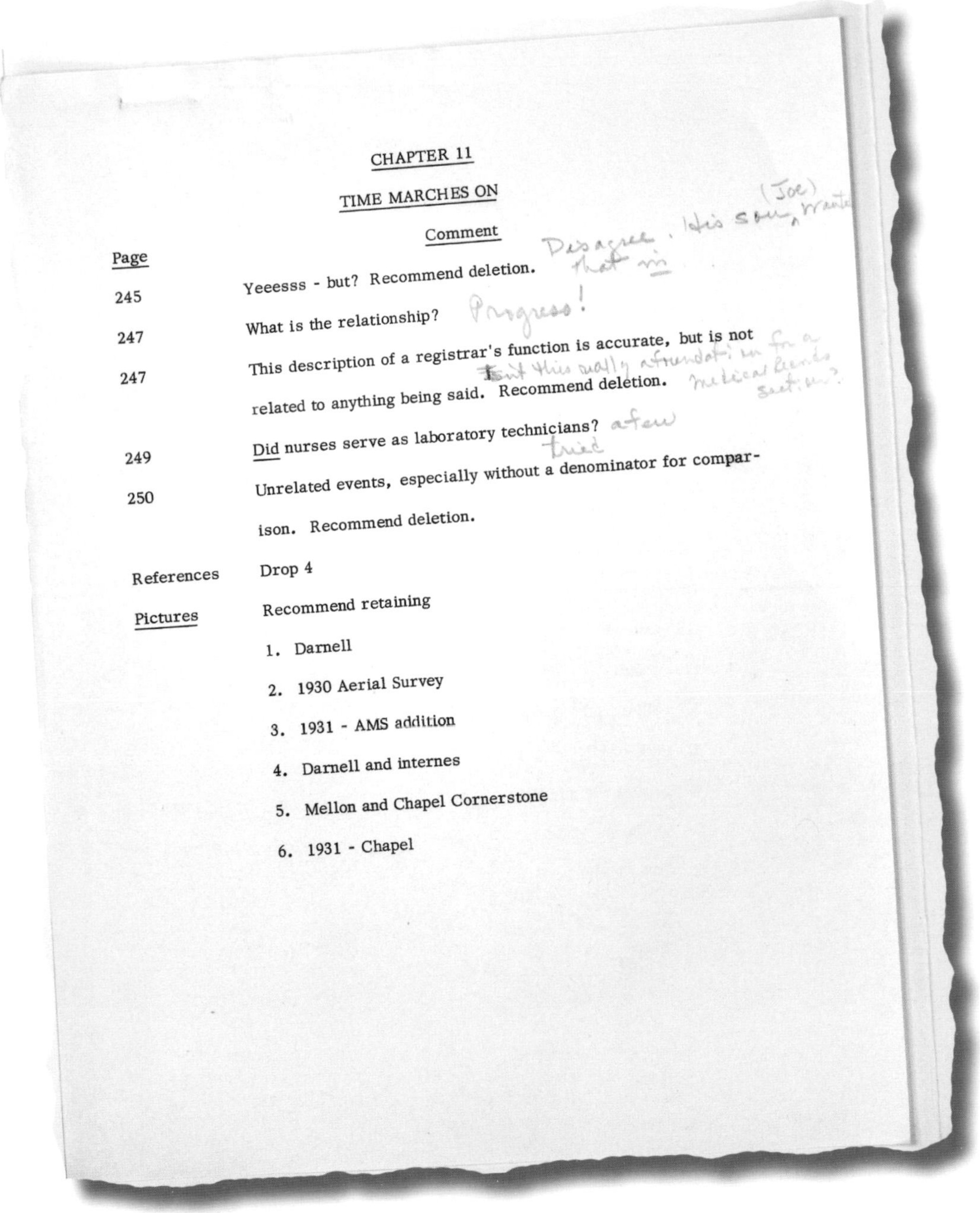

CHAPTER 11

TIME MARCHES ON

Comment

Disagree. It's son, wants (Joe) that in

Progress!

Isn't this really a foundation for a medical records section?

a few tried

CHAPTER 12

REPLACING THE OLD WITH THE NEW

[handwritten, top right: My edition of Webster's first definition of that word is maggot — Shades of Dr. Wagner — a "judgment word.]

Page	Comment
267	Non sequitur? Recommend deletion.
276	It didn't work. Recommend deletion.
276	Not related to WRAMC. Recommend deletion.
277	Kelser's work was done in the Philippines, not at WRAMC. Recommend deletion.

[handwritten left: True, but he was a stem from the AVS Tree. they tried hard for recognition]

| 278 | (Mawkish.) Recommend deletion. |

[handwritten right: no more irrelevant than "Pawnee Sawyer" or "cupid" —]

| 279 | Mawkish, sentimental, and irrelevant. Recommend deletion. |
| 278-280 | I just rearranged the Kimbrough stuff in chronological order. *[handwritten: agreed — over]* |

There is a bit too much of "Uncle Jim" here. I knew him when

I was in intern. He <u>was</u> a colorful character, but I think he has

bigger share of the pie here than I think is warranted. What do

you think? *[handwritten: Don't know how to "cut" him without diminishing his professional personality,]*

[handwritten left margin: Local color; there was never another one like him — as an intern would you have known him very well?]

References   #1 - need full citation *[handwritten: Same problem as with the Haylett — notes burned —]*

#41, 42 - delete

#51, 52 - reposition

Pictures   Recommend retaining

1. Truby

2. 1933 - Gymnasium

3. Rea pool

4. Gas station

5. Lounge, 1933

6. Recreation at ARC Hut

7. Kimbrough

287   There is no evidence that the depression began to wane by 1938 (see J.K. Galbraith's book "The Great Depression"). Recommend deletion.

288   This is pure speculation and isn't really required in this excellent sketch of DeWitt. Recommend deletion.

290   What a delightful touch!

291   Verb change to match 1976 publication.

292   Should these pages on COL Keller be moved back to Chapter 8 to tell the whole "Keller" story in one swell foop?

per page → 294   What does "defensive championship" mean? Was the other selectee a pet of a Board member?

300   Trivial. Recommend deletion.

302   In 1923, the "Army Medical School" became "The Medical Department Professional Service School." It was never officially plural, but in AR 350-1000, 20 June 1942 the plural was used. On 27 July 1949, COL DeCoursey asked that the plural be used in the new (since 1947) title of Army Medical Department Research & Graduate School. This was refused by COL Tynes (for TSG) because of the requirement for separate administrative staffs for each "School." Thus, although the "schools" <u>functioned</u> as "schools", there was only a "school" by General Order. No change needed in text - these comments could be foot note in the references if you wish.

303   Is this what was meant?

304   I think George Deshon organized that first Company. I will look it up.

305   Wrong reference. The Hoff medal correspondence is in the WRAIR archives; I will supply the reference.

305   There were two Sternberg medals and the first award was given by Sternberg himself around 1910. I will provide the dates and a sentence or so on these medals. We can rely on E.E. Hume's little book for the history of these medals.

References -   Recommend changes as described in text and above.

Pictures -   Recommend retaining

1. 1932, Laundry and Bakery
2. 1930, Main Operating Room

References -   Recommend changes as described in text and above.

Pictures -   Recommend retaining

1. 1932, Laundry and Bakery
2. 1930, Main Operating Room
3. COL Keller (move to Chapter 8?)
4. BG Metcalfe
5. Delano Hall, 1939
6. Hoff Fountain

CHAPTER 14

Remarks

Page

316   "blood substitutes" has a very different technical meaning in 1976. My change specifies what these IV fluids were in 1941.

319   This AGO "nutrition" school is new to me. Why would AG and not Quartermaster run such a school? Clarification, please?

320   Penicillin in 1942? Seems to be at least one year early. Have you a reference for the quotation? Any reference for its use by the Orthopedic Service? My references suggest that Penicillin was not generally available until 1943.

References: No recommendations

Pictures: Recommend retaining:

1. 1940, Bergonie Chair (with caption explaining its use in neurological *and neurosurgical patients)*

2. COL Stout

3. MG Marietta

4. Main Entrance, Forest Glen (but get a summer picture from the files at WRAIR)

5. Exterior View, Forest Glen (Castle Picture)

6. Recreation Room, Forest Glen

7. Reviewing the Lady Soldiers

CHAPTER 15

Remarks

334-6

The comments on military-civilian relations are general observations, have nothing specifically to do with WRGH, are all true, and don't especially advance the story. The top paragraph on page 336 cannot be published in a DA book in 1976. Recommend deleting marked paragraphs on pages 334, 335, and 336. The second paragraph on page 336 is a fine lead into the discussion of increased civilian employment.

338

How does gasoline in stoves get transformed into reagents? Please clarify. Does this thought go with the next following paragraph?

345

My records indicate that Strong was a recalled retired (resigned?) ex-Regular officer.

References: Delete reference #7

Pictures: Recommend retaining:

1. Mrs. Rea and Grey Ladies

2. COL Strong

CHAPTER 16

Page

Remarks

358

I got lost on this sentence; must be unusually thick-headed today. Please clarify.

364

Interesting, but not especially germane. Recommend deletion.

References:

#8 - Mrs. Sommers could not have retired in 1947, spent ten years with her husband, and have his death date be 1949. Was it 1959?

#26 - Delete, as referenced material should be omitted.

Pictures:

Recommend retaining:

1. When heroes meet (with new caption)

2. President Truman

3. Milton Berle (isn't that Rita Hayworth next to TSG Kirk?)

4. Cadet Nurses

5. The Wounded Walk

CHAPTER 17

Page	Remarks
375	This sentence should be in the Author's Foreword.
376	This implies that the 8-hour schedule was a <u>new</u> event. Was it?
380	What is a "pathological hospital"? (And don't tell me it's a sick hospital!)
381	Not sure what this means? A separate Pediatric Service?
382	Insert this paragraph on page 381, as indicated. It flows from the School paragraph.
384-5	Move these paragraphs also, same reason. All these paragraphs should be consecutive, as in the present text, on page 381.
386	Move to the consolidation on page 381 of all this School data.
387	Move to School section beginning on page 381.
References:	#12 - Delete; not germane in 1976.
	#54 - Deleted sentence recognized present status of National Library of Medicine.
Pictures:	Recommend retaining:

1. BG Beach
2. Fever Therapy
3. Callender and Plotz
4. LTC Thomson
5. C.O. Jan 1949 (MG Striet-needs new caption)

Note: The picture of COL Morgan fascinates me! Who were (are) the participants and what are they doing with the tulips at the Hoff fountain.

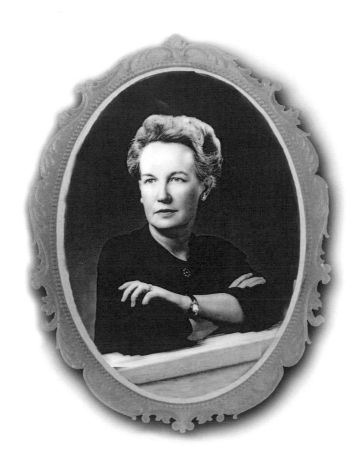

Mary Walker Standlee

1906–1985, Author of *Borden's Dream*

The author, Mary Walker Standlee, undertook the extensive task of compiling and writing *Borden's Dream* while working at the library of Walter Reed General Hospital. She received her master's degree in education from the University of Texas at Austin and was married to an Army physician, MG Earle Glenn Standlee.

This is an unedited publication of Standlee's 1952 manuscript, a vibrant historical account based on interviews and documents. It chronicles the realization of Borden's Dream, "an Army medical center incorporating a hospital, school, library and museum."

Photograph: Mary Walker Standlee, c. 1948, courtesy of Lieutenant Colonel Robert Buechler, US Army, Retired.

ISBN: 978-0-9818228-4-6